D1388093

Praise for The Healing Promise of Qi

"A fine comprehensive overview of Tai Chi and Qigong theory and practice. I look forward to referring to this book—and using it—for years to come."
—James S. Gordon, M.D., founder and director, Center for Mind-Body Medicine, Washington, D.C., and author, *Manifesto for a New Medicine*

"A timely book . . . with easy-to-follow instructions to guide the readers, step by step, toward the success of achieving health and well-being."
—Chungliang Al Huang, Living Tao Foundation, author, *The Essential Tai Ju* and *Embrace Tiger, Return to Mountain*

"Dr. Jahnke's *Healing Promise of Qi* unlocks the practical and profound secrets of Tai Chi and Qigong, China's ancient self-healing tools."
—Kenneth Pelletier, M.D., author, *The Best Alternative Medicine* and *Mind as Healer, Mind as Slayer*

"*The Healing Promise of Qi* is comprehensive, clear, and engaging. I highly recommend it."
—Kenneth S. Cohen, author, *The Way of Qigong: The Art and Science of Chinese Energy Healing*

"Roger Jahnke's writing touches and resonates with the deepest threads of traditional East Asian medicine."
—Ted J. Kaptchuk, O.M.D., author, *The Web That Has No Weaver*

"A most comprehensive and clearly structured presentation of contemporary Qigong practice. It includes numerous sets of concrete instruction on the gathering and moving of Qi in the body, making ample use of the author's extensive clinical experience."
—Livia Kohn, Ph.D., author, *Daoism and Chinese Culture*, *Taoist Meditation and Longevity Techniques*, and *Early Chinese Mysticism*

"Roger Jahnke is the real thing. His work comes from the heart. He gently heals through the heart center—with his brilliant integration of the ancient wisdom of Qigong, Tai Chi, and Western mind."
—Barbara Brennan, author, *Hands of Light and Light Emerging*

"[Dr. Jahnke's] insights on Tai Chi and Qigong are inspiring and philosophical yet very practical—ancient ideas that are solutions for modern times."
—Chi-hsiu Weng, Ph.D., founder, Cardio Tai Chi Monkey System, and author, *Ch'ang Style T'ai Chi Ch'uan*

"Dr. Jahnke's book on Qi and Qigong has a very genuine and inspiring perspective on Chinese medicine and the Daoist cultivation arts."
—Dr. Chang Yi Hsiang, founder, Tai Hsuan Foundation College of Acupuncture and Herbal Medicine, Honolulu, Hawaii, and author, *Ch'i Kung: Art of Mastering the Unseen Life Force*

"Roger has joined ancient wisdom with immediate experience, inspiring stories with hands-on instructions, poetry, and ordinary talk in a page-turner that will guide you toward balance and healing in your day and life."
—Cyndi Lee, director, OM Yoga Center, New York City, and author, *OM Yoga: A Guide to Daily Practice* and *Yoga Body, Buddha Mind*

"With the growing emphasis on personal responsibility for health and personal evolution, Roger Jahnke's fine book creates practical access—for everyone—to the how and why of the ancient healing arts of Tai Chi and Qigong."
—Valerie V. Hunt, Ed.D., author, *Infinite Mind: Science of Human Vibrations of Consciousness*

"Dr Jahnke's new book is a powerful yet practical exploration into many of the parallels that link Chinese medicine and Qi cultivation with Western metaphysics."
—Charles Thomas Cayce, Ph.D., president, Association for Research and Enlightenment (ARE) and the Edgar Cayce Foundation

"Roger Jahnke, O.M.D., is one who can make the profound benefits of Qigong and Tai Chi accessible to *everyone*! . . . Roger's efforts to demystify Qigong and Tai Chi, so that millions more can access self-healing power, are a great service to humanity."
—Bill Douglas, founder, World T'ai Chi & Qigong Day, and author, *The Complete Idiot's Guide to T'ai Chi & Qigong*

"A wonderful summary of this ancient Chinese healing art, accessible to all!"
—Wayne B. Jonas, M.D., director, Sammuelli Institute, and editor, *The Essentials of Complementary and Alternative Medicine*

The Healing Promise of *Qi*

Creating Extraordinary Wellness Through Qigong and Tai Chi

Roger Jahnke, O.M.D.

New York Chicago San Francisco Lisbon London Madrid Mexico City
Milan New Delhi San Juan Seoul Singapore Sydney Toronto

The **McGraw·Hill** Companies

Copyright © 2002 by Roger Jahnke. All rights reserved. Printed in the United States of America. Except as permitted under the United States Copyright Act of 1976, no part of this publication may be reproduced or distributed in any form or by any means, or stored in a database or retrieval system, without the prior written permission of the publisher.

16 17 18 19 20 21 22   QFR/QFR   1 9 8 7 6 5

ISBN 978-0-8092-9528-9
MHID   0-8092-9528-8

Library of Congress Cataloging-in-Publication Data

Jahnke, Roger.
       The healing promise of Qi : creating extraordinary wellness through
       Qigong and Tai Chi / Roger Jahnke.
             p.   cm.
       Includes bibliographical references and index.
       ISBN 0-8092-9528-8
       1. Qi gong.   2. Medicine, Chinese.   3. Medicine—Religious aspects.
       4. Tai chi.   I. Title

       RA781.8 .J34   2002
       610'.951—dc21   2001047390

Interior design by Hespenheide Design
Interior illustrations by Susan Spellman
Calligraphy by Jian-ye Jiang

McGraw-Hill books are available at special quantity discounts to use as premiums and sales promotions or for use in corporate training programs. To contact a representative, please e-mail us at bulksales@mcgraw-hill.com.

To the Qi (Chi) masters of all
cultures and all times.

To my parents for providing inspiration
and support for this fascinating work and play
with the essential energy of the universe.

Qi
*A resource so essential it is impossible to
define or translate*

 Gong
To cultivate—a practice or methodology

 Tai
Supreme, absolute, immense

 Chi
Ultimate balance and harmony

Before the Beginning

Before we begin, it is inspiring to know that healing and empowerment in the ancient traditions that honor Qi (Chi) are rooted in nature and the cycles of the seasons; the rising and setting of the sun, moon, and stars; and fire and water in their multiple manifestations. Qi infuses all of life—humans, plants, and the transformation of the caterpillar into the butterfly.

The extraordinary concepts and methods you are about to explore have origins so ancient that there is no written history of the first several thousand years of their development and use.

The practical act of cultivating the Qi for healing and healthy life is deeply rooted in the very nature of the earth and the immense universe in which it spins. When people cultivate Qi through Qigong (Chi Kung) and Tai Chi (Taiji), they are purposefully accessing and then circulating natural healing resources in such a provocative way that contemporary science has only begun to explain it.

Tai

What you are about to learn and practice is a technology so profound yet so practical that its arrival in our culture could easily go down in history as one of the primary medical breakthroughs of the new millennium.

Chi

It is valuable to know in advance that this immersion into the cultivation of Qi may often seem fantastic and even paradoxical. Qi is not only energy but also the quintessential foundation of the universe. Qigong is not really just an exercise; it can become a powerful way of being. Tai Chi is much more than a martial art; it can actually be defined as a method of accessing and sustaining harmony with the universe.

Qi

Gong

The beautiful Chinese characters in this section provide the perfect inspiration to launch our journey together:

Qigong means "working and playing with Qi, refining inner resources." Some forms of Qigong are so easy to learn that they are being used in clinics, schools, churches, and community centers.

Tai Chi means "supreme ultimate." When people practice Tai Chi, which was originally developed in the thirteenth century, they are not only getting excellent exercise, they are also investigating the nature of their relationship with superior personal energy, maximum endurance, and healthy longevity, as well as the essential nature of the universe.

May this journey into the domain of Qi be a memorable contribution to your life path.

Contents

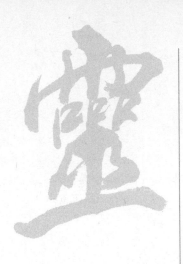

Acknowledgments

Especially to those who catch the vision of this and other works on the mindful management of essential life force—Qi (China) and Prana (India). Qigong (Chi Kung), Tai Chi (Taiji), and their sister Yoga, stand to alter the nature of life, health, learning, and community in this provocative time when the purposeful cultivation of inner peace and personal stamina are so necessary. May you be inspired to use and share these tools and ideas for the benefit of all people—body, heart/mind, and spirit—in all communities of every nation.

To my teachers, some for years, some for months, some for particularly inspiring moments: Master Weng Chi Hsiu, U.S.; Master Chang Yi Hsiang, Hawaii; Dr. Feng Lida, Beijing; Master Zhu Hui, Tian Tai Mountain; Dr. Liu, Hangzhou; Master Huang Jun, Hangzhou; Dr. Tang Yu Fan, Hangzhou; Master Zhang, Guanzhou; Professor Tang You Yue, Hangzhou; Dr. Pang He Ming and Teacher Yu, Qinghuangdao; Drs. Zhang, Li, and Cai, Xi Yuan Hospital, Beijing; Yuan Zheng, Cancer Recovery Society, Shanghai; Zhang Yu, U.S.; Master Sun, Beijing; Dr. Sun, Hangzhou; and too many others to name.

To the writers, physicians, and researchers who made the breakthroughs that allow for complementary medicine, Chinese medicine, Qigong, Tai Chi, Yoga, and meditation to thrive in this new era: Chopra, Dossey, Weil, Ornish, Borysenko, Northrup, Benson, Eisenberg, Gordon, Siegel, Shealy, McGarey.

To the ancient Qi masters: Master Yu, Huang Ti, Lao Zi, Confucius, Zhuang Zi, Zhang Dao Ling, Ge Hong, Wei Bo Yang, Tao Hong Jing, Sun Simiao, Zhang San Fen, Lu Dong Bin, Wang Chong Yang, Zhang Bo Duan, and other luminaries who gave birth to and nurtured the Qi cultivation arts over the centuries.

To those who carried the amazing Qi cultivation arts to America: Chung Liang Huang, Chang Yi Hsiang, Cheng Man-Ching, Yan Xin, Hua Hsing Ni, Mantak Chia, Yang Jwing Ming, Luke Chan, Effie Chow, Jian-ye Jiang, Nan Lu.

To the new Qi masters of the Western world, particularly those men and women whom I have worked with to create the National Qigong Association, who have provided insight for this book or who provided support for the Qi revolution in America—MacRitchie, Garripoli, Johnson, Stewart, Towler, Jarboux, Winn, Kali, Cohen.

To my favorite scholars of Chinese culture, with deepest appreciation for opening up the Chinese classics to Qi-hungry Western readers: Richard Wilhelm, Joseph Needham, Livia Kohn, Bob Flaws, Eva Wong, Isabelle Robinet, Thomas Cleary, and the many, many translators and interpreters of the *Dao De Jing*.

To my allies in the publishing world: Jane Dystel and Judith McCarthy, who are genuine, warm, and wholesome people in a complex and constantly changing profession, and all the folks at Contemporary Books—Michele, Marisa, Katherine, Lizz, and John—whose handle-with-care approach has made it possible to persevere in this fascinating and demanding project.

To the participants in the arts and graphics components of this book for their careful design. Especially to Susan Spellman, illustrator, for her excellent work and patient nature, and to Jian-ye Jiang, the master calligrapher who did the beautiful, classic Chinese calligraphy, and Tom Bishop of Wen Lin Institute (Wenlin.com), for additional help with the calligraphy. To the modern-day centers of learning that have so kindly supported me in sharing the Qi with hungry learners—Esalen, Omega, Kripalu and Naropa.

To my students throughout the world who have so radically accelerated my own learning—from the Santa Barbara College of Oriental Medicine and the International Institute of Integral Qigong and Tai Chi. A special thanks to the instructor training class at Omega Institute who test drove this material in September 2001.

To Rhonda Richey, my personal associate, who is so helpful with the endless list of details and so positive with our alliances in this good work. And Anne, our assistant.

To my family for their love and support, particularly my wife and cocreator Rebecca—a Qi master in her own right—who is ever clear that direct association with nature and Spirit is our highest priority.

Introduction

The Most Profound Medicine

Over thousands of years, the ancient Qi (Chi) masters discovered many treasures that we in the West are only now beginning to appreciate. They knew that *the most profound medicine* costs nothing—it is created naturally within the human system. We in Western cultures, in a kind of disbelief about such a possibility, have been slow to understand and use this extraordinary medicine.

The effect has been immense and painful. In the final years of the last millennium research revealed that both negative drug interactions and medical errors were among the most common causes of death. At the same time the U.S. Department of Health and Human Services announced that 70 percent of disease and the associated medical expenses are preventable.

How can this be? How can such a huge percentage of disease be preventable while at the same time several of the most common causes of death are attributed to the health-care system itself? Citizens have panicked, reaching out to sources of alternative medicine and spending billions of dollars. An act of Congress created the National Center for Complementary and Alternative Medicine and increased its budget 3,000 percent in ten years. The White House created a special commission to explore options to resolve this confusing challenge. Dozens of agencies and foundations have published reports citing more and more reasons why it is reasonable for individuals to take charge of their own health care.

All the while and almost totally overlooked—in parks, community centers, schools, churches, and certain innovative hospitals—small groups of people have begun to gather to produce and utilize that remarkable inner medicine the Chinese discovered so long ago. A rapidly expanding group of people has already felt the benefit of taking weekly or daily "doses" of this medicine within, which has no negative side effects. Is it possible that small groups of average citizens have begun to solve some of the health-care problems that Congress, several presidents, and the nation's health insurance companies have found insurmountable? Not only is this possible, it is very likely happening in your own neighborhood.

You can't buy this miraculous internal medicine; it is free. You can't go somewhere and get it; it is produced within you, wherever you are. What about the programs to organize these activities? Surely they must be developed and managed by huge institutions at great expense. On the contrary, the self-healing practice group that I am involved with has been meeting weekly for more than twelve years in a Santa Barbara, California, community center. A group of several facilitators with some good-hearted, community-minded supporters has sustained this process for the entire twelve years. Your nearby opportunity to become involved will usually cost you between five and ten dollars.

A revolution gave birth to this nation more than two hundred years ago. Thomas Jefferson predicted that occasional smaller revolutions would be necessary to resolve problem areas in the future. Until recently no one would have guessed that our health-care system would be the setting for a very necessary revolution. Fortunately, producing free medicine in the human body is very easy for us to do.

The Promise of This Book

The teachings in this book have been handed to me by an amazing group of teachers. Some have traveled to the United States, but many I met in the hospitals and institutes of China. Others are from temples and sacred sites in China's mystical mountains. Some of these teachers have passed from this life. In almost every case they have said, "This is a transmission of profound and powerful wisdom that has been refined and then passed down for thousands of years. It is intended for the good of all beings. When it was given to me, I committed to care for this information to assure its transmission into the future. Now, the transmission is passing into your care. Please honor, protect, and refine these methods so that the transmission of healing and empowered Spirit may continue for all time."

As you will see, the extraordinary innovation of purposefully producing a profound inner medicine for no cost is only the beginning. By the time you have gotten into the heart of it, you will find yourself in a domain that is boundless. In this book, you will find three special "promises of Qi" that will alter your life. But as you progress, you will find promise upon promise. Once you enter the domain of consciously working and playing with Qi, something fundamental shifts and your new life begins. Where there was discomfort or desperation, the power to become new or healed or wise appears. Where there was no path, a pathway opens. I am deeply honored to meet you here.

My intention, in the tradition of those who taught me, is to support you in accessing a life-transforming experience. As you explore these ideas and implement these practices, realize that you are being flooded with wisdom so rich and so ancient that no one knows just how it came to be. As soon as you can, begin to experience that this transmission is coming to you from the mysterious and infinite source of the Qi itself.

Using This Book

There are lots of opinions about how the Qi is transmitted and how one "should" learn about Qigong (Chi Kung) and Tai Chi (Taiji). The views expressed in this book, and by most of the teachers that have transmitted their wisdom to me, are to follow the Qi itself. Simply use the book or any teaching as a way to gain direct access to Qi.

The Healing Promise of Qi is laid out in a logical order, but you certainly don't have to follow it sequentially. The structure allows you to find things easily.

- Part I is foundation material.
- Part II is an in-depth set of tools and methods of Qi cultivation, from the simple to the sublime.
- Part III supports you in deepening your understanding and practice; it includes the latest science of Qi and explores the deeper meaning of Tai Chi.

If you are new to this territory, begin with Part I and explore the fundamentals and guiding principles underlying Qigong and Tai Chi. If you want to begin with the actual practices, leap ahead to Chapter 3 and Part II. For insights into how to practice and benefit from Qi cultivation methods, explore Chapter 15. If your mind needs to be satisfied with a scientific framework before it can absorb information and experience the Qi, then read some of the science in Chapter 16. Refer to the Recommended Reading and Resources sections for access to additional guidance.

My intent is to inspire and guide you in your practice. This material has been used in lectures, workshops, and professional training for years. The absolute beginner and the advanced practitioner of Qigong and Tai Chi will both find this book useful—but for different reasons.

Traditional Sources

There is significant diversity in opinion about most of the origins and traditions of Chinese medicine, Qigong, and Tai Chi. This, in addition to the teaching and encouragement of great Qi masters plus my own personal insight from a life of practice, has given me permission to carefully distill from diverse sources a dynamic and practical view of Qi cultivation, one that is both traditional and contemporary.

Sincere and experienced scholars may not fully share some of the perspectives that I have followed as my guidance. Others will shout "Yes! My insights, exactly." This scenario is consistent with millennia of history filled with both revelation and commentary. For example, some may reflect that the most important center for Qi cultivation is below the navel, yet others will affirm the meeting of Heaven and Earth in the area of the heart. If we were living in a former time when the martial arts were necessary for survival, I might agree with the first view. However, the critical need is for peace of mind, peace in the world, health improvement, and a sustainable capacity to master stress. In this context I feel that the deepest insights of the ancients and the practical applications of Chinese medical theory suggest that the "center" is in the area of the heart and solar plexus, as you will see.

I draw heavily upon the *Dao De Jing* (*Tao Te Ching*), from the ancient Qi master Lao Zi. Scholars may feel that my choices for how to translate his characters (Chinese written concepts) are actually more like interpretations. This is absolutely correct. I have elected to use my study of many English translations and a long-term investigation of Chinese calligraphy (brush and ink characters) to embrace the spirit of the old master's teaching, in keeping with creating a resource for you that is relevant and empowering today.

A Note to Experts, Scholars, and Advanced Practitioners

You will find that I have carefully selected from the ancient, immense, and diverse body of Chinese knowledge and tradition to distill a user-friendly bridge to Tai Chi and Qigong for a wide audience. As you know, there are levels of depth and subtlety that I could only allude to and levels of detail that can be confusing. As you also know, any one perspective on Qigong, Chinese medicine, or philosophy is at best an informed opinion. Perhaps the openness and diversity in Chinese tradition is our gift from The Mystery. I am making a humble bow to all who explore or foster the Qi cultivation arts for the great service that you render.

Our Qigong and Tai Chi Community

I am in a state of inspired celebration as I place the finishing touches on this project. Qigong and Tai Chi are playing a major role in the contemporary revolutions in health care, education, social services, and business. Everyone that I have met who actually uses these tools seems to be celebrating as well. We are involved in a vital and momentous era of human history, a major turning point. My vision of the future is quite optimistic. The community of people who are working and playing with Qi is no less than astounding.

—Roger Jahnke, o.m.d.
  Santa Barbara, California, USA 2001
  Hangzhou, China, 4,699th Year of the Chinese Calendar

PART I

The Promise

Undifferentiated presence,
  spontaneously arising
  before heaven and earth,
  still and silent, infinite, virtual,
  eternally present
  through interminable cycles.
It gives birth to the Cosmos,
It is impossible to name,
  so I call it pure boundless immensity.

—LAO ZI, *DAO DE JING*, #25

The Promise of Qi

*There must be some primal force,
    but it is impossible to locate.
I believe it exists, but cannot see it.
I see its results,
    I can even feel it,
    but it has no form.*

—ZHUANG ZI, *INNER CHAPTERS*, FOURTH CENTURY B.C.E.

D avid was living in what many call "the zone." His work was perfect—it gave him the opportunity to serve the public, be in constant contact with nature, and make a very good living. How many people are that lucky?

In 1994, with so much going his way, David began to experience severe nervous system attacks—unusual for someone working in a natural setting in a relatively low-stress job. Though he sought assistance from a number of health-care professionals, the symptoms progressed. When David suffered a major epileptic seizure, he sought immediate medical attention from a neurologist. The physician's report after an EEG and a biopsy was catastrophic: brain cancer, an inoperable tumor—stage two astrocytoma with rapidly dividing cells—usually terminal, with negligible chances of survival past two years.

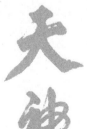

Promise

3

Astrocytoma—literally star tumor—is like a starfish with long slender fingers that wrap around and compress portions of the brain. In David's case the astrocytoma gripped his motor cortex, the portion of the brain that operates body movement. Given the site and size of the tumor, surgery posed a significant risk of irreversible motor impairment—paralysis. David's physician informed him that astrocytoma rarely goes into remission. It grows steadily and is eventually terminal. In David's case chemotherapy was not a reasonable option. Radiation could be used for temporary relief, but could not resolve the case. "If we attempt surgery," the doctor said, "you will likely never walk again."

Stunned, David found himself wrenched out of the zone of security and fulfillment into the zone of alarm and imminent death. Although his basic nature was upbeat and positive, he was caught off guard. As he went about his work with the forest service in the beautiful Montana wilderness, he confronted the fact that medical experts were sure he would die.

David recalls being in shock and deeply depressed. "I had based my life on a career where you walk and climb and work in the forest. This was my preference, my choice. The doctor's diagnosis was devastating." When this traumatic medical opinion was confirmed by a second neurologist, David reached a turning point. "It may have been rebelliousness, anger, or disbelief," he explains, "but I actually feel it was my faith that pulled me up out of my chair. I reached out and shook the doctor's hand, saying, 'I will be alive when your grandchildren graduate.' I walked out. It was as if I had declared out loud what my inner sense had been saying all along—that not only the information I was receiving but also the tone in which it was delivered was inconsistent with my intuition and my values. I had a strong internal feeling that it was possible for someone—me—to recover from this disease."

Believing that there had to be a way to regain his health and his life, David explored many strategies for treatment and personal empowerment. At one point he heard of a form of meditative exercise from China, known as Qigong (Chi Kung). He began to study and practice Qigong and was immediately inspired; this method of personal practice was so much in keeping with his ideals and philosophy. A practice of purposefully accessing the energy of nature to accelerate natural healing seemed more promising than surgery that guaranteed paralysis or radiation that could only postpone death.

Just then he met Karen. She was a total believer in the capacity for self-healing. She had never experienced Qigong but found it to be a wonderful personal discipline that matched her ideals as well. "I had an immediate sense that this was not only a healing practice but a spiritual path. I said, 'David, if you are going to use this ancient Chinese art to heal this tumor you should go to the heart of Qigong.' And, just like that, we were on our way to China, the motherland of Qigong."

David and Karen located a wonderful teacher in Beijing. Dr. Sun, a soulful, positive teacher and doctor of Chinese medicine, taught them Qigong based on a famous system developed in the 1970s by a renowned woman artist who had recovered from cancer. Guo Lin had developed her Qigong especially to meet her own needs, drawing from traditional Qigong forms that she had learned from her grandfather.

Karen reflects, "We learned and practiced and became very enthusiastic about this Chinese healing art with its ancient roots. The most fascinating thing was that Qigong was not complex, it was actually easy to do the practices. The concept that nature heals is just so reasonable. We learned that through Qigong we can tap directly into the power that operates the entire universe. Just think of that. Given the awesome power of the universe, we understood that a tumor could be healed."

Karen and David were practicing Qigong every day, often more than once a day. On their return from China, David had several MRI scans. When a fourth MRI showed definite reduction in the size of the astrocytoma, the doctors were amazed and a bit confused about how to proceed. But one doctor, a neurosurgeon at the University of California Medical Center in San Francisco, felt that the tumor had shrunk enough to be safely removed surgically.

When David had the surgery, in December 1998, everyone was astounded. An inoperable, terminal, class two astrocytoma had converted to an operable, class one astrocytoma. This was a complete reversal at the cellular level; David had gone from having dangerous, rapidly dividing cancer cells to showing absolutely no sign of dividing cells. Amazingly, David had used no chemotherapy and he had had no radiation treatment. The only medical follow-up he had was occasional acupuncture. When David asked what he could do to support his positive progress during his postsurgical recovery, the neurosurgeon answered, "Keep doing Qigong." Instead of the usual medical rehabilitation program, David's physicians agreed that he should follow his inclination to practice Qigong in nature.

Health

A year later, David was able to return to work. He now looks at his illness differently. "This is a quest—a spiritual quest, an opportunity to be of service," he says. "My dream is that people with frightening diseases, and even mild discomforts, will be as lucky as I was. They'll find their way to understanding the Qi [Chi] through Qigong and get swept into a process that leads to a new life. Qigong is not a cure; it is a tool for healing and empowerment. It may seem like a paradox, but I have to give thanks for this tumor also. I am still getting used to being thankful for a life-threatening disease. It introduced me to Qigong and gave me access to the mysterious, vital resource that is Qi."

David's story is not unusual. Many people in China share similar stories of Qigong and its popular offspring Tai Chi (Taiji). In the United States a remarkable revolution is happening in medicine and health care, triggered by people of great conviction and personal fortitude—people like David, Karen, Dr. Sun, and a growing community of innovative physicians and medical providers. The era of the passive patient is over. At the same time, there is a tremendous urge to reduce stress and access inner and outer peace. You, too, can access the healing promise of Qi. For people with health challenges as well as those who simply wish to increase their personal energy and inner calm, ancient Chinese Qigong could be the gift of a lifetime.

The Call of Ancient Medicine

A mysterious vital resource, naturally circulating within us, that we can use for self-empowerment and healing? Surely, we've all wished for this at some level—for a loved one, for a friend, or for ourselves. Many of us have hoped or prayed to uncover such a resource in our lives. Could the formula for healing and personal breakthrough possibly be so simple and yet so profound?

Very early on in my own quest for wisdom and understanding one of my first teachers deeply impressed me with the declaration, "Study and come to know the *one essential* thing that pervades and surrounds all things." This person used herbs and talked about and practiced meditation, prayer, breathing practices, and a fresh-food diet—just like an ancient Chinese Qigong master. This woman—my first teacher in the healing arts—was my grandmother. She was a lot like a hermit in a monastery, living alone in several small rooms that smelled of herbal salves. Like a Qigong master she was immensely humble and spilling over with radiant spirit expressed as love and humor.

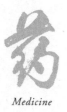

Medicine

At a very early age I began to ask myself what *one essential* pervades and surrounds everything—from the trees, mountains, and stars to life, birth, disease, and death. I asked myself this question as a youngster watching clouds pass over on a summer day, and I asked it when my father passed away before he was forty. I asked again when my children were born, and I asked again when we entered the new millennium. Through this book, I continue to investigate this question with you.

When I was eleven years old my father went into a hospital. He did not return healed as I supposed he would. I never saw him again. As a child I had wanted to be a cowboy or a firefighter when I grew up. Now, suddenly, I wanted to be a doctor. I knew intuitively and through the influence of my grandmother that the primary solution to our diseases is not somewhere outside of ourselves but within us. My whole adult life has been a search for the secrets of healing and personal empowerment that could save people from pain, disease, loss, sorrow, and untimely death. In preparing for a medical career I worked in nearly a dozen hospitals, in numerous departments. At its core, I believe much of my professional journey has been a quest to discover what happened to my father.

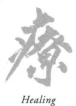

Healing

In the 1960s, long before the era of complementary and integrated medicine, I became discouraged in my pursuit of a role in the medical profession, sensing that something was missing in the way Western medicine was practiced. Gradually, I shifted the focus of my study to comparative world philosophies, mining the ancient traditions for evidence of the inherent self-healing capacity. As a Christian I found myself resonating with the truths of many traditions, including the secrets of the Native American shamans, Hebrew Kabbalah, Hindu Vedas, Sufi mystics, European alchemists, and the Chinese Daoists. In the basement archives of the library at the University of Cincinnati I found the most amazing collection of rare and ancient books. The volumes on those dusty shelves fed a raging hunger in me; I devoured them.

At the time I had experienced very little of Chinese culture beyond that offered by a restaurant near the library. But as I read and read, two profound statements stuck so hard in my consciousness that I still remember them today. One was a question from the ancient Chinese philosopher Lao Zi, who asked "Can you master your wandering mind and realize the Original Unity; can you adjust your breath, cultivate essential energy, and sustain the suppleness of a newborn with no cares?" Standing there in the university library archive I declared out loud, "I want to be a doctor of this!"

Then just days later, I read another line from the notebook of a Christian missionary working in China in the 1920s that opened the gateway to my personal and professional future: "Mind the body and the breath, and then clear the mind to distill the Heavenly elixir within." I didn't know when or how, but I was certain that I would someday be a doctor who would understand and prescribe this inner elixir.

During this same period, I had the opportunity to learn and practice Tai Chi, one of the many forms of Qigong. The instructor taught the very things that had caught my attention in the old books: manage the body and the breath and calm the mind to produce a powerful medicine within. Inspired by these experiences, in 1971 I began the study of Chinese medicine in Vancouver at one of the few schools of Chinese medicine in all of North America. I studied with wonderful teachers at additional schools in Hawaii and California. In 1977 I began my clinical practice as a Master of Acupuncture (M.Ac.) and in 1983 qualified as a Doctor of Oriental Medicine (O.M.D.).

Meeting a Chinese Master

Perhaps the most meaningful moment for me in my quest for the *one essential*, was the day in 1973 that I met Chang Yi Hsiang at the Tai Hsuan School of Chinese Medicine in Honolulu, Hawaii. At the Tai Hsuan Clinic, the air was filled with the powerful scent of herbal medicines. The fragrance alone allowed me to feel healing resources stirring within me. A thin haze of sweet-smelling smoke drifted from several treatment rooms where heated herbs were being used. Sunlight filtered through the window, casting a templelike glow. In a small office near the waiting room, I sat before the headmaster of the college, a woman small in stature but with tremendous presence. Around us were bookcases filled with volumes covered with Chinese characters, which, I guessed, described ancient medical secrets and strategies for healing, longevity, and inner peace. I avoided the headmaster's gaze by directing my focus to the items on her desk—a lidded teacup with a painting of two dragons playing with a flaming pearl; a container with a large calligraphy brush and a neatly tied bundle of stalks of some sort of herb; a white porcelain bowl filled with cotton contained what I estimated to be two hundred neatly aligned acupuncture needles.

"We have your letter of application and your statement of purpose for the study of Chinese medicine," Dr. Chang began. She had an excellent command of the English language and a charming accent. "It is agreed, what you say here is true.

Master

Acupuncture, herbal medicine, and Chinese massage are among the most eloquent, gentle, and profound medicines in the world. But medicine is not our ultimate focus here. We are involved in exploring the essence of life as understood by ancient scientists, physicians, and philosophers. Natural healing treatment is just one of the most practical expressions of this study. Personal Qi cultivation, Qigong, is our primary focus."

I knew that Chinese diagnosis looked for signs of health and disease by reading one's Qi through the skin color, speech, posture, and other signs. As Dr. Chang regarded me silently, I wondered if she could see my energy field. I guessed that she was observing the whites of my eyes for brightness or dullness, additional information on the state of my vitality. I remembered that even in my own culture the eyes were thought to be a window into one's soul.

Some gentle influence from her was causing me to feel more comfortable. My hands began to tingle. She was smiling. I relaxed a little.

"Before the world was," she continued, "before the multitude of things, the primordial universe was a vast undifferentiated ocean of potential—a boundless 'no thing' known as Wuji. This eternal cosmos, the origin of all events, beings, and things, is infused with a subtle, pervasive, invisible resource—Qi. Deep within this endless, seamless pool of no actualities and infinite possibilities stirred an impulse, which excited the 'no thing' to differentiate and become 'something.' Suddenly light emerged in contrast to darkness. Emptiness and material were born and permeated with the ever-present Qi. First, in its becoming there were cosmic gases, stars, and planets. Much, much later came the living beings."

When she said this, I couldn't help but think of God's breath upon the water that created the world in the view of the Western cultures and the declaration, "Let there be light." Her account also reminded me of the Big Bang theory. I knew in the instant that she began to speak that I had come upon a real treasure. Imagine my excitement to discover that the entire Chinese culture had long loved, honored, and investigated the *one essential* thing—and now I even knew it by a name: Qi.

"Even now the stars, the planets, the elements, the plants, the creatures, and ourselves; all of these move within and are penetrated and influenced by that original field of Qi. Qi is what causes the planets to maintain their orbits around the sun. It is the Qi that causes each snowflake to be unique and the Qi that shifts the moon phases and the tides. Qi sustains our health and Qi is the force behind intelligence and emotions. Qi is the vitality that causes the evolution of a tiny embryo of dividing cells to mature into a full-size human. The longing of the Qi of the earth to reach up and merge with the Qi of heaven drives a small sprout out of the seed—upward in spite of the force of gravity—to become a giant tree. Qi is known from the expressions that it embodies: the process of healing, the creativity that generates poetry and art, the transformation of tadpoles into frogs and caterpillars into butterflies. Qi is life force, energy, and consciousness—it is the essence behind all effects, influences, and events as well as all elements, materials, and objects."

Heaven

Earth

I sat in a kind of wonder and remembered those special moments with my grandmother and those times watching clouds or walking in the woods when I had journeyed about in my own heart and mind seeking clues to the essence of all things.

I was indescribably fulfilled hearing Dr. Chang refer to Qi as this essence. "At this school," she went on, "cultivating the Qi in our lives is the primary training for the art of healing. Medical skills spring from this art. As a physician of Chinese medicine, through your own cultivation you will always be in an intimate relationship with the Qi and therefore within constant reach of mystery, healing, benevolence, and peace. I sense that Qigong will become a primary life focus for you. This is a great fortune for your patients; your ability as a physician will spring from understanding Qi."

Amazingly, just as Dr. Chang predicted, Qigong and Tai Chi have become my primary focus. I have been gently drawn deeper and deeper into their secrets. Now a doctor of Chinese medicine for more than two decades, I have practiced cultivating Qi almost every day and taught thousands of people, who now teach many thousands of people, how to access and cultivate Qi through Qigong and Tai Chi. I have been to China seven times, where millions of people practice Qi cultivation every day in hospitals, parks, and temples.

Doctor

There are now more than forty schools of Chinese medicine in the United States alone. I have lectured for audiences from diverse professional and personal backgrounds. In 1997 *The Healer Within* was published to bring the basic concepts of Qigong and Tai Chi to a wider public. I am pleased that it is now used by hospitals, schools, community agencies, churches, and even prisons. I understand that clinics give it to patients and that people give it to their doctors. It has helped to create numerous small groups of community practice throughout America, Canada, and Australia. It has now been thirty-five years since I first heard the word *Qi*, and though it remains the foundation of my work, I am still filled with amazement and questions.

The Ancient Science of Personal Energy Management

My story and your story may not be so different. Perhaps you have felt the pull of destiny in your life too. We are honestly seeking health and vitality. Through personal mastery of the practice of Qigong and Tai Chi, I have been able to help build a bridge between ancient Chinese tradition and the millions of people in contemporary culture who want and need to improve their health, vitality, and personal capacity.

You are beginning, or perhaps you are continuing, your own discovery of the essential underlying forces of nature, which enliven, heal, empower, and inspire us all. We each have been called to investigate what in China has been known for centuries as *Tai Xuan* (*Tai Hsuan*), "the Great Mystery." Qigong is one of the most eloquent, poetic, and effective tools in our quest for personal breakthrough and peace of mind.

Wuji,
Primordial

This ancient investigation into the nature of the world, the discovery of Qi, and the evolution of Chinese medicine took place along with other advances in arts, astronomy, mathematics, and agriculture among some of the world's first scientists—a community of people known as the Daoists. Originally these communities were focused around observatories (*Guan* in Chinese). We now call them Daoist monasteries, due to the later introduction of religious themes into Daoism. Typically, Daoist communities were protected environments located deep in the mountains. The observatories were devoted to the focused exploration of nature, the cosmos, and the inner realms of human experience.

Daoist masters, among them the renowned Lao Zi, author of a classic Qigong primer entitled *Dao De Jing*,[1] first explained the interaction of nature's forces within the human body. They located the primary storage centers of Qi, the channels or passageways for the circulation of Qi, and the acupuncture points where Qi is concentrated. These ancient findings are only now beginning to be embraced by the Western world. However, they were the basis for a powerful system of medicine, longevity, and empowerment five to ten thousand years ago.

The *Huang Di Nei Jing*, or *The Yellow Emperor's Classic Book of Medicine*,[2] one of the most ancient medical texts in the world, is still revered in traditional Chinese medical education and practice thousands of years after its first publication around 300 B.C.E. Legend holds that Huang Ti, known as the Yellow Emperor and one of China's founding rulers, gained access to knowledge of supreme health, hearty longevity, and eternal truth by learning secrets of the ancient Qi masters from his trusted master teacher and spiritual minister Qi Bo. *The Yellow Emperor's Classic Book of Medicine* is one of the earliest books that suggests that the most profound medicine is produced naturally within us.

On the first page of the first chapter, entitled "Universal Truth," Huang Ti says to master Qi Bo, "I understand that in ancient times people lived well into the hundreds without showing the usual signs of aging. Have we lost the correct way of life?" "In ancient times," Qi Bo answers, "people practiced living in accordance with nature, called adhering to the Way of Life [*Dao* or *Tao*]. They understood balance as it is expressed in the transformation of universal Qi. They formulated and utilized practices such as *Dao Yin* (the ancient word for Qigong) including gentle body movements, self-applied massage, breath practice to promote Qi flow, and meditation to harmonize themselves with nature and the universe. They lived a natural life with balanced diet, sufficient rest, avoidance of the effects of stress on body and mind, and careful refraining from overindulgence. They purposefully maintained well-being and harmony of the body, mind, and spirit—it is no surprise that they lived in health over one hundred years."

Huang Di Nei Jing, with its focus on health improvement and the prevention of aging and disease through inner resource and energy management, provides an immensely insightful view of Chinese medicine. For your whole existence, according to Chinese tradition, from before your birth through this present moment and into your future, you always have been, are now, and always will be infused with the essen-

Mystery

tial unifying feature of the universe—the Qi. It is never not present, you are swimming in it. It bathes you, internally and externally, constantly fueling, cleansing, healing, rejuvenating, and enlightening you. Neither money, position, education, nor political power makes Qi more available. You cannot buy Qi. It is the birthright of all beings.

You can, however, become more capable of accessing, utilizing, and managing Qi. You can accomplish this through Qi cultivation—or Qigong. It is no surprise that Qigong, Tai Chi, acupuncture, and other ancient Asian sciences are beginning to gain great interest. For many, accessing the raw power of the universe through a self-healing empowerment system that has been refined and improved for thousands of years is like discovering an extraordinary treasure.

Ancient Formula for Flow

Ancient Qi masters developed a formula for health and longevity based on the Qi:

Inner Harmony = Qi Flow = Health and Longevity

This formula is the foundation of all Chinese medicine, acupuncture, and herbal medicine. Concepts in Western science such as coherence, resonance, and integrated body/mind function are parallel to the concept of harmony in China. In the West science points to numerous forms of flow including blood, lymph, brain chemical distribution, nerve transmission, and the movement of ions.

When they added the capacity to purposefully cultivate inner harmony through personal practices the ancients created this formula:

Practice + Intention = Inner Harmony = Qi Flow = Health and Longevity

Exploring Qi and Qigong is like opening a marvelous Chinese puzzle box—boxes within boxes, secrets within secrets. Think of yourself as having just reached a gateway where, only a moment ago, no gate was visible. According to Chinese tradition, if you open this gate and enter the realm of Qigong—with sincerity—a multitude of practical benefits will be yours. And the best news is that it is very easy to open the gate through a process that leads naturally to greater skill and mastery in a comfortable and phased process over time.

The First Promise of Qi

Secrets of ancient masters, formulas for healing and longevity, the gateway to personal breakthrough, and the way to understand the essence of the universe—these are big promises. On the surface it may seem as if such prizes must require travel to exotic places, lots of leisure time, access to special instruction, and great expense. But the truth is that Qigong is not complex and, as you will see, anyone can take the first steps.

Health, healing, power, sex, wealth, opportunity, pleasure, and inner peace all require one thing: essential life energy. Imagine trying to work, play, make money, have sex, or heal disease with deficient life force and depleted stamina. It can't happen. This fact is so obvious that we usually overlook it. Does the fish notice that she is moving in water; do humans notice that they are swimming in air?

The Chinese *did* take notice. Thousands of years ago they noticed that we are surrounded and bathed and infused with Qi. They made understanding the workings of this universal essence into a primary discipline—Qigong. Their findings are the subtle secrets of the Qi masters. These concepts and methods—developed and carefully guarded by emperors, physicians, monks, philosophers, and military experts— revealed the promise of the Qi. Then for hundreds of generations they refined that understanding, as if they were polishing precious jade.

Cultivating Qi will make you more vital, magnetic, and productive. Ample and harmonious Qi enhances brain power and clarity of thought, which nourishes the capacity to learn new things and pursue intentions and goals. People with ample energy create opportunities and innovation. Harmonious Qi will make you more resilient to stress and less vulnerable to negative situations. With healthy and vital Qi you will have the stamina and clarity to purify and release the emotions that perpetuate stress and sabotage productivity. In relationships you will become a more dynamic, more empowered, and less dependent partner. You can learn to access the universal source of energy rather than depending on someone else to be your source. Energetic people are more interesting, more tolerant, more fun, more sexual, more creative, and more productive.

Consciously Connect to the Force That Runs the Universe

Every level of Qigong is based in the process of intentfully choosing where you place your attention, focus, and purpose. Through this focus you can choose to connect with a wide array of different potentials or frequencies. The ultimate Qigong goal is to plug directly into the force that runs the entire universe.

Certain activities, events, people, and thoughts are draining. They exhaust your vitality and dim your radiance. Likewise, certain activities, events, people, and thoughts empower and energize. They enhance your vitality, and your inner light radiates.

Feel the difference within yourself. Visualize experiencing the restoring natural influence of a waterfall deep in a lush rain forest or pristine mountain wilderness. Then picture yourself experiencing a hectic, crowded airport full of frustrated travelers. Notice the difference within yourself. Visualize connecting with sources or influences of rejuvenation and inspiration. Then imagine connecting with their opposites—stress and exhaustion. This observation itself is a form of Qigong, simply noticing where you gain and where you lose Qi. Waterfalls and sunsets give you energy, power, and increased capacity. Crowded airports and traffic jams put your whole system on alert, drain your life force, and leave you exhausted.

Through Qigong, you can purposefully create a direct channel into an unlimited field of ever-present nourishing resources. The origin of this energy is the universe itself—the sun, the earth, the boundless field of potential (sometimes called the quantum field). The same astounding resource that regulates the seasons, causes plants to grow, and creates stars and galaxies is available to each of us. This resource is Qi.

The Qi Matrix

The extraordinary system for absorbing, circulating, and refining Qi in the body is called the Qi Matrix. The Qi Matrix is a pervasive network, the subtle circuitry of your life force. The channels or pathways of Qi (*Jing Luo*) deliver the life force to every part of the body as fuel or resource for every function. The Qi Matrix interfaces with the living physiological matrix. It vitalizes the blood, enables nerve conductance, sustains organ activity, and provides functional capacity for every cell and tissue in the living process. The bioenergetic interface between the Qi Matrix and the physiological matrix is emerging as a key area of twenty-first century science.

Contemporary biophysics and new era cell biology are confirming much of what the ancient Daoist investigators of Qi seemed to intuit. We know that the universe is alive and dynamic with various forces including gravity, cosmic rays, and the energetic frequencies of the sun. In Qigong theory a profound force enters into the human system from the universe—Qi of Heaven. An equally potent and subtle force enters the human body from the earth, which we know is a huge magnet—Qi of Earth. As you can imagine the resources of Heaven were conceived by the ancients to gather in the Qi reservoir of the head and influence particularly the upper body. The resources of Earth gather in the lower-belly Qi reservoir and influence the lower body.

The Heaven and the Earth link together through what is often called the Central Tai Chi Channel. You will notice right away that this channel has the same name as the beautiful form of Qigong known as Tai Chi. While many people know Tai Chi as an exercise practice, a moving meditation, or a martial art, it was originally an explanation of the formation of the universe and the foundation of human life. The connection of Heaven and Earth in the human system, through the Central Tai Chi Channel, parallels the vertebral column, and the central flow of blood, lymph, cerebrospinal fluid, and neurological activity.

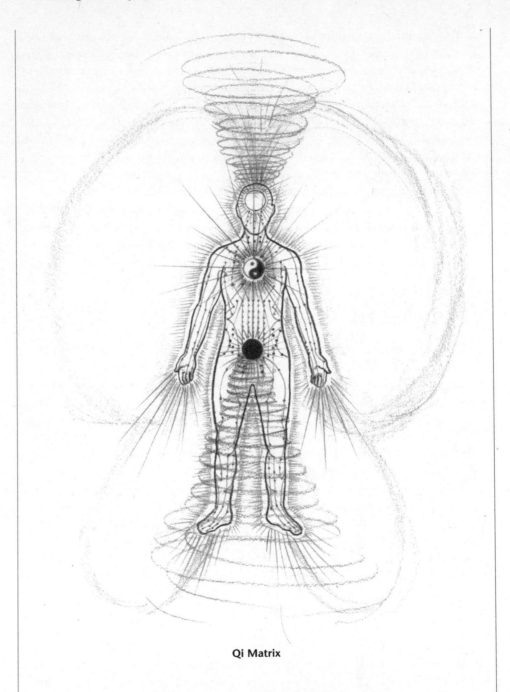

Qi Matrix

The interaction of Heaven and Earth is the basis for life and the foundation of the whole system of Chinese medicine and Qigong. This life force infuses everything living and infuses the natural influences that create and sustain life, such as water, air, and sun. In addition to absorbing the Qi of Heaven and Earth, we can absorb Qi from the field of life as well. Gathering the Qi of life from trees, crowds of enthusiastic people, fields of grass or flowers, as well as bodies of water and mountains all can contribute to the quantity and quality of our personal Qi.

In Qigong the goal is to open the Qi Matrix and maximize the dynamic interactivity of inner and outer Qi forces through the Qigong state. Qi cultivation practices reduce inner resistance and create optimal Qi circulation—flow. By using Qigong to cultivate and enhance the Qi, the most highly refined resource—the healer within—is being created and circulated to foster maximal healing and peak personal performance. This is the elixir that I read about in the basement library so many years ago. "Mind the body and the breath, and then clear the mind to distill the Heavenly elixir within." At the more advanced levels of Qigong this is known as the Golden Elixir of Life. It is a medicine that can heal not only the body but the mind, emotions, and spirit as well.

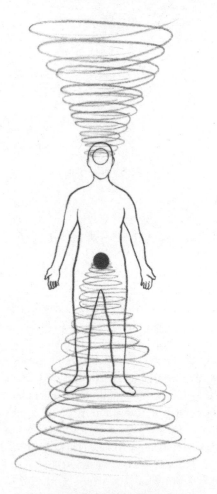

Heaven and Earth Qi Reservoirs

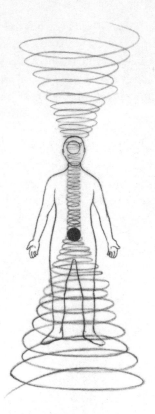

Central Tai Chi Channel

The Qi Paradigm: A Way of Being

Qigong asks us to lighten our grip on how we perceive the world and how we approach our lives. To get into the Qi enhancement state means that you will relax when formerly you have become tense. You will be electing to breathe deeply when you formerly have held or constrained your breath. The Qi, mysterious and invisible, is ever present though not obvious. Qi creates a whole new view of life.

You probably would not consider living in a house made of mud or grass to be a measure of great success. Yet, in some parts of China and the cultures of the South Seas such a dwelling is indeed highly esteemed. Similarly, one person may see a certain plant as a weed, while others honor it as an important medicine or nutritious food. These contrasts represent different ways of seeing, different ways of being—different paradigms.

The Qi paradigm may seem strange to you at first. Fortunately it is neither painful, complex, nor expensive. The Qi is always present and it is free. Begin to notice it around you. Step outside, plant your feet firmly on the ground, think past the sidewalk or the grass to the soil, the rock, the planet below you. Look up into open blue

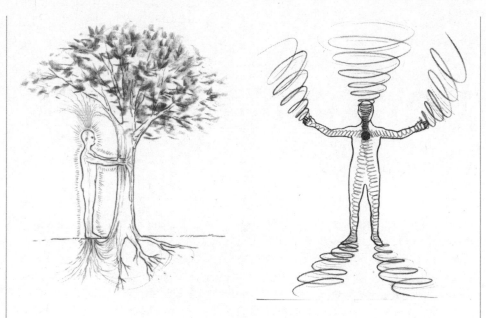

Accessing Qi from Nature

sky or the black night and speculate on the boundless nature of the cosmos. Take on the thinking of the ancient Qi masters, sincerely penetrating nature to understand and align with the forces of Heaven and Earth, which rush together and merge within the vessel of the human body.

Imagine deciding not to think or worry about the details and complexities of your life for an extended time. Let go of work, errands, frustrating feelings about people and things, and your endless to-do list. Imagine being in this state for thirty minutes or more every day. A hundred million people do this in China through the practice of Qigong and Tai Chi. They purposefully disassociate from the complexities and challenges of their personal situations and take up an intentful association with the powerful and invisible resources of nature.

There are a variety of ways to manage life and perceive the world. Historically our Western paradigm has not embraced the concept that the function of the human system is driven by an invisible and pervasive essential force. Can we grasp the idea of allowing Qi to operate within its natural realm, rather than trying to incorporate it into our familiar Western point of view? When you let the Qi be what it has always been, a kind of radical magic arises.

In my teaching it has been inspiring to watch people awaken to the possibilities of cultivating Qi. Many gain access to healing. Others are empowered with a new vision of the world that triggers personal transformation. It is easy to become addicted to Qi. It has no cost. Though it makes you feel high, it is completely legal. It gives you access to greater energy, maximizes your potential, and creates empowered self-reliance.

Understand Qi. Access Qi. Cultivate Qi. Master Qi. It is the essential fuel behind all intention and action. It is the power of the universe within you. This resource creates supercharged potential, optimizes your creativity, and nourishes your ability to overcome obstacles and gain success. Qi is your edge in sports, business, relationships, and personal performance. Qigong is a power tool, profound yet simple, that will assist you in fulfilling your intentions, needs, goals—even your dreams!

Qigong Methods

Open

HISTORICAL REFLECTION Every form of Qigong or Tai Chi has initial movements that commence the practice. In ancient times the practitioners from the temples and armies used openings that were quite detailed. From the way in which practitioners opened their Qigong or Tai Chi form you could tell who their master was, their lineage, or their alliance in a particular political or martial conflict. Such openings were highly secret and frequently very complex. The opening described here is simple and practical; it is similar to the opening used by many practitioners in contemporary Qigong and Tai Chi. We will use it to open any set or combination of methods for our practice.

INSTRUCTION Standing with your feet together, toes ahead or just slightly turned out, sink your weight and bend your knees comfortably. It is customary in many forms to step out to the left, but please feel free to step either way and mix it up over time. Shift your weight to one foot so that you are balanced with your weight completely on that foot. Step out. Usually the distance is about shoulder width. For those just beginning,

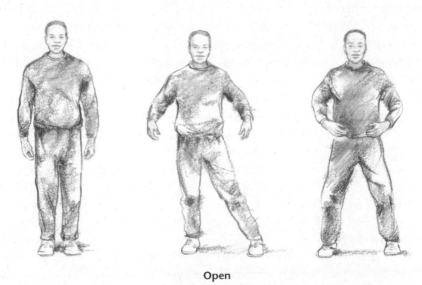

Open

this could be a little less; for those more advanced, a little more. As you sink down and shift your weight, your arms open outward. Inhale.

Redistribute your weight evenly to both feet and settle. Check to see that your lower back is somewhat elongated, as if it were pressed against a vertical wall. Position your head on top of your upright spine. Allow your arms and hands to move together gently as you exhale—as if you were cradling an invisible ball of Qi. The ending position of the hands will depend on whether you intend to use this posture for a meditation or to move into other methods of practice. The posture that you are in after the opening movement is a classic standing meditation posture. You could simply remain in this posture and enter into the Qigong state: "Mind the body and the breath, then clear the mind to distill the Heavenly elixir within." Or you might proceed with a Tai Chi form or a Qigong method.

Close

HISTORICAL REFLECTION It is customary to add a closing gesture to all forms of Tai Chi and Qigong. Like the opening, this movement is often associated with certain rituals or secret information about a practitioner's rank and position in a certain lineage or school. More important for our considerations, it closes the form that you are practicing and is intended to be a signal to yourself to conclude your practice.

Because Qigong practice is intended as a method for life improvement, the close is a moment in which to simply thank yourself for taking the time to take care of your health. In addition, it is an opportunity to remind yourself of the value of taking the benefit of your practice into your day. Qigong intends to be more than a few minutes of practice in an isolated corner of your life. It can become a way of being, choice making, and consciousness. In the closing you can declare internally that you intend to implement a Qigong approach to life and take a moment to count your blessings or confirm your highest intentions.

INSTRUCTION From whatever method of Tai Chi or Qigong you have just finished practicing, open and outstretch your arms. Breathe in. Both the movement and the breath suggest gathering Qi. Shift your weight to one foot. As you reach out imagine you are gathering healing and empowering resources from the whole cosmos—Heaven and Earth. As your hands come over the top of your head begin to exhale; bring the extended foot in to rest next to the weighted foot.

As you exhale slowly allow your hands to come drifting downward, passing the face, chest, and abdomen—it is as if you are bathing yourself in the healing Qi of the universe. Visualize that you are filling the Central Tai Chi Channel and the Qi Matrix with powerful resources. Finally, place one hand over the other and rest your hands on the lower abdomen, your thumbs resting over the umbilicus. In this position your palms rest on the Earth Elixir Field, a powerful storage area for the inner elixir. Allow yourself to drift gently here until you feel that you have concluded and are ready to move gently into your day or the next chapter of your life.

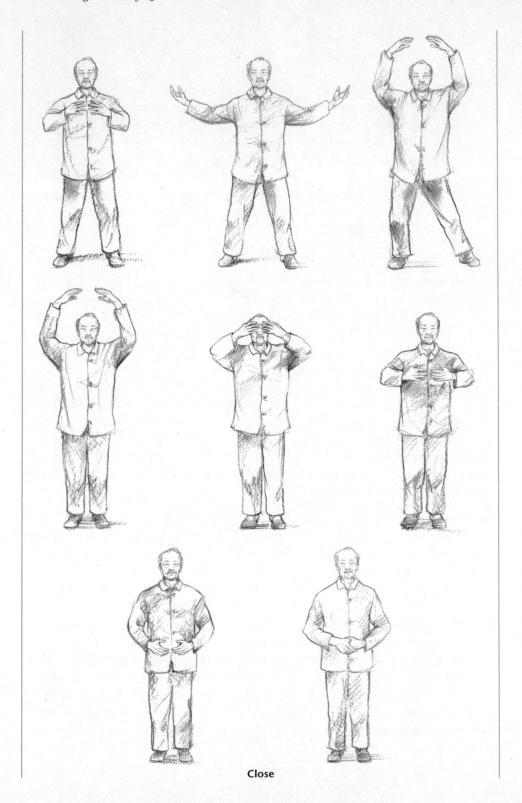

Close

Simple yet Profound

For the Universe
even the most difficult things
occur spontaneously.
The largest result
is composed of countless minute elements.
The master understands,
in the Universe and in life,
great achievements may easily be accomplished
by starting with small actions.

—LAO ZI, *DAO DE JING,* #63

Purple Bamboo Park

Take a deep breath, adjust your posture, relax your shoulders, and visualize yourself entering Purple Bamboo Park in Beijing, China, at 6:00 A.M. It is a cool morning in May. There is a misty vapor in the air that glows with the sun's early light. The air carries the fragrance of spring flowers and the freshness of new grass and spring growth on willow trees and pines. Ancient trees, huge areas of bamboo, and the lake thick with lotus plants are all like guardians committed to protecting and maintaining this natural sanctuary in the northwest corner of China's capital city.

Profound

Bamboo

You are acutely aware of your own sense of awe and wonder as you step deeper into this famous park, which has been carefully tended for centuries. Almost immediately, along the bamboo-lined corridor of the entry walkway, you note faint figures moving silently, almost floating in the mist, in one of the grassy open areas. Your first impression, judging from their gestures, is that these are large birds, stepping deftly in shallow water. Finally you realize that these graceful creatures are people engaged in the mysterious fluid movements of Qigong (Chi Kung). This particular form, its original roots deep in the rich shamanic traditions of Chinese philosophy, medicine, and culture, is likely the offspring of the bird forms of ancient Qi (Chi) masters who enacted the forces of nature through dance.

This group of about thirty people seems to be inhabited by the spirit of majestic cranes in a uniform and synchronized ritual of intentful movement. They ruffle their wings, they turn, and advance—they fly without leaving the ground. Touching their wing tips purposefully to their backs, they turn and advance again. The intensity of their practice has an effect on you, even though you are just observing. For nearly an hour they continue in silence until, as the mist is clearing, the practice is complete. The group breaks into random clumps of people chatting happily. For another half hour most of the participants linger in a lighthearted social exchange.

I have visited Purple Bamboo Park many times to have conversations with the Qigong practitioners. Imagine we are there together, you and I.

"Why do you come to the park every day?" we ask. "We are the Flying Crane Longevity Group," a cheerful older woman answers. "We come here to cultivate health and vitality. My family has historically suffered from severe arthritis; I have prevented this disease in myself through this practice."

A much younger woman dressed in very modern Western attire adds, "I work near this park. If I ride my bicycle here at six, I avoid the bus and truck fumes, have a nice wakeup practice, and then go to work knowing I have enhanced my health and my thinking."

A man between thirty-five and forty comes forward, "I always thought that Qigong and Tai Chi [Taiji] were for older people. But my productivity at work has increased significantly since I started with this practice. Because I have the aspiration to start my own business in our new economic era, I need the extra energy while I am working a second job. I actually do a second practice—a short form of Tai Chi—in the afternoon, following a brief nap, before I start my computer job."

A gentleman of about fifty joins the discussion. "We come to the park early in the morning. Most of us need to be at our work by seven or seven-thirty. The hours around the sunrise are associated with rich resources of nature. The dew on the ground becomes mist as the sun rises and evaporates the moisture. We believe that this is nature making a medicine for us that we breathe in and bathe in, both internally and externally. The night is Yin and the day is Yang, sunrise is the harmony point between night and day—this represents our own inner harmony—as we transition from our resting to our active self."

Throughout Bamboo Park groups are practicing—large groups on the sidewalks and grassy areas, smaller groups and individuals on plazas and among the trees and shrubs. There are several thousand people here every day. Several hidden areas with water nearby give the classic mixture of natural elements so important to the Chinese for health and tranquility. There are rocky grottoes, small meditation areas, all around the lake and an island with traditional round Chinese bridges, which, together with their reflection in the water, create a beautiful circular image.

My favorite Qigong and Tai Chi spot in Purple Bamboo Park is a complex of traditional Chinese buildings. You enter through a round moon gate, walk along a passageway that borders a peaceful pond, and arrive at a terrace or plaza that offers a perfect practice area for Qigong and Tai Chi. Several willow trees surround the pool. Willows are the perfect example from nature of reaching to Heaven (the trunk) and relaxing down to Earth (the graceful branches). Beyond the pool is a meeting hall much like those in a typical Daoist temple, which is very conducive to deep Qigong practice. Once late at night, I was there at just the right moment to catch the reflection of the full moon in the pool surrounded with willow branches. How many of China's greatest poets tried to capture such a moment and how many enlightenments were triggered by such an image?

Qigong Breakthrough

The human system produces the most profound medicine naturally within. Qigong and Tai Chi are time-tested tools for activating this incredible human capacity. And the range of application is immense, from personal challenges such as disease and fatigue to cultural challenges such as violence, learning disabilities, and addiction. From health care and personal productivity to education and spirituality, the Qi cultivation arts are a remarkable breakthrough.

However, Qigong is often overlooked as a tool for fitness and empowerment because, ironically, to some it seems too simple. It is true that certain forms of Qigong are quite simple; that is their beauty. Such methods can be accessed by anyone. I have had the opportunity to teach simple Qigong and modified forms of Tai Chi to kids and teachers in schools, recovering drug addicts, executives seeking stress relief and greater effectiveness, and inmates at Folsom Prison. It is also true that some forms are quite esoteric and more difficult to grasp. But in the park every morning in China, millions of people practice forms of Qigong and Tai Chi that are very simple and practical, targeted toward basic energy enhancement and healing.

The wonder of this ancient, multilevel system of mind/body enhancement is that it can contribute benefit for diverse situations and needs. There are no boundaries to who can benefit—the very old and the very young, people who are extremely ill and those who are well and want to stay well. The simplest forms of Qigong allow easy access in the beginning. Those who wish to evolve their practice can advance to levels

Longevity

that naturally suit them. Even the ancient masters will reveal that there is not really a limit—one can always go deeper.

In China, when the physician recommends the practice of Qigong or Tai Chi, the patient can simply go to the park in the morning and find an instructor. A physician or a friend may say, "In Purple Bamboo Park, go to the small island in the part of the lake where the lotus grows. Teacher Shi is just across the bridge to the left. His method of Tai Chi will be excellent for your condition." These morning classes are the foundation of the Chinese public health system.

Several prominent ministers of health from the Chinese government have confirmed this to me personally, saying that those millions of people who go to the parks to sustain their health and vitality cost the government and the health-care system nothing. Besides the Chinese people's natural love for vitality, the popularity and success of Qigong health and longevity practices lie in the strength of numbers. Any one person is inspired to do Qigong or Tai Chi because there are millions of other people doing it and a mountain of research on the benefits has accumulated in recent years.

In the United States, it has until recently been more difficult to direct a patient to a Qigong or Tai Chi class. Fortunately, this situation is rapidly changing and many hospitals, health-care organizations, schools, churches, and community agencies have begun to offer classes in Qigong and Tai Chi. An array of excellent books in English, including *The Healer Within*,[1] have introduced Qigong and Tai Chi to the American public, who are more interested in vitality, longevity, and stress management every day. As we delve deeper into the philosophical foundations and practical applications of Qigong and Tai Chi, you will see that there are many paths to investigating the promise of the Qi. (See Recommended Reading for more resources.)

The Two Kinds of Medicine and the Three States of Qi

One of the most powerful features of Chinese medicine is that for thousands of years it has been accessible to the average citizen. Traditionally, everyone learns a little Chinese medicine to apply: nutrition, the self-massage of Qi points, and the practice of Qigong or Tai Chi. Many doctors in the West consider it inappropriate for their patients to do minor medical procedures at home. They do not encourage people to self-prescribe medicines. However, in China anyone can walk into a pharmacy with an herbal formula written by a grandparent and walk out with a mild, natural remedy without the recommendation of a doctor. It is very typical for family members to massage each other using a few commonly known acupuncture points. This great accessibility of self-directed health care to the average person allows self-reliance to be the foundation of the traditional Chinese health-care system.

Cultivation

As you practice Tai Chi and Qigong you will benefit from these insights into traditional Chinese medicine. A little bit of knowledge will allow you to conduct a simple assessment of your own health using the very same framework that Chinese doctors use. This will allow you to gain a preliminary understanding of how Qigong may be used alone as a tool for self-healing or as a complementary method along with acupuncture or whatever medical regimen you follow.

Exploring the basic concepts of Chinese medicine that emerged from the original understanding of the Qi in very ancient times will inform your own Qi cultivation. These are ideas that everyone knows about in China. They are fundamental and commonly understood, as we in the West understand the value of grandma's chicken soup and vitamin C. The "two kinds of medicine" and the "three states of Qi" are theories that are easy to understand. They help to reveal why Qigong and Tai Chi remain so popular in China, thousands of years after their origin in ancient times, and why the Qi cultivation arts are so rapidly gaining momentum in America, Europe, and the rest of the world today. You can share these concepts with family members and associates. The essence of Chinese medicine is not complex. It was originally developed by kind-hearted grandparents, the elders of China's ancient communities.

The Two Kinds of Medicine

In the West, traditionally, we have had only one kind of medicine—the treatment of disease. Unfortunately, in our culture we wait until we are sick and need to be cured before we think about medical treatment. Our Western medical heritage has historically taught us very little about using personal methods of disease prevention, health enhancement, or self-potentiation. In fact until recently, in Western medicine, even prevention has usually been characterized by clinical procedures—immunization, mammography, etc.—that are employed to fight or screen for disease. In the Chinese approach a key aspect of prevention is accomplished by enhancing general health with behavioral activities including nutrition, meditation, Qigong, and Tai Chi.

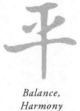

Balance, Harmony

Most ancient cultures have a strong tradition of prevention. For example, Native Americans talk about "big medicine," referring to an individual's personal capacity, strength, or power. While big medicine can be focused on disease curing, its primary focus is the enhancement of inner potential for daily life and for enhancing intuition. In China this kind of personal radiance and stamina—big medicine—would be called big Qi (*Da Qi*). It is the obvious presence of individual energy and life force—a robust field of personal power. The Chinese would say, "He or she has big Qi."

In Chinese culture, from the very beginning, the concept of utilizing medicine for longevity and personal optimization has held equal weight with the use of medicine for the treatment of disease. Because they enhance inner harmony and balance, such practices as acupuncture and herbal medicine can be used equally for preventive health care as well as for disease treatment. As we saw earlier, the *Huang Di Nei Jing*, China's most ancient and revered medical resource, begins not with a focus on disease curing, but with a focus on well-being and long, healthy life.

True, Righteous

The superior physician, that text suggests, honors the unique inner spirit in each person and renders health-enhancing treatment while people are healthy to keep them well (usually through nutrition and Qigong), rather than merely treating them after they have lost their health. The foundation of Chinese medicine is health improvement, rather than disease curing. There have always been physicians in the West who share this view. Dr. William J. Mayo, of Mayo Clinic fame, said, "The ideal of medicine is to eliminate the need for a physician." William Osler, a Canadian physician who was famous for advocating warmer relationships between patient and physician, likewise stated, "It is not just important to determine what disease the person has, more it is important to determine what sort of person has the disease."

The earliest mention of these ideals occurred in the first writings of the Han dynasty (200 B.C.E.–200 C.E.). Most scholars agree that these writings indicate concepts so well defined that they may have been in existence thousands of years before they were written down. In the centuries since, many accounts reaffirm this philosophy in texts that are revered as medical classics, books with wonderful titles like: *Compendium of Essentials on Nourishing Life, Prescriptions Worth a Thousand Ounces of Gold, The Great Clarity Discourse on Protecting Life, Record on Nourishing Inner Nature and Extending Life, Book of the Master Who Embraces Simplicity,* and *The Visualization of Spirit and Refinement of Qi.*[2]

Like Western medicine, Chinese medicine includes a component related to disease curing called "attack the disease" or "address the pathology," which has a long history of effectiveness. However, it is the Chinese category of medicine that is directed at potentiation and disease prevention that is such a revelation and a breakthrough to us here in the West. Known as "enhance the righteous" or "support the natural self-healing capacity" (*Fu Zheng*), this approach aims to maximize what is right rather than trying to fix what is wrong. This is an extraordinary gift to us in the Western world at a time when our health-care system is in serious distress. The complementary utilization of these two forms of medicine—attack the disease and enhance the righteous—is the foundation of the current breakthroughs in complementary and alternative medicine (CAM) and integrative medicine in the United States.

Qigong can be used to cure or heal, but it does so by maximizing naturally occurring inner resources. For example, there are two ways to kill bacteria. With a medical antibiotic the goal is to kill the bacteria, an "attack the disease" strategy that may cause side effects as well. Alternatively, boosting the immune system with acupuncture, herbs, massage, and Qigong is probiotic—the healthy immune system is programmed to kill bacteria. In this case, the benefit is achieved through an "enhance the righteous" strategy—typically with very few side effects.

Until recently, cardiac medicine had only "attack the disease" methods such as bypass surgery and cholesterol-reducing drugs. We now know that heart disease can be reversed through "enhance the righteous" behaviors such as enhanced nutrition, stress mastery (including Yoga, Qigong, and meditation), and support groups.[3] In a complementary system of health care the most appropriate strategy is chosen depending on the case. The clinical choices are based on using the least invasive and least expensive measures that are in the highest and best interest of the patient.

Certain Qigong forms, known as medical Qigong, are specifically targeted at healing disease. However, they are not purely "attack the disease" approaches because the personal practice of Qigong always unleashes maximum potential with no negative side effects. Most Qigong traditions are focused primarily on longevity and the development of maximum human function, focusing on "enhance the righteous." That these forms can also help to cure disease is a beneficial side effect. When grandma said, "an ounce of prevention is worth a pound of cure" she was referring to the concept of "enhancing the righteous" or "supporting the natural self-healing capacity."

When you come to understand Qigong in the context of the "Two Kinds of Medicine," it becomes obvious that the scope of Qi cultivation is broad. In the "attack the disease" context, Qigong is a tool that is complementary to any treatment plan, whether of Western medicine, holistic medicine, or Chinese medicine. In the "enhance the righteous" context, Qigong becomes a tool for personal optimization that can be applied to work, play, decision-making, stress mastery, energy management, relationships, and personal empowerment. Qigong transcends the limited realm of disease and treatment to become a powerful tool for life mastery and personal transformation.

The Three States of Qi

To further understand how we can use Qigong to heal disease and optimize function we can turn to a basic theory in Chinese medicine that declares that Qi exists in three possible states in health and disease: harmony, deficiency, and stagnation. This is common knowledge in China—the Chinese know the states of Qi as we in the United States know that baseball season starts in the spring or that children love ice cream. In harmony, the life force is ample and in balance—the individual is in a relative state of health. In this context, Qigong is used to prevent disease, maintain health, and enhance function. Deficiency means that the person's Qi is insufficient. The purpose of Qigong in this context is to access and gather Qi to build and circulate an ample and robust supply. In stagnation, the Qi flow is blocked, stagnant, erratic, or toxic. In this context, Qigong is used to manage the Qi, neutralize or break through stagnation, and regain the optimal state of inner flow.

This system for describing health status is one of the first things that Chinese doctors learn. It points directly to the value of Qigong in your life and can even help you determine your need for additional medical treatment with acupuncture, herbs, massage, or conventional medicine.

Assess Yourself

Using the two lists that follow, you can do a preliminary Qi assessment of yourself. It is likely that you will show some signs of ample and harmonious Qi from the first list below. At the same time, you will likely find in yourself some signs of either deficiency or stagnation from the second list. If you find that you express most of the qualities from the first list, you are among the few very fortunate people who can simply use Qigong for health maintenance, longevity, and empowerment. In such cases, an "ounce of prevention" will sustain health and build personal power. If you find that you express more than three or four of the qualities from the second list, this suggests that you have either Qi deficiency, stagnation, or both and will need the "pound of cure." Fortunately, the pound of cure can be provided through Qigong by activating the profound medicine that is produced naturally within our own bodies. A pound of Qigong is definitely preferable to a pound of surgery or drugs.

Signs of Ample and Harmonious Qi

Review the following list. If you recognize these signs as part of yourself, you have some of the qualities associated with ample and harmonious Qi:

- little or no pain
- normal body temperature
- normal pulse rate and volume
- pink tongue
- feeling rested
- good stamina
- productive
- creative
- energetic
- humorous
- happy/peaceful
- imaginative, curious

If you exhibit six or seven of these qualities you have ample Qi. Your Qigong practice will be geared less toward accessing and building Qi and more toward attaining the ability to manage Qi. Ample Qi can help improve the imbalances that you may find in the list on page 29. In this case an ounce of prevention is all you need to sustain your health. However, many of you will be so fascinated with Qi cultivation, and the possibility of sharing Qigong and Tai Chi with others, that you will be compelled to deepen your practice as a way of reaching toward higher levels of personal performance or spiritual clarity. People like this are fondly known as Qi lovers. They tend to have more vitality, which translates into more accomplishment, more fun, and more peace.

Signs of Deficiency or Stagnation of Qi

Almost everyone exhibits some signs of Qi deficiency or stagnation, even relatively healthy people. Signs such as these serve as a gentle wakeup call at first. If you respond quickly, you can resolve minor health challenges before they become major illnesses— often by simply enjoying Tai Chi or Qigong. Otherwise a louder, more serious wakeup call may sound later. The ancient Qigong classics say, "Disorder is easiest to overcome before it starts; prevent problems before they arise." The following list shows some of the most common signs of deficiency and stagnation of Qi:

- fatigue
- stress, tension
- pain—joints, head, neck, back
- digestive and bowel problems
- anger, fear, worry, panic
- sickness and disease
- frequent colds, flu
- sexual or menstrual difficulties
- lung disorders
- allergies
- overly emotional states
- forgetfulness
- depression, lethargy
- anxiety, restlessness
- frustration, violence
- laziness, procrastination
- difficulty regulating body temperature
- sleeplessness
- red, pale, or coated tongue
- slow, fast, weak, or erratic pulse

If you express three or four of these symptoms, an ounce of prevention is not enough. Begin with a lighthearted, preventive practice of Qigong to neutralize health problems while they are minimal. If you have five or more of the signs on this list, I would suggest a more accelerated approach to Qigong. You will find everything you need in this book—except perhaps for some good friends to enjoy your practice with, your Qi community.

For thousands of years, doctors of Chinese medicine have diagnosed health problems without the use of Western medical technology by simply watching and listening for these signs of Qi imbalance. There are, of course, many symptoms that are not mentioned here. The goal is not to create a conclusive medical diagnosis, but instead to help orient you to your own level of need for Qigong and to create an understanding for taking action to "enhance the righteous." In China millions of people use Qigong and Tai Chi to balance their body, mind, and spirit and to reduce or eliminate health problems. This is why the parks in China are so full of practitioners at six o'clock every morning. You will likely find that the regular practice of Qigong resolves health challenges that once would have required a doctor visit or medication.

If you have the unusual state of both ample Qi (six to seven signs of ample and harmonious Qi) along with signs of deficiency and stagnation (three to four signs of deficiency or stagnation), you are fortunate. Most people with many signs of deficiency and stagnation do not have so many signs of ample and harmonious Qi. The time to improve is now while your vitality is high.

Your Qi Cultivation Prescription

Take your time getting started. If you force yourself to do too much it will just take the fun out of it and sabotage your progress. If you are well and want to remain well, do fifteen to thirty minutes of Qigong or Tai Chi each day. If you are well but you want to be *supremely* well, extend your practice to forty-five minutes or an hour. If you are experiencing symptoms that you wish to resolve, build up slowly to thirty minutes or more—up to one hour.

Secret

If you are seriously ill you may need to spread your practice out to sustain your strength. Try to become aware of when Qigong is enhancing you. Notice when it becomes important to rest or to sleep. An hour or more of practice is not too much, especially if it is spread out to three or four sessions of fifteen minutes throughout your day. In some of the famous Qigong hospitals in China there are Qigong practice sessions available throughout the day. Some people with cancer or paralysis practice in little bits every hour or so.

For those who are well, the practice helps to sustain health and maximize the potential for attainment of the highest personal goals. For those who have lost their health, the practices can help to build up inner reserves of life force, which decreases signs of disease and discomfort. In more advanced Qigong your practice will evolve to become a moment-to-moment experience using awareness of breath, mind focus, and posture throughout the day. This powerful program for self-improvement can operate almost all the time.

These ancient Chinese medical theories are completely complementary to Western medicine. No matter what discomfort or diagnosis you are working with, or what sort of treatment you are receiving, information from the two kinds of medicine and the three states of Qi can help you to improve or heal yourself using Qigong or Tai Chi. All of the health challenges you noted in your self-assessment can be positively modified to some extent with Qigong. As you move deeper into your practice, you are likely to find yourself having insight upon insight.

The Second Promise of Qi

In the Chinese tradition it is believed that it is the automatic function of Qi to teach, heal, and empower anyone who accelerates and refines his or her relationship with it. In my own practice I have continued to experience such break-throughs on a regular basis. One of my own first insights was that every Qigong or Tai Chi prac-tice session where I reached either genuine relax-

> ## THE SECOND PROMISE
>
> Every person who uses Qi cultivation methods consistently experiences some form of health improvement and personal access to greater energy and power.

ation or uninterrupted gentle movement for even a few minutes gave me a sense of subtle inner improvement. Much later I came to understand the fascinating physiol-ogy behind this phenomenon—another revelation. Even now, thirty years after my first experiences with Qigong and Tai Chi, new insights continue to flow in.

People who are consistent in the use of Qi cultivation methods, even if their approach is quite humble or simplistic, get results. Sophisticated practice is less impor-tant than sincere practice. It is not enough to enjoy the idea of Qi cultivation. When Qigong is implemented the second promise is fulfilled. Sometimes these results seem miraculous. More often they are simply a gratifying reflection of slow but sure per-sonal improvement. With consistent Qigong you will never know what disease you might have had. And you won't care. People don't notice the pains and diseases that they aren't having.

As you develop your Qi practice, particularly if you are consistent, you will find less need for medications, physician visits, and medical procedures. You may find that you sleep better, have more stamina, or experience less pain. With just a small but con-sistent contribution of time and attention you can be a healthier person, which means you will also be a happier person. By "enhancing the righteous" you improve your capacity for creativity, insight, clarity, and energy. This is the second promise of Qi.

Easing into Qigong

The first breakthrough in your practice of any Qi cultivation method is simply to decide to do the practice. Whether you take a deep breath and relax for a moment, go down to your Tai Chi spot in the park, or attend a Qigong class at the local hos-pital, electing to "do it" is the gateway to the benefits of Qigong. This decision is what makes your practice so profound and powerful. Turning your attention to the prac-tice of Qigong initiates a major shift in consciousness, which in turn triggers the benefits. Qigong implies a progression, a path, a way. Whether you are at the very beginning, exploring the possibility of engaging in intentful practice, or you are a sea-soned practitioner, the conscious act of deciding to practice makes all the difference.

Having a practice does not imply that your Qigong or Tai Chi will automatically be perfect; it doesn't need to be. In the growing of a great garden there is a tremendous amount of cultivation before the harvest: preparing the soil, selecting the best seeds, planting, watering, tending, and waiting. Similarly, in cultivating Qi there is the constant return to the essential components of cultivation to gain the harvest of inner harmony and vitality.

The Three Intentful Corrections

Fortunately, taking the first step is easy. In Qigong the all-important first level of practice is called the Three Intentful Corrections. They are so accessible that you can begin these without even leaving the comfort of the spot you are sitting in right now. And interestingly, no matter how far you progress or how complex and esoteric your practice becomes, these Three Intentful Corrections will always be an integral part of it.

THE THREE INTENTFUL CORRECTIONS

- Adjust and regulate the body posture or movement.
- Adjust and regulate the breath.
- Adjust and regulate consciousness.

Given the inspiration that I felt reading those dusty old books in the basement of the university library, you can imagine how inspiring it was later when numerous Chinese teachers taught me the Three Intentful Corrections as the foundation of Qigong and Tai Chi. I recalled that single line I had read in the journal of a missionary, who had most likely copied it from one of the ancient texts or heard it from a Chinese teacher: "Mind the body and the breath, and then clear the mind to distill the Heavenly elixir within." He had clearly described the Three Intentful Corrections as the formula for making a healing elixir within our own bodies. So simple, yet so profound.

The Three Intentful Corrections, also known as the three regulations, the three adjustments, or the three focal points, are the bedrock of every form of Qigong and Tai Chi. You will notice that to take a deep breath, you must adjust your posture. And you will notice that to adjust the posture, it helps to take a deep breath. Once you adjust the posture and the breath it becomes natural to relax and clear the mind/consciousness. In the thousands of Qigong practices, including all of the styles of Tai Chi and even Yoga, the Three Intentful Corrections are repeated constantly, from moment to moment.

This elixir has implications for healing every level of our being. And yet we don't have to wait for some ambiguous future to make this medicine. It begins with the very first lesson, with the simplest first level of practice—the Three Intentful Corrections.

Posture and Movement

In every form of Qigong and Tai Chi, posture is primary. Even if you practice Qi cultivation while lying in bed, adjusting the posture will enhance the practice.

Adjusting the posture optimizes all aspects of natural inner flow. The Qi flow is assisted by adjusting the body posture and relaxing purposefully. The blood and lymph, which are the fluid media in which the Qi circulates, are both enhanced when the posture is optimal and the body relaxed.

Imagine you are the lungs trying to get a full breath in a person who is under the pressures of stress or gravity. Imagine you are the kidneys trying to filter the blood, and instead of having plenty of room your inner pipes and vessels are restricted because the posture is contracted or collapsed downward. Imagine you are the liver trying to process the blood and remove metabolic or toxic waste, but your owner is frustrated, tense, and slumped in his or her chair. Now shift your posture to give the lungs optimal space and breathe deeply. You undoubtedly will find a major difference in volume. The organs operate at their best when they are suspended in their spacious, naturally designed environment where the Qi and fluids can freely circulate.

In either the sitting or standing posture, visualize a connection from the crown of your head up into the celestial realm—Heaven. Through this connection a gentle force lifts your head upward, which straightens and lengthens your spine. Relax your shoulders completely. Now visualize a connection from your sacrum to the center of our

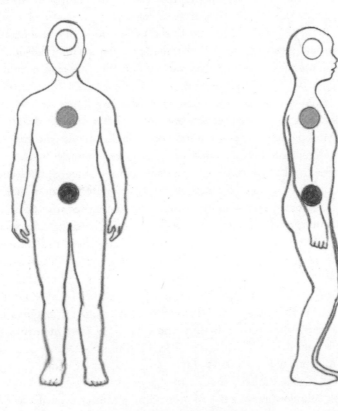

First Intentful Correction—Posture

planet. Through this connection a force gently pulls the lower part of your body downward, which straightens and lengthens your spine. The upward lift and the downward pull opens the center of the body, from the umbilicus to the heart, which fills with water (blood, lymph) and is infused with Qi.

This posture is the initial position—called Align or the Preliminary Posture—for almost every practice in this book and most Qi cultivation practices. The feet are about shoulder width apart with the toes pointing forward. The knees are slightly bent. The bowl of the pelvis turns gently on the hips so that the lower back flattens, the pubic bone lifts toward the chin and the abdomen automatically pulls in. Another way to think of this is that the pelvis is a bowl and the organs are like fruit. In most people the bowl spills forward and the fruit rolls out, causing an expanded belly and a forward curved lower spine. Straighten the spine and readjust the pelvis so the fruit is balanced in the bowl. The spine is erect and straight, with the head on top. The shoulders are relaxed and the arms and hands dangle downward completely relaxed; if you're sitting, they can rest in your lap. Finally, the elbows move slightly away from the body, creating an opening under the arms as if a small balloon has inflated there.

Movement in Qigong pumps and diffuses the body fluids and contributes to all aspects of the function of the Qi. Movement and breath combined are the primary beginning Qigong tools for learning to gain control of the acrobatic mind. Giving oneself something positive to focus on is the beginning of all systems of personal empowerment and transformation. Some Qigong teachers promote the idea that inner practice (meditation), with no external movement, is superior to moving practice. However, only for very advanced practitioners, who have achieved the ability to control the busy mind, is external movement replaced with stillness.

As you begin your Qigong practice, you will find that most Qigong methods are quite mild. Movements in Qigong must always be limited to those that heal and improve. Some more provocative forms of Qigong are intended to facilitate changes in the body structure by affecting the connective tissue. Try to get more familiar with Qigong before investigating such practices. Do not execute Qigong practices that are uncomfortable unless you are working with a very experienced instructor. When you bend, sink down, and stretch, be particularly careful for your neck, back, and knees. Stay in the comfort zone.

Breath

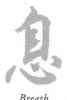

Breath

The breath is the most powerful tool for gathering, circulating, purifying, and directing Qi. Your first act upon birth into the world is to inhale. One ancient Qigong practice is to begin your day as if it is a new birth, by simply becoming conscious of the breath and taking a few deep, purposeful breaths, before you launch into your usual first practical thoughts. Rather than counting your projects, take a moment to count your blessings. End the day with conscious breathing as you surrender to the mystery of sleep. You can complement this with a list of things for which you are grateful. Is there anything more worthy of your attention as you drift into sleep? The breath is the easiest of the Three Intentful Corrections to practice. Changes in posture and movement are obvious but you can adjust your breath in meetings or in public places as a momentary Qigong practice without attracting attention.

On the inhalation the air enters the lower lungs first, expanding the abdomen. Then the continuation of the inhalation expands the chest. During the inhalation you are gathering resources with the air—oxygen and Qi. The pores are also breathing in. The skin is like a second set of lungs. On the exhalation the chest and abdomen empty simultaneously. Waste air and spent Qi are expelled while oxygen and fresh Qi are gathered from the air and environment and circulated within.

Inhale slowly and deeply. Hold your breath for a count of one, one thousand; two, one thousand; three, one thousand. Then exhale very, very slowly through your nose, unless it is more comfortable through your mouth. Feel if you can, or even visualize, that when you inhale, Qi is pouring into your lungs. Then on the exhalation feel the

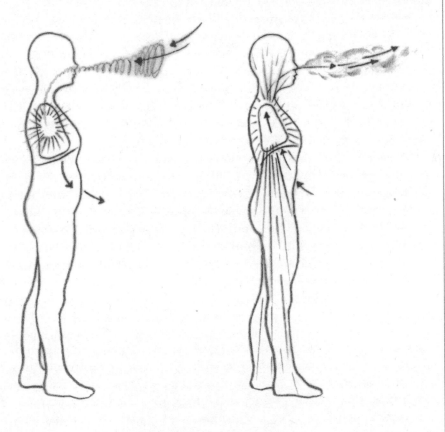

Second Intentful Correction—Breath

sensation of healing resources circulating throughout your internal environment. If you focus carefully inward without distraction you will very quickly feel what is called the Qigong state—a subtle sense of inner flowing, warmth, or tingling.

Do it again; inhale slowly and deeply. Hold your breath for the count of one, one thousand; two, one thousand; three, one thousand. Then exhale very slowly through your nose. What do you feel? When I ask this in workshops and lectures I get a wide variety of responses, such as "I feel tingling in my chest or my hands" and "I feel myself drifting toward peace." See what happens if you do this for just a few minutes. Each breath takes fifteen seconds so you can do eight in two minutes. If you can stay focused you will feel something. It is the medicine within, the elixir, the Qi.

Most people learn to perceive this sensation pretty quickly; however, if you do not immediately experience it, do not worry. Worry is the enemy of the Qigong state. In this case simply use your imagination or visualization to get a mind's eye view of Qi circulating internally as you exhale. Repeat the intentful breath correction whenever you have time. Do you have fifteen seconds? Set your intention to repeat soon—every fifteen minutes or every hour—whatever you can manage.

It is worthwhile to note that one of the definitions of the Chinese character for Qi is "breath," and Qigong is often translated as "breath practice" or "breath exercise." However, beginning students can become overwhelmed by detailed Qi cultivation instructions that include extensive suggestions for the breath. While many teachers insist breath focus is central, others insist it is not. After many years of investigating all of these perspectives my response has been to develop this guideline: In the beginning the breath is not important, in the middle the breath is very important, and at the end the breath is not important.

This means that, when you begin to practice Qigong you should keep it simple; just breathe naturally. Whenever you remember to, take a full relaxed breath. As your skill progresses you will enter a stage of your practice, the middle, where the breath is very important. In many of the classics of Qigong it is noted that "the breath is the handle." How do you use a door or a hammer without a handle? The breath is the handle that makes the tool of Qigong more effective and more influential.

As you advance, much of the particular detail of breath practice becomes second nature and no longer requires conscious attention. At this point Qi cultivation effects can be achieved without thinking about the breath. As your practice matures, breath focus will become less important; the breath is naturally integrated.

While many teachers insist that the benefits of Qigong are attained with the mind, Dr. Felix Chang, a physician from New York, opposes this view. "Stop breathing and focus the mind for three minutes." He challenges, "What happens? You die or pass out. That doesn't really suggest that the mind has a more powerful effect than the breath; in fact it is the opposite. Now, breathe in deeply; it makes you strong. We do this when we lift things. In Kung Fu we deliver the punch with the exhalation. Now, breathe out completely, and hold the breath out—feel how quickly you start to get weak and need to breathe. The breath is a master key in Qigong." This is a very insightful lesson from a sincere Qi cultivation practitioner and instructor.

Mind and Consciousness

Without the cooperation of the mind or consciousness, only conditioned responses can come about. Little or no choice or creativity can occur in the absence of the intentful mind. To elect to adjust your posture you use intention. Without intention the breath becomes shallow, unless you are exercising vigorously. All of the Qigong and Tai Chi benefits that can be attained through movement and breath must happen with the permission and cooperation of the mind and intention. In fact the Chinese language uses a unique character (word, concept) to represent the presence of conscious choice and purposefulness—mind intent (*Yi*).

The problem is that our poor minds often are the home of lengthy lists, limited views, judgments, trauma, memories, and habitual behavior patterns. Focus, direction, concentration, clarity, and intention are not easy to sustain. If the most refined levels of Qi cultivation depend on an advanced capacity to manage the mind, most of us have our Qigong work cut out for us.

If your mind is distracted by internal circles of thought about old grudges, transgressions, aspirations, creative tangents, or lists, your evolution to more advanced Qigong may be stalled. In Qigong it is ultimately through the mind and consciousness that we seek to achieve the capacity to control, focus, and direct the Qi. Without the deep mind focus of Qigong and Tai Chi, the breath and movement are really more like calisthenics. In Qigong, breath and movement are the tools we use to help the mind to attain effective and clear focus for cultivating and enhancing the Qi and accessing the power of the universe.

The features of your mind that show up over time as difficult to clear or control will serve as a diagnosis of what might be a useful remedy in addition to your Qigong or Tai Chi. If you find yourself thinking in circles about your work, it may mean that you will have to communicate with someone at your job to clear the mind snag. If you find your mind returning again and again to a certain relationship where someone has transgressed against you, you may need to communicate with that person or engage in some counseling to reach forgiveness or to let go. If you find yourself making certain lists over and over, you may have to find a way to accomplish the things on that list, to cut some things off that list, or to work with a professional to help you to discover why that list keeps coming up.

When it is not distracted, the mind is a power tool in Tai Chi and Qigong. One of the ancient, anonymous Qigong proverbs is, "When the mind is distracted the Qi scatters." Because the mind is difficult to tame or manage it is very useful to practice Qi cultivation methods that include movement and breath to give the mind something to do. Literally hundreds, maybe thousands, of people have complained to me that sitting meditation has been impossible for them. For many the gentle focus and moving meditation of Qigong and Tai Chi have finally made it possible to quiet the thoughts. Inner tension restrains the circulation of Qi. Mind focus can be used to achieve and sustain relaxation, releasing inner tension. Or, you may use more vigorous Qigong methods to shake out stagnation and release stress. The most important

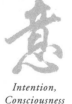

*Intention,
Consciousness*

key to circulating the Qi is to relax. Relaxation cannot occur in the absence of the willingness of the mind.

In the domain of Qi cultivation the Chinese point to three states of mind—conditioned mind, focused mind, and clarified mind. The day-to-day business of life with all of its excitements, hopes, frustrations, and fears stimulates the conditioned mind. When you initiate the Qigong process of intentfully managing what the mind is doing—for you and to you—this engages the focused mind. In your transition toward a more conscious, healthier, more empowered life, the practice of Qigong, Tai Chi, Yoga, or meditation can be used as a tool to coordinate and direct the conditioned mind to become a more focused mind.

Clarified mind is a little like the Qigong jackpot—attainable and of great value but often out of reach. Most people can get to pure clarity of mind for just a few moments. Lao Zi asked, "Can you coax the mind from its wandering?" With any more than a brief connection with clarified mind, we begin to have spiritual revelations. Prolonged association with clarified mind is called Nirvana in India. In China it is associated with enlightenment and immortality, which is the state of full and prolonged awareness of your eternal nature. The most practical application of Qigong is to attain and utilize the focused mind with all of its health and performance benefits. Should you find your way to clarified mind, the gifts of the transcendental life will begin to manifest for you.

Inner light is an image that is often used for intentfully focusing the mind. Some form of spiritual light is referred to in most cultures. It is prominent in the Chinese tradition of Qi cultivation to refer to "turning to the light" or Circulating the Light.

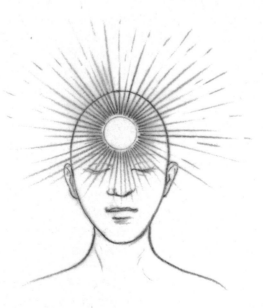

Third Intentful Correction—Mind

Interestingly, Western researchers have discovered that human cells emit biophotons—and have determined that the human system stores energy as light.

Close your eyes and look for that inner light. For some this is easy; for others it takes some practice. You will find through practice and over time that the light and distress are incompatible, they cannot exist simultaneously. Turn to the light, and simply declare to yourself that you will do this again and again for the rest of your life.

You may also turn your attention to calming the pace of your breath or noting the sensation of the breath entering and leaving your nose. Or you can simply focus on the sensation of your body's self-healing capacity working—the inner feeling of flow. Particularly, as you exhale, you can literally feel this flow. It may occur as a sensation of spreading warmth internally or a tingling sensation. The point of the Third Intentful Correction is to hold the focus on something simple that does not produce stress or resistance in your body.

The Three Intentful Corrections and the High-Performance Zone

Interestingly, the Three Intentful Corrections are used by champions and superstars to initiate or prepare to participate in everything from giving a lecture or winning a world championship to practicing Kung Fu and making executive decisions. Imagine it is your turn to bat in the World Series. You step up to the plate, carefully plant your feet, position your body to maximize the force that may be brought to bear on the ball with the bat, take a deep breath, relax, and focus. This sets you up to be in the high-performance zone—identical to the Qigong state. To get there you used the Three Intentful Corrections.

Imagine you are going to sink a prize-winning golf putt or shoot the winning basketball free throw—millions of dollars and fame ride on this moment of truth. You carefully adjust your feet and your body posture, you deepen and relax your breath, and you clear your mind to a sharp focus and drop into the zone—the Qigong state. The Three Intentful Corrections get you there.

The essential foundation of Qigong happens to be the very same essential foundation for any sort of high-performance activity. Daily Qigong is like constantly sharpening your capacity to an optimal level. In *Seven Habits of Highly Effective People*,[4] business guru Steven Covey identifies a high-performance technique called "sharpening the saw," which allows for constant self-rejuvenation and personal enhancement. Qigong is one of the oldest and most refined methods of sharpening the saw. Whether you are going to address a large audience, give the performance of your lifetime, or fight a serious health challenge, the Three Intentful Corrections will become a supreme tool for maximizing your internal resources—your Qi.

The Simplest Form of Qigong

To demonstrate how very easy Qigong practice can be, try this basic exercise. Simply adjust your posture so that your body is upright and your spine is straight, deepen your breath, and direct your mind to a simple image such as clouds drifting across the sky. You see, it only takes a moment to initiate the Three Intentful Corrections. You may wish to close your eyes and drift here in a state of quiet for a few moments.

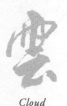

Cloud

If you are very new to the idea of practice or cultivation, you may need to take a few breaths to really relax. You may have to remind yourself every few seconds of what you are doing because the mind is addicted to its usual pattern of bouncing around. If you have decided to focus on clouds in your mind's eye, then you might just say to yourself every few moments, or on the exhalations of the breath, "clouds," "clouds," "clouds."

That's it. You are in the practice of Qigong. You have initiated the Qigong state. In this very simple practice you are using the Three Intentful Corrections as a Qigong method.

While you are in this state, you are enhancing your internal functioning. This potentiates the health, peak performance, or peace of mind you seek. More importantly, this state can lead you to pure wonder. Check in again—this time lead with an intentful breath—breathe slowly, deeply. Notice that it is difficult to take a really full breath unless you bring your attention to the body posture—make that correction. Now, adjust your consciousness to a single focus, such as billowing clouds. Let this displace, for a few moments, all of your stresses and worries. Take a few breaths and continue. Now, declare to yourself, "I can do Qigong anytime." If you really begin to know this, it will change your life.

There are two major challenges in this preliminary exploration of the Three Corrections that make it more advanced than it at first appears. One is that it is simply not all that easy to remember to use the Three Intentful Corrections. The other is that it is difficult to sustain this state. The practice is easy but life is complex. We get busy. There is always something that "must" get done before we allow ourselves the liberty to take better care of ourselves.

The solution to these two challenges is really what having a daily Qi cultivation practice is about. This is why 100 million people practice Qigong and Tai Chi in China every day. This is also why so many Qigong methods were developed. The variations of posture and movement, breath and consciousness or mental focus that make up the thousands of forms of Qigong provide the busy and distractible mind with numerous and various activities. Daily focused practice, whether for a fifteen-second round of the Three Intentful Corrections, or for an hour of various practices, helps us begin to remember to use the practice throughout the day. Ultimately it helps us learn how to extend and sustain the Qigong state and gain the awesome benefits.

You will learn, as the mind and your Qi come more and more under your management, that your practice will need to have fewer components to occupy the consciousness. The most advanced practices are largely quiescent meditations with minimal external activity. But these are not particularly useful if the mind is busy doing something else, or as Zhuang Zi (Chuang Tzu) the famous student of Lao Zi, wrote, "The lack of authentic internal stillness is called sitting while wandering."[5]

As a practitioner of Qigong, you will repeat the Three Intentful Corrections thousands of times. In any form of Qigong or Tai Chi practice of fifteen minutes, you will likely do the Three Intentful Corrections thirty to fifty times or more. Master Zhu Hui, one of my favorite teachers from Tian Tai Mountain in Eastern China, told me, "A person who makes wise use of the Three Intentful Corrections a few times a day will resolve their pains, cure their diseases, and achieve longevity—a person who makes wise use of the Three Intentful Corrections a hundred times every day will become a sage." In the beginning it is a huge step in the direction of a successful Qigong practice to simply do the Three Intentful Corrections whenever you can remember to, even if it is only once or twice a day.

Invent some ways to remind yourself to do this practice. You can set several appointments with yourself and have your watch remind you with a beep. Some computers can be programmed to sound a signal every half hour or so. If there is a church bell that tolls near your workplace, use that prompt as a reminder. Or you might decide to initiate the Three Intentful Corrections whenever you answer the phone.

The Simple, Most Difficult Path: Natural Flow Qigong

There are thousands of schools of thought in Chinese history that have created a multitude of methods and techniques of Qigong and Tai Chi. As an ancient scholar wrote in the Tang dynasty, a renaissance period in China, "May a thousand flowers bloom." These thousands of schools or approaches are like flowers—beautiful expressions of Chinese wisdom and creativity. Each of those schools has a set of methods for cultivation and mastery of Qi.

Among these many Qigong paths a particularly unique one is worthy of mention here—the nontechnique or nonmethod known as Natural Flow Qigong. In many years of study, practice, and teaching it has become obvious to me that this is one of the richest secrets in all of Qi cultivation tradition. Natural Flow Qigong is a kind of advanced practice that even the great masters refer to as mystical. Even those of you who have studied quite a bit of Qigong, Tai Chi, or Yoga will appreciate Natural Flow Qigong.

This is not a form that can be taught, it is not a set of movements, nor are most of the practitioners of Qigong and Tai Chi in the parks of China typically aware of this method. I learned of this Qigong path from several personal encounters with master teachers and traditional written sources. Natural Flow Qigong is a version of the Qigong revealed in *The Secret of the Golden Flower*,[6] a beautiful merging of Daoist and Buddhist Qi traditions. It is also revealed in the intriguing tradition known as

Guarding the One, which we will explore in Chapter 3. Natural Flow Qigong assumes that the conditions and situations that spontaneously arise in our experience and in our world are the natural expression of the force and power of the entire universe, equal to the sun rising, an eclipse of the moon, or the order of the solar system.

In Natural Flow, rather than determining how you think things should be, you carefully honor how things are. Rather than trying to make something happen, you become more focused in this practice on purposefully participating in or aligning with what is already occurring—what is spontaneously arising around and within you. In one of the streams of ancient Daoism, the School of Complete Reality or Perfect Truth (*Quan Zhen*), a primary focus of Qigong is to reach a state of "flow" where acceptance of "how it really is" with an open, grateful, cheerful heart is the essence of the practice.

Many of the practices that follow in our study of the phases of cultivation are methods with specific steps. Natural Flow Qigong is more like a nonmethod—how to be. Even though this can become a very advanced practice, it is appropriate to reveal this method to you here, before we begin methods and forms. As you advance in Qigong, this approach will always be a path that you can turn to. Natural Flow Qigong is really at the core of all of the deepest and most profound Qi cultivation practices. As you advance, this becomes a natural aspect of all Qigong and Tai Chi and is woven into the fabric of your moment-to-moment life.

Throughout this book, references to Natural Flow Qigong are intended to remind you of this path of no particular method. If you find yourself thinking that one of the phases of cultivation discussed in Part II is a little beyond your reach, just think "Natural Flow." When you become stressed but cannot practice a method that requires movement or overt breathing practices, turn your focus to Natural Flow Qigong.

Many people inadvertently tense up during normal activity—the neck and shoulders, the digestive system, the lower back, or the muscles around the jaw. When you engage Natural Flow Qigong you relax and release your habitually contracted muscles and turn your attention (or as much of your attention as possible) to allowing the Qi to do what it is naturally programmed to do. This process elicits both the first and second promises of Qi and activates the elixir within.

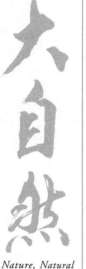

Nature, Natural

Natural Flow Qigong is often called the Simple, Most Difficult Path because it is easy to understand and easy to do for a few moments. The difficulty is to be able to remember to use the practice and then to sustain it. One of the most renowned of the ancient Qi cultivation masters, Master Ge Hong, describes Natural Flow Qigong in his third century C.E. treatise *The Book of the Master Who Embraces Simplicity*: "It is not hard to know, but to be persistent is difficult."[7] In the lighthearted tone that is always encouraged in Qigong, practitioners occasionally say, "Gotta Flow" or "I am better off if I go Natural"—meaning that the situation has reminded them to engage in Natural Flow Qigong. You will notice over time that this kind of language makes it easier to bring Natural Flow Qigong practice to life.

You can learn how to use the momentum of the powerful natural forces in the universe to assist you. You have seen hawks rise upward without using wing strength by finding naturally rising invisible air currents. That is Natural Flow. You've probably noticed that worry doesn't really change much. Turning your attention to flow is at least as useful, and it protects and conserves Qi. Anger stalls Qi, but honest communication and forgiveness create momentum. You've also probably noticed that you can try to accomplish something for a long time with only marginal results. Then later, after you have given it up, it happens just the way you wanted it to—all by itself. Timing is another expression of Natural Flow. These are all expressions of the principles on which Natural Flow Qigong is based.

Natural Flow Qigong, sometimes referred to as the Water Method (or the Watercourse Way), achieves results by simply allowing the innate nature of Qi to express. As Lao Zi says, "The most supreme is like water, water achieves all the things that it does without trying."[8] In Natural Flow Qigong you allow yourself to participate, without effort, in what is naturally occurring. By doing so you cooperate with the power of the entire universe. In Natural Flow Qigong your only assignment is to eliminate as much inner resistance as possible, to use your intention and concentration to get out of the way of what the Qi has the natural capacity to "do" for you. Those who master Natural Flow are seen as lucky, intuitive, psychic, and blessed.

Water

One Version of Natural Flow Qigong

Many ancient writings in the Daoist canon[9] and in Buddhist scripture are devoted to explaining Natural Flow Qigong. The paragraphs that follow are a contemporary interpretation of these texts assisted by the thoughts of many revered teachers. As you grow into Qigong, teachings such as these will start to take on significance. When you use this approach to Qigong it is helpful and appropriate to use the Three Intentful Corrections as well.

"Bring yourself into optimal mental, emotional, and physical position in relation to the boundless and infinitely intelligent universe that is richly infused with Qi. Allow yourself to relax deeply and be maximally open to the infusion of healing and empowering celestial resources. Celebrate as you awaken to the vibrant flow of fresh, clean, clear, positive Qi, pouring through your channels, Qi reservoirs, bones, organs, glands, and tissues.

"Understand that this Qi is a rich mix of powerful energies, a multitude of resonating frequencies ranging from the magnetism of your life force to pure heavenly radiance. Saturated with the subtle information and consciousness of all creation, these influences are pouring through your Qi Matrix. These resources are naturally programmed to nourish, heal, and transform every aspect of your being. Open and surrender to this extraordinary state, come to the awareness that the universe is completely oriented, attuned, and coordinated—automatically permeated with perfect wisdom.

Experience a sense of total trust welling within you like a rushing fountain of profound resources that are healing and restoring your heart, mind, and emotions and transforming your body to reflect the essential original blueprint of your soul.

"Relax completely, do not clench or strain anything. Do not force or resist particular thoughts—simply tend toward a mind as open as endless sky. Allow your breath to be natural and when it feels appropriate deepen the breath. Feel how the inhalation gathers supreme potential and how the exhalation diffuses the radical power of the universe throughout your being. Allow the experiences, events, and influences that surround you and are within you to flow with the natural momentum of the entire cosmos. A huge, crashing waterfall of Qi is washing through you—no reaction, resistance, or effect can lodge anywhere in your multidimensional being. You are a completely open system filled with boundlessness.

"Allow yourself to be a thoroughly unobstructed vessel for the expression of the irrevocable presence of pure and exhilarating Qi. Absolutely pristine universal essence flows through and around you, dislodging and discharging all possible accumulation or constraint. You are completely sustained in the safe and comfortable embrace of Primal Origin, radiant and awake to your ever perfect eternal essence."

Because it is not always possible to engage in Qigong practice methods that employ particular movements, Natural Flow Qigong is like prayer and affirmation. It is very useful when you are caught in a stressful situation at work, unable to move in traffic, or worse, experiencing tragedy or trauma. We will refer to the Natural Flow occasionally as we progress into traditional Qigong practices. You can bring this practice with you into any of the methods we will be learning. While it may be a little difficult at first to remember to use this Qigong, you will begin to get a feel for it over time. All that is required is that you mindfully shift your focus.

Qigong Methods

Align

HISTORICAL REFLECTION A preliminary step in any form of Tai Chi or Qigong is to align the body between Heaven and Earth. This can occur before or after the opening, to align for optimal practice. It also typically occurs just after, or as a part of, the closing, to align for the most peaceful or effective day or for an intentful life.

Begin aligning by initiating the First Intentful Correction, then deepen your attention. Align more fully by connecting the reservoir of Heaven Qi in the head and the reservoir of Earth Qi in the lower abdomen through the Central Tai Chi Channel. Most traditions put a major emphasis on aligning as a time to initiate the Qigong state using the Three Intentful Corrections along with a focused awareness of the connection of Heaven and Earth through the harmonizing of one's personal, inner Tai Chi.

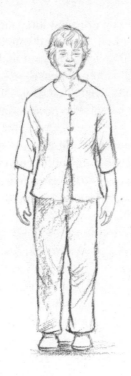
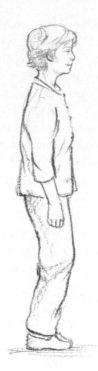

Align

Most Qigong methods have their roots in particular historic eras, traditions, or lineages. Align is so basic and so much a part of every form and style of practice that we can only say its roots penetrate deep into the fertile, original soil of all Qi cultivation.

INSTRUCTION Stand (you can align sitting or lying as well) with your feet close together but not touching; if it is more comfortable, your toes can point just slightly outward. Knees are slightly bent, the bowl of the pelvis is balanced upright, and the organs are in the bowl. This stance causes the lower back to straighten as if you were standing against a wall. To accomplish this you can place your hands on your belly and gently push in, which will cause the lower spine to straighten. Sense that your head is adjusted to be on top of the spine and shoulders.

Your shoulders are relaxed with your arms dangling comfortably at your sides. The Heaven is gently pulling your head and upper torso upward into the universe. The Earth exerts a gentle force, pulling your tailbone toward the center of the planet. The upper body rising and the lower body descending creates an expansion in the center between the umbilicus and the heart. The organs of the chest and abdomen have more space. Physiologically this opening fills with blood and body fluids. In Qigong this openness fills with Qi.

Allow the breath to become more full, not urgent. With mind focus explore the relationship of the body alignment with the alignment of the Qi channels and reservoirs. Enter into—induce—the Qigong state and the practice of Qigong. In a lifetime of Qigong practice a practitioner uses Align in this way thousands of times.

In a gentle internal voice you might say to yourself: "Aligning the body aligns the Central Tai Chi Channel, which aligns the primary energy reservoirs—the primary keys to cultivating Qi and enhancing inner healing resources. When I align to initiate my practice it is a preliminary meditation for setting the tone of my practice. When I align I open to the powerful influences of Heaven, which are pouring down on and through me like a healing waterfall, and the influences of Earth which are rising up within and around me like a gushing fountain. These forces merge within me and flow freely throughout my Qi Matrix to empower my life and health."

You may simply remain in this posture, gently drifting, as a form of Qigong meditation. In most cases, however, it will serve either as a preliminary to the opening movement or as the conclusion of the closing movement.

Walking Qigong

HISTORICAL REFLECTION Walking Qigong is essentially a form of walking meditation. The point is to walk purposefully and, usually, slowly. The movement of the hands and arms becomes stylized. The mind is clear. You are walking but the destination is not a place, it is a state—the Qigong state.

Walking Qigong is sometimes done backwards to sustain a higher level of focus. Learning Tai Chi often includes a very specific form of meditative walking that is a powerful tool for improving balance. Even in the martial arts, the foot work is primary. In ancient times Kung Fu included training in special forms, with a focus on intentful walking gestures on delicate rice paper, where no evidence of the steps was left. A renowned form of Kung Fu Walking, highly stylized and in a circle, is called Ba Gua. In many traditions walking meditation provides for a contemplative or prayerful practice in motion. Walking the Labyrinth is a more European form of Walking Qigong.

The most famous contemporary form of Walking Qigong is Guo Lin Qigong, developed in the 1970s for healing cancer and now used as an easy-to-learn form for all diseases. This was a key component of the Qigong practiced by David in the story at the beginning of Chapter 1. The point in Walking Qigong is to move into the Qigong state and meditate while the body is moving very gently. This is the brilliance of all Qigong; gentle movement in a deep meditation creates the medicine within. Walking Qigong is particularly brilliant because it is very easy to learn and practice. Legend holds that one of the most ancient forms of Qigong is a walking form.

INSTRUCTION A whole book could be written on Walking Qigong. In the interest of making the practice simple and accessible, it is easiest to begin by walking normally, then shift your pace into slow motion. Add a little stylized flourish to the movements.

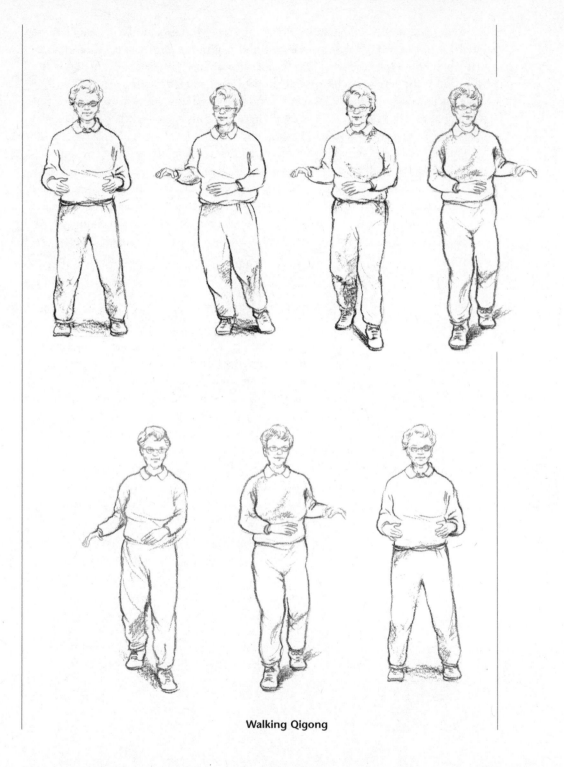

Walking Qigong

If you were to speed it back up it would no longer be your usual walk; it is much more intentful and focused. Practice this for a while. It is not necessary to execute a particular gait or stride; just walk very slowly and purposefully. Work with the breath if you wish. The most important thing to remember is that this is a moving meditation. The mind focus is very important. As you attend to the walking, focus on the breath and repeat a phrase in your mind: "I am walking toward my renewed self" or "Each step that I take in this peaceful state is healing me."

Later you might modify the method. As you are walking slowly "swish" your palms in front of you on each step. As the right foot steps forward and you shift your weight onto it, your hands pass like a pendulum in front of your belly from the left toward the right. Inhale in two separate puffs. As your left foot steps forward and takes the weight, your arms swinging to the left past the belly, release one long exhalation. Think of this as a two-part process:

1. Right foot, inhale two puffs, hands right.
2. Left foot, one long exhalation, hands left.

This is called *Xi, Xi, Hu* breathing. You inhale (Xi) in two puffs. You follow with one long exhalation (Hu). After walking like this for a while, in either the first, more simple version or the second, more specific version, many people have a significant sense that something has altered within them. Because this practice is so simple, many will find it challenging to think that walking could be so powerful. Yet, millions of people swear that doing this practice has literally changed their life and even saved them from cancer and other life-threatening diseases. There are a number of references to such cases in *The Healer Within* along with an introduction to the remarkable China-wide Cancer Recovery Society.

The Three Treasures:
Unity, Harmony, Diversity

Dao gives birth to the boundless, eternal One,
The Two emerges creatively from the One,
The Three arises dynamically from the Two,
The Three gives birth to all beings and things.

—LAO ZI, *DAO DE JING*, #42

Legends abound regarding how the earliest forms of Chinese medicine and traditional philosophy were born. Because the Chinese kept particularly detailed accounts it is clear, from the very earliest writings, that medicine and healing were already well developed before writing—indicating that their origins are veiled by the mists of remote prehistory.

On my first trip to China we were training at a Qigong (Chi Kung) institute just adjacent to the Temple of the Soul's Retreat in a small village in the hills west of Hangzhou and the beautiful West Lake, called the Village of Heavenly Bamboo. Hangzhou, a half day west of Shanghai by train, was the capital of China one thousand years ago and it has a rich heritage in medicine and Qi cultivation tradition. Being at this traditional training center and clinic was like entering a wonderland of Qi (Chi). Outside the gate of the training center, a steady stream of people made their pilgrimage to the mountain where the original founding monk of the temple did his cultivation practices.

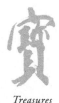

Treasures

Our esteemed teacher, Master Huang, a former monk himself who had lived for years at the famous Shaolin Temple, told one of my favorite Qigong stories, the legend of Master Yu, who is often called the originator of Qigong. Over the years this story has been retold by many other teachers with innumerable variations. Early references to the legend of Master Yu appear in the Daoist encyclopedia *Seven Slips of the Cloudy Satchel*[1] and the earlier *Book of the Master Who Embraces Simplicity*.[2] This legend and the many references to Master Yu in the ancient literature suggest that Qi cultivation is actually the mother of traditional Chinese medicine and healing, appearing several millennia before acupuncture. Master Huang's story:

"In very ancient times lived one of the original Qi masters named Yu. It is of course unknown whether Yu was a man or a woman; there are reasonable accounts for both possibilities. One of Master Yu's most important contributions was a ritual called the Pace of Yu. Along with ancient shamanic dances that imitate bears and birds, the Pace of Yu is the most ancient Qigong. Master Yu developed this walking form of Qigong to call the benevolent forces of Heaven to Earth by marking the designs of the celestial realms, stars, and planets on the ground through a movement set of nine steps and three deeply focused breaths.

"One of Master Yu's students asked for insight as to how to support healing in people who are sick, how to empower people to strength and endurance, and how to help create a pathway to the enlightened life of access to universal wisdom. Master Yu is supposed to have said, 'There are three treasures; the body merges Heaven and Earth into one.' The apprentice asked whether there was any more that the master could teach on the subject. Master Yu answered, 'Three Treasures, humans dance Heaven to Earth.' Bewildered, the student realized that there would be no further discussion.

"The student decided to practice dancing Heaven to Earth to explore what the Three Treasures would turn out to be. During different times of the day, over a period of one hundred days, she created her own dance to reflect the concept of Heaven on Earth. She did it at night and paced out the stars. She did it at sunset on the day of the full moon and danced the sun setting and the full moon rising. She danced sunrise; she danced noon when all of Heaven is full of brightness. During this time she kept asking herself the question, 'What three treasures?' Above is the Heaven, the boundless domain of space, moon, sun, and stars—obviously this is a treasure and a marvelous resource in healing and empowerment. Below is Earth, the concentrated and dense domain of solid soil and stone, the source of food and water and the ground for the rootedness of life—obviously a treasure for health and endurance.

"She wondered about the third treasure. Was the third treasure herself, the dancer, suspended between Heaven and Earth? Every day in her dancing she explored the possibilities. By the hundredth day of practice, she realized that the third treasure was the interaction of Heaven and Earth to create life—all life."

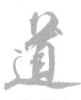

Dao (Tao)

Heaven	Life	Earth
Spirit	Mind	Body
Yang	Harmony	Yin
Shen	Qi	Jing

This idea of the Three Treasures evolved into a primary foundation principle of Chinese medicine. Heaven and Earth merge, and life is created. The Three Treasures—Heaven, Earth, and life—are also the foundation of Qigong theory and Tai Chi (Taiji), representing three aspects of ourselves, known in Chinese medicine as Jing, Qi, and Shen.

Numerology of Chinese Systems

Like every culture, China has its distinctive view of numbers and numerology. As expressed by Lao Zi at the beginning of this chapter, the One (*Tai Yi*—Supreme Unity), the Two (Tai Chi—Great Harmony of *Yin-Yang*), and the Three (*San Bao*—Three Treasures) are fundamental. There are additional important numerological associations—the four directions and four seasons; the five elements (*Wu Xing*) and five energies; the six causes of disease and six levels of Qi; the seven emotions; the eight principles of nature (*Ba Gang*) and eight original Qi channels. One of the most important number concepts for medicine and Qigong is the eight primary aspects of nature reflected in the divine tortoise shell (*Ling Gui Ba Fa*). According to legend, Master Yu, in his revelations of the order of the universe, determined many practical applications for healthy living and medical treatment, as well as engineering and flood control, based on the eight sections around the circumference of the shell of the tortoise.

Nine is one of the most important numbers to the Chinese; it represents the nine bodily openings, the nine inner chambers, and the nine heavens. The "nine times refined Golden Elixir" is a spiritual medicine that is cultivated internally through advanced Qigong called Inner Alchemy or externally in an alchemist's laboratory. The heart of this book explores the traditional system for Qi cultivation which is a progression of the Nine Phases of Cultivation and the Tenth Phase of Compassionate Expression, that are directly associated with the Three Treasures. Chinese numerology continues with the Ten Heavenly Stems and the Twelve Earthly Branches, and so on.

This book's goal is simply to inspire and to guide. There are a great many wonderful books that explore these concepts in detail. To keep our learning and practice simple and applicable, we will focus primarily on the One, the Two, and the Three.

Master Yu's Model of Teaching Qigong

Master Yu revealed the Three Treasures to his students, not through a spoken lesson, but through a kind of cryptic declaration and an assigned experiment. This is the highest form of Qigong. Instead of teaching by telling, the master serves as a living example of how to be and provides suggestions for how others might gain authentic insight. The core of the teaching comes through the individual's practice. My favorite and most esteemed teachers have passed along to me this way of teaching. They have said, in essence, "Take these principles into your practice; the deepest healing and most profound revelations will spontaneously arise." Some teachers insist that you must learn the method and repeat it exactly. This is important for perpetuating a particular lineage, but it is not necessary for authentic Qi cultivation. Master Yu's way liberates us into pure and direct experience of the Qi. It is Master Yu's way that we follow in this book.

Beginning with Master Yu, formulas and methods for producing powerful inner medicine have been passed forward in the traditions of philosophy, medicine, and science. Because of the incredible practicality and insight of the ancient Chinese Qi masters in their refinement of these ideas, the Three Treasures are now experiencing a renaissance as a framework for healing and self-actualization in the twenty-first century.

While in a complete study of Chinese medicine and the myriad approaches to Qigong and Tai Chi one would become knowledgeable about a great deal of numerological theory, you can relax. The Three provides an approach to Qigong and Tai Chi that is deep and rich and relatively easy to grasp. An even easier approach is Natural Flow Qigong, which, as discussed in Chapter 2, is based in simplifying the thoughts and freeing the mind to access the Qigong state naturally. Lists of numbers and esoteric logic can become confusing. From my more than twenty years of teaching, I know that there is a middle path. This path offers enough information to inspire but not so much as to confuse and distract. So, let us investigate the One, the Two, and the Three. Then, like Master Yu's student, you can deepen your experience through your own practice.

Like the air all around you, the One, Two, and Three are irrevocably present. They are embedded in all beings and things, and you are embedded in them. You do not have to make them work for you; they are already spontaneously working. As with graceful birds unaware of the air in flight, in Qi cultivation it is not necessary to focus on the Three Treasures—just enjoy the flying.

If, on occasion, you have a deepening revelation based on this information, that is all the better for every level of your healing and empowerment. However, your Qigong practice will be a powerful tool in your life even if you do not understand or retain any of the poetry or the logic we will now discuss. Rather than trying to memorize it, allow yourself to marvel at the insight of the ancient practitioners who developed these concepts over many centuries.

The One: Supreme Unity, the Dao

Multitudes of Dragons and Tigers guard the One.
The One is eternally secure.
Spontaneous, the One never ceases.
Preserve the One, guard Truth
　　and you communicate with the whole Universe.
The One is not hard to know,
　　the difficulty is persistence.
Guard the One with no distraction
　　and you are eternally vital.

—MASTER GE HONG, *THE BOOK OF THE MASTER WHO EMBRACES SIMPLICITY*,
　　FOURTH CENTURY C.E.

Tai, Supreme

If health means wholeness, then what exactly does this wholeness consist of? Certainly, functional coherence—which implies inner accord, coordination, and harmony of our multidimensional being—is one way to describe health and wholeness. So, what is the best model for wholeness and coherence? The ancient Chinese felt sure that the best model was nature. The foundations of philosophy as well as the practical applications of Chinese medicine, Qigong, and Tai Chi are firmly rooted in this principle. The ultimate picture of wholeness is the coordinated, interactive nature of the universe—the One Supreme Unity (*Tai Yi*).

We often forget that the word *universe*, used so often to describe everything everywhere, means "one song" or "one tone." Long before written history the Chinese embraced the idea that all of nature is one and that we can bring ourselves to health and wholeness by emulating it. When the very early Chinese explored the One, somehow they knew that the universe or the cosmos was essentially not a thing but an evolutionary process of constant cyclical change. They called this whole, singular, unitary process Dao (Tao), which translates as "way" or, more specifically, "the ultimate Way that things work."

In Qigong practice the value of the One is supreme. When you become aware that everything is connected, it is easier to relax and trust. When all the complexity of life—good and bad news, good and bad days, opportunities and challenges—is perceived as an expression of the One, it is easier to feel safe; you can relax and stay clear in your practice.

Primal Origin

When you relax the Qi is unrestrained. When the Qi is unrestrained it can flow freely, and the result is internal coherence and harmony of physical, mental, and emotional function. This inner harmony causes the healing of disease, increased stamina, and creative access to Spirit.

Guarding the One

The most advanced levels of Qigong are based on a sincere and consistent association with the One. At the level of the One you are—and all is—perfect. Each of us is completely perfect in our wholeness, which already exists. The practice in this approach to Qigong, when you are able to engage in it, is to allow that which already *is* to be revealed and actualized. This has been called the release of your imprisoned splendor. In the beginning of your Qigong practice it seems impossible that inner perfection of the One is attainable and so you will most likely use cultivation practices that gather and circulate Qi for healing and empowerment. Later, in more advanced Qigong you will learn "to be." This means to reveal and release the true self that is already there—to reveal and radiate the One from within.

Merging with the One, on a moment-to-moment basis, is actually the easiest and most direct path to the most desired benefits of Qigong and Tai Chi. As the great Qi master Ge Hong teaches: "The One is not hard to know but persistence is the difficulty." This is why there is Natural Flow Qigong. It requires very little exploration of facts and details, it is not a Qigong form with movements to remember. Natural Flow is completely spontaneous and arises naturally, as a way of being, when you vigilantly sustain a direct relationship with the One.

The One Supreme Unity is represented in our universe by the Big Dipper and especially the Pole Star. Master Yu's Qigong method to induce the influence of the stars to the earth represents calling the One in to oneself. Another of the most ancient and respected forms of Qigong is known as Guarding the One (*Shou Yi*). According to the *Book on Precepts*, "The consistent practice of Guarding the One for a long time will bring about a state where the Qi of the One inundates the whole body. As your body and spirit are deeply pervaded by the universe, you will radiate light and undergo transformations without end. This is the benefit of knowing how to properly Guard the One."[3] Guarding the One has a very rich history throughout many dynasties in China. It is a practice that promises healing at all levels of the body, mind, and spirit.

Guarding or attending to the One is a continuous practice. "During all of your activities, in the midst of the thousands of affairs, you must always attend to the One," says the *Scripture of Divine Nature*.[4] "While eating or drinking, attend to the One! When happy, attend to the One! When anguished, attend to the One! When sick, attend to the One! Whether passing through water or fire, always attend to the One! Especially when you are agitated, attend to the One!"

Guarding the One is almost always a form of deep meditation. However, it is typical for the deep state to follow on a set of preliminary practices. In *The Method of Extending One's Years and Increasing Knowing*,[5] there is a practice called "Order Oneself and Guard the One," which includes massage so that the body feels warm and begins to glow; breathing exercises; swallowing of saliva and clicking the teeth with the chanting of invocations. This is followed by the Guarding the One meditation. Practical,

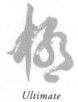

Ultimate

body-focused health enhancement methods are typically associated with transcendental practices in the Chinese Qi cultivation tradition.

The One is Primal Origin, the Source—everything comes from it, is contained within it, and returns to it. However, it is not necessary—nor is it possible—to *understand* the One; it is mysterious and incomprehensible. In the more advanced phases of Qi cultivation the ultimate ideal is to merge with the One—to become the One. Probably the most interesting and comprehensive writing on the One in the contemporary era is an essay by Livia Kohn called "Guarding the One" in *Taoist Meditation and Longevity Techniques.*[6] She writes, "Any guarding, embracing, or realizing of the One as original purity will bring about oneness with the primordial or with the harmony of the universe. Any realizing of the One allows the realizing subject to become what he or she was originally meant to become, to fulfill his or her proper destiny in the cosmos. The true nature of human beings is to be healthy and long-lived, to participate willingly in the changes of the world. Practitioners of Guarding the One become incomparably richer in primordial harmony and they become healthier and increase their life spans, if not become as immortal as the One itself."

The Two: Yin-Yang, Secret of Balance and Harmony

> The method of the Golden Elixir
> concerns one Yin
> and one Yang,
> and that really is all!

—Wei Bo Yang, *The Secret of Life Everlasting (Can Tong Qi)*,
second century C.E.

Though the words *Yin* and *Yang* are often spoken outside of China, they are only rarely understood. The meanings of these words are unique and filled with implication in Chinese culture, yet they are unfamiliar to the Western culture and therefore cannot be adequately translated. These words are key to our understanding of Qigong, Tai Chi, and Chinese medicine.

The concept of Yin-Yang has vast implications. Like Qi, Yin-Yang is representative of an entire worldview. Yin-Yang is the foundation of an essential Chinese theory of how the world was created and how it works. It describes how the One—Dao—operates and is used to create descriptions of the state of the Qi. Thousands of years after its origination the Yin-Yang theory remains the highly respected foundation of Asian systems of philosophy and medicine.

Yin

Simply stated Yin and Yang are opposites. In temperature they are cool and warm or cold and hot. In texture they are smooth and rough. In density they are soft and hard. In their original form as Chinese characters, Yin describes the shaded side of a mountain—the north; Yang represents the slope that gets full sun—the south. Together they make the whole. From practical features—temperature, texture, density—the Yin-Yang concept graduates toward the realms of the profound. Yin is mystery—hidden. Yang is revelation—revealed. Yin is absorption; Yang is radiance. Yin is gravity; Yang is levity. As you can see, Yin-Yang cannot be fully translated into English and yet its place in our quest for power and understanding is enormous.

These secrets will reveal their meaning to you over time, through your practice of Qigong and Tai Chi. Your awakening to these ideas through your experience of the Qi will potentially become keys to deeper secrets. Embodying and experiencing Yin-Yang through your practice can trigger revelation and cause you to evolve in your relationships, your work, your quest for health, and your ability to make decisions based on a growing sense of the deep and subtle workings of the universe.

Zhu Hui, who taught me several of my favorite Qigong forms, was a medical doctor and master teacher. He explained it this way: "First, allow Yin-Yang to capture your attention, then just notice how some simple Yin-Yang aspects show up in the world—like moon/sun, dark/light, and hard/soft. Soon, they will begin to communicate with you. Inherent in the Yin-Yang concept are balance and harmony, which are major keys to our success in cultivating Qi and in life. In health we are neither too

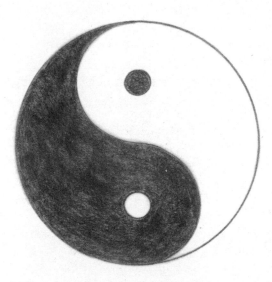

Yin-Yang Symbol—Tai Chi

cold nor too hot, we are neither too asleep nor too awake. Soon, you will find Yin and Yang everywhere—together. Seeing the sun (Yang) we remember the moon (Yin). Feeling cold (Yin) we remember ways to seek warmth (Yang). The importance of rest and restoration (Yin) is implied in every activity and energy expense (Yang). The balance and harmony of Yin-Yang is a primary secret of understanding the function of the natural world, human events, and the health of the human being. Think of your world without the balance of work and play, activity and rest, silence and sound. It is easy to see how meaningful Yin-Yang could become in your life. As you pursue Qigong the teachings of Yin-Yang spontaneously will be revealed to you."

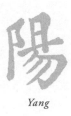

Yang

As is written in the thirteenth century Daoist classic, *The Book of Balance and Harmony* from Master Li, "If one can be balanced and harmonious within oneself, one is clear and aware—awake in quietude, accurate in action; thus one can respond to the endless changes in the world."[7] The state of health and optimal function is based on balance and harmony of Yin and Yang. When one is neither too hot nor too cold one is comfortably balanced. When one is neither too sad nor too happy the nervous system experiences well-being. When one is neither too hungry nor too full of food, one is nourished and energetic. Science calls this homeostasis; the Chinese call it balance. These expressions of balance are necessary for harmony. Using knowledge of Yin-Yang you can enhance your well-being and your potential.

Even the fundamental essence of the universe and yourself—the Qi—has a Yin aspect and a Yang aspect. In fact, the channels that carry the Qi of Heaven into the body are called the great Yang channels (*Tai Yang*). The channels that carry the Yin of the Earth into the body are called the great Yin channels (*Tai Yin*). The body's organs are also considered to be Yin or Yang. When Yin and Yang are in balance, health prevails. The essence of acupuncture, herbal medicine, and massage, as well as Qigong and Tai Chi, is based on recovering and sustaining the state of balance and harmony in the Yin-Yang realm. Together, all that is Yin combined with all that is Yang appear as two balanced aspects—of the One—in the Chinese culture's most famous icon—the Yin-Yang symbol (*Tai Chi Tu*).

The Yin-Yang symbol represents Yin and Yang and their constant interactivity. Seeing this symbol brings the entire philosophy and science of Yin-Yang to mind. This symbol is the best translation of Yin and Yang, it tells the whole story of the universe in one image. The famous physicist Niels Bohr even adopted the Yin-Yang symbol as his personal logo—to represent his theory of the universe. The state of balance in the Yin-Yang symbol, reflecting harmony where the black and the white components are exactly equal, is called Tai Chi.

You already know that Tai Chi is a familiar kind of Qigong. In fact, the concept of Tai Chi, meaning "supreme ultimate" or "universal harmony," is actually the name of the Yin-Yang symbol. Tai Chi the practice is named for this extraordinary concept, where opposites are in a dynamic state of balance and harmony. When people practice

Tai Chi they are actually investigating universal forces and activating Yin and Yang to produce harmony within themselves.

Take a few moments and explore this list of Yin and Yang concepts. It is not important to understand everything here—over time Qigong will teach you these concepts at an intuitive level. I have been involved with these concepts since my first Tai Chi class in 1967, and even now I learn more each day. Just allow yourself to marvel at the nearly boundless range of possibilities associated with the framework of Yin and Yang.

Yin	Yang
Off	On
Cold	Hot
Wet	Dry
Soft	Hard
Empty	Full
Inside	Outside
Back	Front
Near	Far
Slow	Fast
Small	Large
Rest	Act
Conserve	Spend
Confine	Liberate
Dark	Light
Earth	Heaven
Water	Fire
Relaxed	Excited
Sad	Happy
Dense	Diffuse
Substance	Energy
Gravity	Levity
Mystery	Revelation
Absorptive	Radiant
Concentrated	Expansive
Local	Universal
Limited	Boundless

If you're still not sure you understand, don't worry about it. Worry disturbs the Qi and cancels the benefits of the Qigong state and your Tai Chi practice. Let this worry go and simply enter into and enjoy the practice. Without straining to understand Qi or these ideas on Yin and Yang with your mind, you will come to understand them in your being. Simply do the practices, and the obvious as well as the hidden meanings of Yin-Yang will spontaneously arise within you. Follow the direction in Qigong that is easy and fun for you. Enjoy working and playing with the Qi. The rest—health and personal power—will flow from that.

The Three Treasures: Jing, Qi, Shen

Jing naturally transforms into Qi,
*   Qi naturally transforms into Spirit,*
*   and Spirit naturally transforms into pure openness,*
*   uniting with cosmic space.*
This is called returning to the root,
*   returning to origin.*
The path of everlasting life
*   and eternal vision is complete.*

—MASTER LI, *THE BOOK OF BALANCE AND HARMONY*, THIRTEENTH CENTURY

Jing, Essence

Our discussions of the One (unity) and the Two (harmony of Yin-Yang) are aimed at creating a philosophical foundation for Qi cultivation. Qigong and Tai Chi are not just exercises; they are, rather, multidimensional meditations toward empowered and enlightened living, which include health and peak performance as desirable side effects. The Three Treasures (San Bao) concept is a comprehensive and systematic framework that allows us to expand the discussion of Qigong and Tai Chi in more practical terms. It may be easiest, in the beginning, to think of the Three Treasures as body, mind, and spirit. In Chinese medicine and philosophy, the Three Treasures are Jing, Qi, and Shen. However, as you will see, the Three Treasures system is much more. It provides a powerful and systematic way of understanding your personal progress with Qi cultivation in the context of the diversity of life.

Lao Zi declares, "Dao gives birth to the boundless, eternal One." All beings and all things—also known as the Ten Thousand Things—have their origin in the One, but they are birthed into actuality by the Three. The Ten Thousand Things encompass all of the diversity and complexity of life—from the multiple components of your body to the list of things you hope to accomplish. Your health is one of the Ten Thousand Things and so is your state of mind. The implication is that by managing your relationship with the One, the Two, and the Three through the practice of Qi cultivation, the Ten Thousand Things will be most favorably arranged. The promise is that, if we attend to the One, balance Yin and Yang, and mindfully cultivate body, mind, and spirit, we will have more health, more power, more wisdom, and more peace.

In Qigong and Tai Chi, the Three Treasures provide a master key to profound insight. Using the system of correspondences of the Three Treasures provides the foundation for the Ten Phases of Cultivation and Mastery that we will be exploring in Part

II. And like the Yin-Yang system (the Two) that we have just reviewed, the Three Treasures will continue to teach you subtle lessons and provide you with countless revelations through your practice in the future.

Qi and the Three Levels of Being

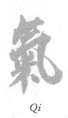

Qi

One of the ways to investigate Qi is to recognize that body Qi, mind Qi, and spirit Qi are simultaneously similar and different. This is an easy way to see how simple, and complex, the Qi can be. These aspects of the Qi are the same—as your body, your mind, and your spirit are the same; they are all you. However, these aspects of the Qi are also different in the same way that your body, your mind, and your spirit are different. Your body is your substance, a network of trillions of molecules creating mass and form. Your mind and emotions are insubstantial but they certainly do affect your body. Just think about the excitement that gives you butterflies in your stomach and the stress of an overcommitted schedule that can give you a headache or make you more susceptible to illness. Clearly, your spirit (which is at least as hard to define as Qi) is neither your body nor your mind, but it is linked to both.

The Qi of your body, mind, and spirit are all Qi, yet they reflect very different expressions of you. Your body Qi is associated with *Jing*, which in Chinese medicine is equivalent to neurotransmitters, hormones, DNA, sperm, and the egg. Jing is the most subtle aspect of the physical self. The body is local and substantial, and it operates through an integrated array of physiological interactions. Mind Qi is somewhat local, is insubstantial, and is not limited, as it operates through memory, emotions, thought, intuition, and creativity. Spirit Qi, known as *Shen Qi*, is transcendental, non-local, and boundless. It is the most incomprehensible form of your own Qi.

Spirit Qi holds the pattern of your eternal being, it is the immortal aspect of what appears to be a mortal self. It implies that you have the quality of individuality while being unified with all that is. It is not necessary to understand this or remember it. Simply being aware of the possibilities of the Three Treasures and engaging in Qi cultivation offers you compelling access to extraordinary benefits.

The Chinese worldview associates the body with Earth and the spirit with Heaven. The current concept of how Qi and Qigong work evolved from an ancient root concept. It originated in the prehistoric Chinese shamanic tradition of Dao way before written history and has been retained in the theory of Chinese medicine and Qigong for millennia. This root concept holds that between Heaven and Earth—in the field of interaction between the expansive forces of the universe and the condensed forces of our planet—there is profound merging, which creates life. Between Heaven and Earth is the domain where living beings arise—plants, animals, and humans.

The most obvious quality of the Heavenly Qi (*Tian Qi*), which is associated with spirit, is diffuse openness—expansion. It exhibits itself through stars, planets, galaxies, and universes. Blue sky, open space, cosmic rays, and all of the mysteries of the

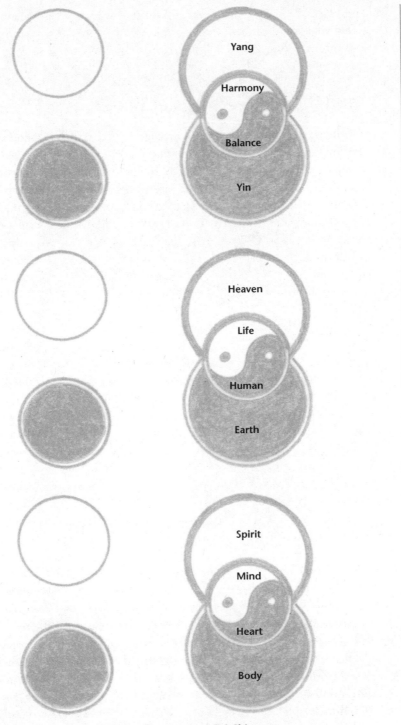

Merging Yin-Yang into Tai Chi

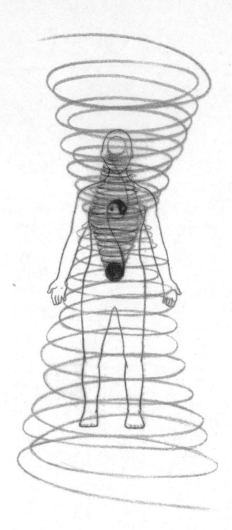

Merging Yin and Yang in the HeartMind

boundless cosmos are expressions of Heavenly Qi, which is Yang. The most obvious quality of Earthly Qi (*Di Qi*) is density and concentration, or contraction. The expressions of Earthly Qi—Yin—are substantiveness as in rock, sand, and soil, as well as condensation of vapor into the water of rain, river, lake, and sea. In the body, the organs and blood are Yin and the Qi is Yang.

The mixing of Heaven and Earth creates neither hard nor soft, neither dense nor spacious, neither compressed nor expansive but the balance of each in harmony. Life, as embodied by plants, animals, and humans, is made of substance but is not purely substantial—Yin. Life forms have energy, emotions, and thoughts, but they are not purely insubstantial—Yang. The mix of Yin/Earth and Yang/Heaven creates the conditions for the existence of a third state—balance and harmony—our delicate, flexible living body/mind/spirit complex filled with vitality and infinite possibility.

In the Qi cultivation context, the Three Treasures (Jing, Qi, Shen) are centered in and operate from powerful reservoirs of resource called *Dan Tian*. Dan Tian is translated as "Elixir Field"—elixir as in inner medicine, field as in the fertile fields where the cultivation of a nourishing harvest is carried out. The Three Dan Tian comprise a central concept in Qigong. These centers are roughly equivalent to the Western physiological structures of the gut, heart, and brain. In advanced Qigong the Dan Tian are the residences of energies, influences, and levels of Spirit—all forms of Qi. They are the location for the making and storage of profound inner medicines.

Earth represents the physical aspect of the multidimensional self, and its Qi resides in the Earth Dan Tian (lower Elixir Field) at and below the belly button at the energy and acupuncture points called Gate of Origin, Sea of Qi, and Spirit Gate. The lower Elixir Field is the residence of Earth Elixir or body medicine, used for healing the physical aspect of an illness or challenge. Heaven represents the spirit component of the multidimensional self, which resides in the Heaven Dan Tian (upper Elixir Field), just below the Point of Celestial Convergence (*Bai Hui*), which is located at the soft spot of your head (when you were born), and behind the area between the eyes, called *Yin Tang*. Heaven Dan Tian is associated with what is sometimes called the third eye or the Dao eye—which sees true reality and is the basis of intuition.

In *The Secret of the Golden Flower* (*Tai Yi Jin Hua Zong Zhi*),[8] one of the most beautiful books on cultivation and mastery (mentioned earlier regarding Natural Flow Qigong), Master Lu Dongbin discusses this area as "the Heavenly Heart, wherein dwells splendor." The upper Elixir Field is the reservoir of celestial resources, medicine that is the elixir of Spirit. Your spirit, because it is transcendental and eternal, is completely healthy, now and forever—it is perfect. Spirit Elixir cannot heal an already perfect spirit; it is intended to merge with Earth Elixir in the middle Dan Tian, associated with the heart and solar plexus, to help heal the mind, emotions, and relationships. This assists in revealing your most radiant self—your spirit—by uncovering or bringing to light your hidden splendor, referred to by Master Lu.

Heaven and Earth naturally reach toward each other like the poles of a magnet. They meet and merge to create your life. That is how your being is sustained from the very first moments when the parental essences merge in the womb. When your life is complicated by social, political, and survival stressors this merging of forces to create your being is at risk for becoming imbalanced, confused, and even diseased. When purposeful cultivation is practiced, however, the mind can act as the bridge between the body and spirit. When the forces of Heaven and Earth are carefully refined through the intentful mind, the Qi of the Earth is purposefully directed upward into the domain of Heaven (upper Dan Tian). Similarly, the Qi of Heaven is purposefully directed downward into the domain of Earth (lower Dan Tian). The Central Tai Chi

Channel (see page 16) is the primary pathway for the rising Yin, descending Yang, and their merging in the middle Dan Tian, in the area of the heart (see page 66).

This process is known as reversal of Yin and Yang. The Yang naturally ascends— fire. The Yin naturally descends—water. Through the application of deep and focused intention Yin and Yang reverse to foster a vital and awakened life. This is a foundation in Qigong. You can't force it to happen. It happens because you cross a special threshold in the process of potentiating yourself through Qigong over time. These details are fun and interesting to know and explore, but intentful practice is the key, not the accumulation of details. However, the details do inform us about the incredible insights of the ancient Qi masters and provide inspiration for our own practice.

When the cultivation occurs and the Yin and Yang penetrate each other, life, vitality, and creativity are reinforced. The flash point for the merging of Yin and Yang is in the middle Elixir Field, which parallels the physiological location of the heart, the thymus gland, and the solar plexus. When these forces meet in the middle Elixir Field,

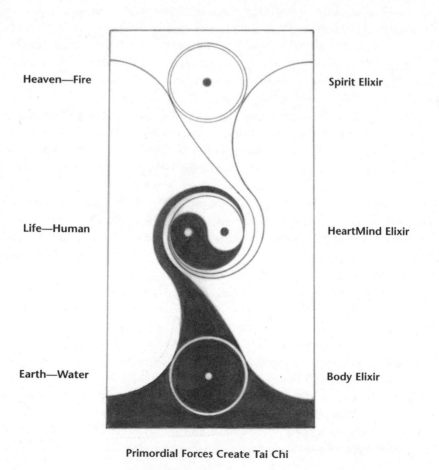

Heaven—Fire   Spirit Elixir

Life—Human   HeartMind Elixir

Earth—Water   Body Elixir

Primordial Forces Create Tai Chi

we experience the true Tai Chi within the human, the balance and harmony of the two primary forces—Yin and Yang. This is the identical phenomenon that occurred when the primordial cosmic forces merged to create the Tai Chi at the birth of the universe. Our immense cosmic universe and our small personal universe were conceived and born through the same process.

Xin, HeartMind

The middle Elixir Field, sometimes called the heart Dan Tian, is the residence of the mind and spirit according to Chinese medicine and philosophy. In Chinese, there is no discrete concept for *mind*, nor is there a discrete concept for *heart*. One single concept, *Xin* (pronounced "shin"), embraces both. Confused Western translators have struggled with this, often translating Xin only as "heart" or only as "mind." There is no heart and there is no mind, there is only Xin—HeartMind.

This is one of the most important keys for deepening your Qigong practice; it could be the master key. The conditioning of life and all its traumas causes us to believe that the brain and mind are the directors of life, but when the thinking self is allowed to be integrated with the feeling self in the HeartMind, everything changes. As you begin your practice you will find that the HeartMind is typically busy and distracted. With cultivation this is resolved through HeartMind Elixir, the harmonious blend of the Earth and Heaven elixirs in the middle Dan Tian. This level of medicine is far superior to Earth Elixir. In Chinese tradition this HeartMind Elixir heals emotional trauma and mental distraction. Even Western science agrees that approximately 70 percent of illness is related to stress. These kinds of diseases are healed with HeartMind Elixir. At some point in the future of your practice, through sincerity and intent, you will find that you are thinking with neither the mind alone nor the heart alone—you will understand that the HeartMind is directing your thought and your life. The ultimate goal of Qigong is to clear the HeartMind, to empty it of worry and judgment.

When this integration occurs, Yin-Yang/body-spirit come into balance. Some ancient sources call this Jing Shen. Your being radiates. When the HeartMind is clear your Shen, or Spirit, is revealed. Chinese tradition holds that even if a person is not cured, he or she may be *healed*. In fact, with Qigong, even people who are terminally ill are more peaceful; they experience less pain and use fewer drugs. This, it is suggested by Qigong researchers, is because the body is only one aspect of the whole person. It is possible for the body to die while the integrated and harmonious being is liberated.

Shen, Spirit

Initially, it challenged my thinking to learn that in Chinese medicine the mind and spirit are thought to reside in the heart. However, there is now a huge wave of breakthrough research demonstrating that the heart, even more than the brain, expresses the state of the mind. In acupuncture and herbal remedies from Chinese medicine, the Xin (HeartMind) is a predominant target for treatment of imbalances such as anxiety, depression, sleeplessness, and addiction. Yet, in the West these diagnoses have been associated with the mind and nervous system.

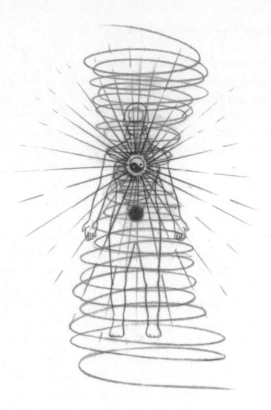

Radiant HeartMind

My grandmother, who was also my first Qigong master, told me repeatedly, "Your body is the temple of your spirit." The most effective Qigong is actually focused primarily on the eternal self, where our highest expression of perfect health already exists. The promise of Qigong is that if you focus on cultivating and expressing Shen Qi—revealing the latent presence of your spirit self—then health and productivity will arise spontaneously as side effects of your practice.

If these ideas seem elusive or mysterious, don't worry. The practice of Qigong will deepen your understanding over time. Following many pilgrimages to China to get a better understanding of Qi, I can tell you that it is not by using the reasoning mind of our Western tradition that we gain access to the brilliance of the Chinese worldview and the benefits of cultivating Qi. Rather, it is by purposefully overruling the confused and anxious mind and intentfully exploring the strange and wonderful HeartMind that we penetrate the remarkable wisdom of China's ancient scientist monks.

The Three Treasures Correspondences

The Three Treasures penetrate all aspects of our lives. The list of the correspondences of Three Treasures is not conclusive. It is intended to give a feel for the Three Treasures and provide a reference that you can return to occasionally to deepen your exploration or confirm insights that arise through your practice. Over time instead of finding new ideas on this list you will find yourself adding to it. As noted earlier, the Three Treasures are not something that you must understand. Like Qi, Yin-Yang, and the One, they are always present and dynamic resources. Through your practice and your intention you will uncover them, exactly as you uncover a marvelous treasure.

Three Treasures Correspondences			
	Earth Treasure	**Life Treasure**	**Heaven Treasure**
In Chinese Medicine	Jing	Qi	Shen
Domains of Being	Body (Earth)	Mind (HeartMind)	Spirit (Heaven)
Elixir (Dan)	Earth Elixir	HeartMind	Heaven Elixir
	Jing Dan	Xin Dan	Shen Dan
Elixir Field (Dan Tian)	Earth Elixir Field	HeartMind Elixir Field	Heaven Elixir Field
Kind of Qi	Jing Qi	Zhen Qi	Shen Qi
Three States	Yin	Harmony	Yang
Physics	Electron	Neutron	Proton
Practice Method	Kung Fu, Calisthenics	Qigong Mind Focus	Alchemy, Meditation/ Stillness
Cultivation Intention	Heal Body	Clear Mind and Emotions	Radiate Spirit
Lifestyle Focus	Nutrition, Exercise	Emotional Resolution	Spiritual Practice, Meditation
Nourishment/Fuel	Food	Qi	Spirit
Three Realms of Dao	Earth	Human	Heaven
Three Buddhist Realms	Earth	Atmosphere	Heaven
Transformation Symbol	Caterpillar	Cocoon	Butterfly

Reflections from Two Chinese Masters

I want to share two stories that are reflective of the ideas in this chapter. The first is from Master Zhu Hui. The second is an ancient tale of transformation as retold by Yuan Zheng.

Master Zhu Hui's Story

At a training at the Nine Clouds Mountain Qigong Sanatorium near the Six Harmonies Pagoda in Hangzhou, Zhu Hui told the following Three Treasures story one morning during a tea break. Master Zhu's home in Tian Tai Mountain has a strong heritage of both Buddhist and Daoist monasteries and temples. A practitioner of Chinese medicine for nearly fifty years, Master Zhu always taught with a rich blend of influences—medical, Daoist, and Buddhist.

"A young monk felt he was prepared to deepen his cultivation practice and his master gave the assignment to cultivate inner quiet and discover the secret of the source of life and the preservation of health and vitality. He gave the suggestion to focus on the Earth Dan Tian. After some months of practice the young monk reported to the master that he felt sure that the secret of the source of life was nourishment, rest, and the conservation of Qi and inner resources. The master encouraged the young monk, but let him know that his search was not over. 'You have found the secret to preserve the Jing and sustain the body, but you have not found the source of life.' The master asked the young monk if he was still interested in pursuing the deeper secret. The monk nodded and the elder gave him the suggestion to focus on the HeartMind Dan Tian.

"This time it was considerably longer before the younger monk visited the elder. When he returned, now older, he responded that the secret of the source of life and its preservation was accepting what naturally arises and bringing love and compassion into the world. The master agreed and encouraged the monk to continue his good work of compassionate service. The monk said to the master, 'I know that I have penetrated the secret of the highly refined interactions of Qi and the opening of the HeartMind. It has inspired me to the service of my fellow humans. It is clear that this sustains life—my own and others. But I have not determined the secret of the source of life.' The master suggested, 'Now, focus on the Heaven Dan Tian.'

"Some years passed. When the younger monk returned he was much older. The elder monk said, 'Tell me in one word.' The younger monk said, 'Unity.' They both smiled quietly. The two then parted knowing that even though they would not meet again they were always together at the source."

Stories such as this suggest that our practice can operate on three levels, each associated with one of the Three Treasures. When people turn to Qi cultivation in their lives it is not unusual for the process to evolve. The beginning focus is almost always on health and the body or on the desire for greater productivity or performance. When people discover the magnitude of the power of the Qi (after all it is the energy that runs the universe), body health and longevity frequently become secondary benefits of attaining peace of heart and mind.

The tradition of Qigong tells us that once we taste one of the treasures, we are destined to pursue its cultivation. As you begin to have an awakened experience of your body essence (Jing), your HeartMind (Xin), or your Spirit (Shen), you will be compelled to deepen your exploration of the treasures. When you cultivate body essence, you feel vitality. When you authentically cultivate HeartMind, you gain peace of mind. When you cultivate the treasure of Spirit, you experience miracles.

The Transformation of the Butterfly

Stories about healing in Qigong and Tai Chi often make poetic references to the Three Treasures. The three stages of the life of a butterfly are often used to represent the transformation from body, through mind to spirit. Yuan Zheng, a highly regarded teacher of Walking Qigong in Shanghai and one of the founders of the Cancer Recovery Society, told this story during a lecture about the use of Qigong for recovery from cancer and other diseases:

"When people are diagnosed with a life-threatening disease they are often exhausted in body, mind, and spirit. It is as if they are forced to crawl slowly and begin to think of their world as a terribly limited place and their experience of life as scary and depressing. I liken this to the body level of the Three Treasures, the stage of the caterpillar. At this level we are simply looking for a way to survive. We focus on the body, the most limited aspect of ourselves. When we start to do Qigong we begin to change because we get a sense that our self is not limited. The simple practice of Qigong begins a process in the body that is wonderfully healing. The pressure of the experience of the disease plus the support of Qigong friends create the permission to take on the challenge of becoming a new person.

Butterfly

"The caterpillar uses the Qi to spin a cocoon. In our group work with Qigong we use the building up of the Qi to create the safety and courage to be reborn. This is our cocoon. We meet to do our practice of Qigong and we have tea and discussion afterward that we call social oncology. You know that when the caterpillar is in the cocoon its former self is transformed to a new being. In our process of recovery from disease we often explore uncomfortable things about our lives, talk about things we have kept hidden, and improve our sense of humor. Through this transformational process we create a new self. Just as the caterpillar constructs a cocoon to become a butterfly.

"Eventually, we emerge with wings to fly. Many in the Qigong groups recover their health and are reborn as new people who have a completely different attitude about life. Some of our members do not recover but through the Qigong process and group support they become butterflies too, and fly free in a different way. The goal in our work is not just to cure diseases, but to heal. Sometimes healing does not accomplish a cure. But still the person is like a butterfly because he or she has the love of the Qigong group to support a needed transformation. Through Qigong and the love and support of our friends we gain the courage to transform from a caterpillar, to enter the cocoon and be liberated as a butterfly."

Qigong Methods

Three Warm-Ups

The following methods are classic practices with prehistoric roots. No one knows who developed them, and they are used in medical, Daoist, and Buddhist Qigong as well as many Tai Chi traditions. The primary purpose of the warm-ups is to awaken, excite, and accelerate your inner self-healing resources—Qi, blood, and internal water—as a prelude to deeper cultivation practices.

Repetitions and focus. Do as many repetitions as you feel will awaken and accelerate your Qi. Six or nine repetitions to each side is in keeping with traditional numbers from ancient Chinese philosophy. After some time of using these or any similar method most people will tell you that they can tell when the practice has done its job. You will soon gain a sense of this. Start with mild sessions and pay attention. You can feel the benefits of these methods. Always go for the very clearest state of mind. Alternatively, you could choose a specific focus, such as clouds drifting or waves crashing—something simple from nature. Just counting the repetitions or focusing on the breath is a reasonable starting place. Eventually you will want to advance to a quiet, calm focus on nothing in particular, mental neutral, or cheerful indifference.

Ringing the Temple Gong

HISTORICAL REFLECTION   This practice is used by almost every practitioner of Tai Chi or Qigong as a beginning warm-up to get inner resources circulating. It has a powerful effect on the spine. Notice that it is very rare to actually make this movement under normal circumstances. This suggests that the movement was designed for us by the architect of the universe to allow us to improve our health. The twist sends a strong stimulus into the connective tissue of the spine, which fosters flexibility and generates very low level electrical potential. As the hands strike the body, it sends a mechanical stimulus to the organs.

INSTRUCTION   After aligning and opening, begin to twist at the waist. In Tai Chi it is a key principle to lead from the waist. Do this first by simply turning to face the right or left with the arms dangling from the shoulders. Initiate the movement from the waist; do not lead the movement from the arms or the shoulders. Notice that the shoulders move automatically and that the arms and hands follow. Do this movement a few times. Now begin turning rhythmically to the left and right. At the last instant add a little hand power, or lift the body slightly, to make the hand strike to the body in front and back with either loose open hands or with fists. Experiment to find a comfortable breathing pattern. This may differ from time to time.

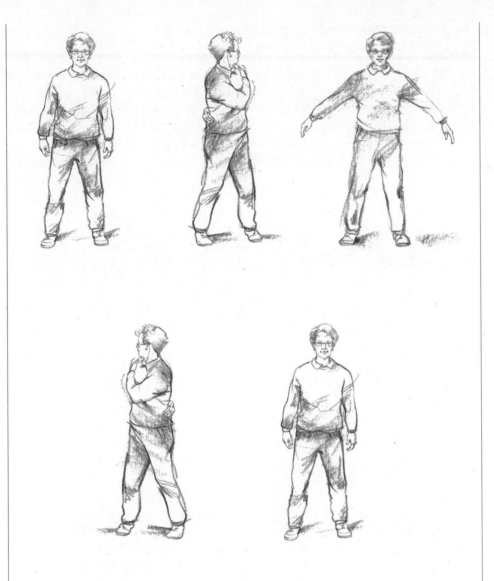

Ringing the Temple Gong

When you turn to the left, your right hand should strike the lower rib cage on the left, stimulating the spleen and pancreas. A variation on this would be to strike the chest near the left shoulder, which sends a healing impulse to the lungs. Your left hand should strike the kidneys in the back. When you turn to the right, the left hand strikes over the liver at the lower rib cage. Alternatively, you can strike the chest near the right shoulder and stimulate the lung point. The right hand would then strike the kidneys in the back. Do this gently at first. As you progress, increase the vigor of the gestures and turn to look behind you.

Beating the Heavenly Drum

HISTORICAL REFLECTION This is another classic warm-up that is timeless and shows up in all traditions. Many of the temples in China have a huge drum that is housed in a tower. This drum is used in ceremony and as an alarm. In both cases the intent is to bring those who hear its sound to a higher level of alertness. The reference to Heaven is always related to Yang as well as the celestial and spiritual, however, it is important to remember that drums are representative of the powers of the Earth in all original cultures. This practice awakens the Qi and the Spirit. After you have done the move-

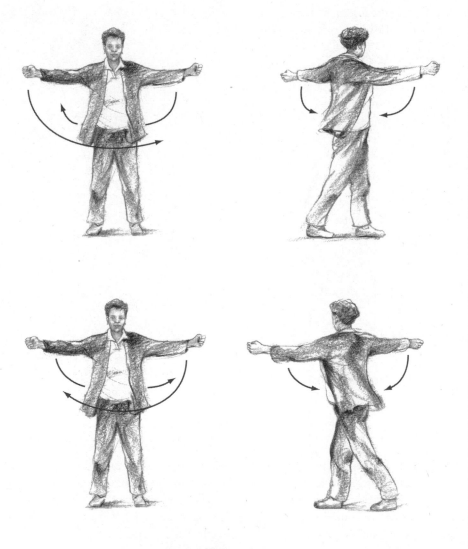

Beating the Heavenly Drum

ment for a while you will understand this. It is often used as a first exercise of the day—not just to warm up but to wake up.

INSTRUCTION Starting from the opening posture lift the arms out to the sides at shoulder level and form fists. To beat the drum, drop both arms, which will swing downward as you turn the body. When you beat the drum to the left with the right fist, it passes downward in front of the body. The left fist passes behind you. Exhale vigorously. Then return to the starting position, inhaling. To beat the drum to the right, the left fist passes in front and the right fist to the back. Exhale vigorously. Repeat. Make the sound of a drum if you wish, "boom." Or make any sound that suits you and gives you the feeling of alerting or awakening your Qi: "woosh," "ho," "uhh." It's your choice. Kids like to do this because the sound makes it more fun.

Warrior's Breath

HISTORICAL REFLECTION The warrior—warrior athlete, warrior for peace, warrior for life—is constantly working to enhance his or her function. This method was often used by martial arts warriors as an early morning warm-up. In contemporary time this practice is very well suited to starting one's practice because it provides the opportunity to detoxify and dispel accumulated factors that might compromise function or

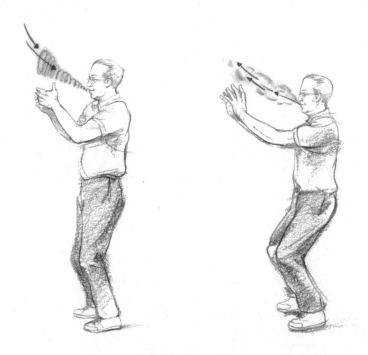

Warrior's Breath

performance. Visualizing the image of dispelling inner sludge and stagnant Qi from the channels brings the mind and imagination into the practice. The sharp exhalation is a powerful tool for clearing the body as well as the emotions.

INSTRUCTION Standing in the opening posture, breathe in deeply and raise the hands to heart level. Unbend the knees a bit, raising the whole body slightly. Right away or after holding the breath briefly, quickly sink down while extending the palms forcefully and exhaling sharply. Then drop the hands below the waist (not shown), breathe in, and use the hands as if you were clearing cobwebs or sludge from the Qi field in the front of the body. At the top of the breath, when the hands again reach the level of the heart, repeat the Warrior's Breath with a sharp exhalation. This clears the lungs and dispels stagnant or toxic Qi.

You can make a sound on the exhalation, such as "ho," "ha," "he," "yah," "yo," or any other. It is very satisfying. In addition, experiment with pushing forward from different levels on the exhalation. At the lower level you are clearing the gut (associated with the organs). At the heart level it is more like clearing feelings or stuck emotions. A sharp release from the head level can help clear tangled thoughts and open your system for the influx of your spiritual nature.

PART II

Cultivation and Mastery of Qi

Health, well-being, and long life can only be achieved by
    remaining centered with one's spirit,
    guarding against squandering one's Qi,
    using breath and movement
    to maintain the free flow of Qi and blood,
    aligning with the natural forces of the seasons,
    and cultivating the tranquil heart and mind.

—*THE YELLOW EMPEROR'S CLASSIC BOOK OF MEDICINE*,
    HAN DYNASTY, 200 B.C.E.–220 C.E.

The Ten Phases of Cultivating and Mastering Qi

Cultivation of the Fullness of Life
*   is like sowing grain,*
*   success is in the harvest.*
No matter how impressive your farm
*   you will reap little*
*   unless you sow select seeds*
*   in perfect timing*
*   and then cultivate intentfully to assure*
*   fertile soil, ample water*
*   and maximum care.*

—MASTER GE HONG, *THE BOOK OF THE MASTER WHO*
EMBRACES SIMPLICITY, FOURTH CENTURY C.E.

Cultivation of your health, of your true nature, of your inner potential, and of the light of your spirit may all be accomplished through cultivation of Qi (Chi). Careful tending of Qi through Qigong (Chi Kung) or Tai Chi (Taiji) yields a bountiful personal harvest for the body, mind, and soul, in tune with the dynamics of the seasons and the elements of nature.

The concept of Qi cultivation is abundant with references from nature. In my earliest training in Qigong, the imagery for the practice of Qi cultivation was based on knowledge from an ancient Daoist community in China called the Celestial Teachers

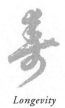

Longevity

77

(*Tian Shi*). Early in the first millennia this stream of Daoism based in family and community developed in their secluded mountain centers a beautiful and rich approach to Qi cultivation.

Cultivation as Inner Farming

The Dan Tian—Earth, HeartMind, and Heaven—your Elixir Fields, are the areas of your body where potent healing resources are cultivated and stored. The Chinese character for *field* (*Tian*) represents a symmetrical agricultural plot of land, which produces nourishment for self, family, and community. It also represents any area in which an interaction of forces or resources creates a positive result. This would include magnetic fields, information fields, and fields of consciousness as well as fields of abundant crops.

Cultivation, whether of the garden or of the self, can only begin when you consciously decide to do it. Our garden can flourish with diverse crops or lie empty and parched, depending on whether we elect to cultivate it. Consciousness and intent are key. Many people have satisfactory lives without Qi cultivation, but that level of existence is more like survival. It is acceptable. Clearly, you are attracted by life's possibilities. You want something more than mere survival; you are intentfully seeking to fulfill the promise of the Qi.

Reaching for the fullest life—the enriched and potentiated life—demands purposeful cultivation of inner and outer resources. Cultivation cannot occur until the field is prepared. Just as agricultural fields must be cleared of boulders, brambles, and weeds, our inner fields must be cleared of obstacles to cultivation that can range from the conditioning of old habits and attitudes to actual blockages of internal Qi. Some people can move through this clearing with ease, others may have significant work to do.

Given the major differences among the Earth, HeartMind, and Heaven fields, each will likely be cleared and prepared for cultivation at different times. For example, clearing the Earth Field (Di Dan Tian) may require dietary change or added rest. Clearing the field of the HeartMind (Xin Dan Tian) may require forgiveness, clearing of long-held grudges, or releasing stored-up anger, worry, and fear. The Heaven Field (Shen Dan Tian) is inherently clear. Spirit is like light. Clearing the Earth and HeartMind will allow the influence of Heaven—the light of Spirit—to shine through. The work that we do to clear and cultivate these inner fields is a kind of profound farming of the body, mind, and soul.

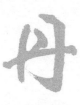

*Elixir
Field*

The True Seed

If cultivation is the way to create your bountiful inner harvest, it is essential to know what you intend to grow. The ancients in all cultures point to the seed as a kind of magical source of life and a symbol of the mystery of transformation. In Chinese tradition the image of the seed is an honored focus in the teaching of Qi cultivation. Why would you cultivate the field if there were no preferred crop that you intended to cultivate for harvest? In the phases of cultivation that follow, your Elixir Fields are the sites for cultivation, but it is this wondrous seed and its promise that is your ultimate focus.

There are several powerful interpretations of the true seed as represented by the tiny grain you may choose to plant, cultivate, and harvest. Early in the first millennium the Celestial Teachers held that certain true and righteous individuals (*Zhen Ren*) were seed people who would help to create and sustain a safe and honorable world. Seed people carry within them the best of what might be cultivated. A seed person, a righteous woman or man, is honest and hardworking with the intent to cultivate the personal self to a heavenly and virtuous state. She or he is the hope of the world.

A second interpretation of the meaning of seed is that we each have a "true seed" within. This seed represents our absolute highest possible state of being. It is the seed of the self that could become. It has been in existence since before Yin-Yang was born from the One. Cultivating the true seed is akin to Guarding the One.

Seed

> The true seed is the point
>   of spiritual light
>   which existed
>   prior to the separation
>   of Yin and Yang.

—MASTER LI, *THE BOOK OF BALANCE AND HARMONY*, THIRTEENTH CENTURY

In Qi cultivation we tend to plant this seed purposefully, using time-tested tools. We create the proper conditions. We use knowledge of nature to choose the timing for each phase of cultivation. We ensure that the soil is nourished with nutrients and moisture and warmed by the fire of the sun. Every aspect of farming is an aspect of self-cultivation—careful planting, tending, harvesting, and storing. Both vigilant work and enduring patience in careful cultivation help one to harvest a bountiful and rich yield of inner medicine (*Dan*), which can heal the self and be shared with others through compassionate service.

Cultivation as Inner Alchemy

Another traditional Chinese image for Qi cultivation is the process of using heat and fire to refine raw ingredients. In Qigong, this cooking, known as firing, is like the alchemy of refining raw inner ingredients to create pure gold or a marvelous inner elixir of supreme vitality. As the level of cultivation advances or evolves through numerous firings, the ingredients are transformed; they become precious. The elixir that can be cultivated is more and more highly refined as the alchemy practitioner cultivates and refines the different levels of the self—Earth level, HeartMind level, and finally Heaven level—making medicines for the Body, Mind, and Spirit.

This alchemical fire burns away the illusions of our conditioned life, self-sabotaging habits, and compulsions to reveal what the ancient life scientists called true reality (Quan Zhen) and the true person (Zhen Ren). At this point, in the highest levels of Qigong, pure spirit is revealed and the practitioner is considered an immortal or a fully realized being. In chemistry, in the purification of gold, fire is used to burn off all impurities. In Inner Alchemy, all of the complexities and conditioned factors of the self are refined in the fire of personal cultivation to reveal the pure gold of the essential nature.

Distilling the Traditions of the Ancients

We are about to begin our exploration of the Ten Phases of Cultivation and Mastery of the Qi. This is a framework for learning and practicing Qi cultivation that is a representative distillation of all of the ancient cultivation traditions, including Daoist, Buddhist, Confucian, medical, and martial.

As a student myself—learning, practicing, and then teaching the cultivation arts over a period of thirty years—I present this approach to working and playing with Qi as a sincere offering for your own journey of healing and empowerment. I am not presuming to speak for any particular traditional school or lineage. The Ten Phases of Cultivation are the result of a kind of alchemical refinement. I have, with the greatest respect for the origins of the Qi cultivation arts and sciences, distilled this framework with input from hundreds of colleagues, masters, teachers, and scholars; insights from both ancient and contemporary written literature; my own personal practice; and the guidance of the Qi itself.

Whether your focus is to heal yourself, help others, merge with nature, accelerate productivity and performance, maximize intuition and creativity, attain inner peace, or intimately touch the mysterious fabric of the cosmos, these ten phases, with their roots in ancient tradition, are tools with extraordinary power to release your inner potential.

The Ten Phases of Cultivating and Mastering Qi
1. Discover Qi.
2. Gather Qi.
3. Circulate Qi.
4. Purify Qi.
5. Direct Qi.
6. Conserve Qi.
7. Store Qi.
8. Transform Qi.
9. Dissolve in Qi.
10. Transmit Qi.

Phases one through nine involve the personal cultivation of Qi. In phase ten the influence of your cultivation spills over into compassionate service, a transmission of outflowing influence to help and to heal others. The nine phases of personal cultivation and the tenth phase of compassionate expression—the Ten Phases of Cultivating and Mastering Qi—can be approached in numerous ways, always with a light heart and a sense of wonder. Investigating the phases is a lifetime process. Do not feel that you have to follow a particular order or fully master one level before you explore the next. You will likely make advances in purifying Qi and conserving Qi before you become fully adept at gathering Qi.

From simply becoming aware of the existence of Qi in the world and within yourself, you may eventually be able to learn directly from the Qi itself. While you already know this as a theory, one of the rewards of Qi cultivation is that, over time, you can go beyond mental concepts. You may evolve or mature to a deep knowing or an experiential grasp that Qi is the essence of everything. It will become clear that you *are* Qi. You are primarily energy and consciousness, and your body is a vehicle for your multidimensional self. This is challenging. The invisible part of your multidimensional self becomes more dominant than the visible part of yourself. The physical and physiological selves become secondary to the energetic self, the mental/emotional self, and the transcendental or spiritual self. These realizations are the essence of Qi cultivation and Qigong. The ten phases are the tool kit for understanding how to use this information for the good of yourself and others.

Human, Person

The ancient wisdom traditions and the contemporary science community already agree—the universe is an undifferentiated continuum, a unified whole. Using Qigong, we can now personally begin to embrace and apply practices that address these important findings. When you enter the Qigong state you step closer to your essence of personal wholeness and unity with nature. Qigong is literally a method for awakening to the fact that you have radical access to the power of the entire universe. You are filled with and swimming in this power. The Ten Phases of Cultivation and Mastery promise to lead you, not only to healing and empowerment, but also to a state of understanding, aligning with, and utilizing the forces of nature.

Ancient Secrets of Qi Cultivation Accessible to All

This knowledge of the Ten Phases of Cultivation and Mastery is a profound gift from the ancients. Over the millennia this system of cultivation was kept as a secret in only a very few families, imperial courts, or monastic lineages. Most frequently, students received only parts of the teaching. In many cases the only people lucky enough to receive the deepest secrets were the elder male offspring or one single monastic disciple. Those elected in this extremely exclusive framework were then sworn to reveal the cultivation system to only one carefully chosen follower. Others would glimpse bits and pieces of the whole and were taught primarily the "form" of the practice rather than the essence and principles of the "Way." Many of these carefully guarded principles are presented here in the Ten Phases of Cultivation and Mastery.

In former times a number of reasonable excuses existed for keeping such secrets. For one, during many eras in ancient history, the schools of inner cultivation were forced by recurrent and severe political challenges to direct the power of their transcendental knowledge into martial applications. Unfortunately, it was necessary for the survival of the lineage to protect the secrets so that the school or family could remain invincible to attack from competing forces. Most of the key Daoist and Buddhist monasteries have been destroyed several times in the last 1,500 to 2,000 years. Such cultural trauma, common in Chinese history, created a very closed and secretive context for the evolution of Qigong and Tai Chi.

In the contemporary era two factors have made it less necessary to keep these self-energizing and empowerment systems as warrior secrets. While postimperial China has social and political challenges, the New China culture has definitely created the possibility for less internal strife than in former dynasties. This climate has allowed average Chinese citizens to access Tai Chi and many other forms of Qigong. In addition, modern warfare has eliminated the practical need for hand-to-hand combat where the cultivation of Qi and secret martial applications would determine the victor. In the current era the most appropriate applications of the Qi cultivation arts are for health and healing and the maximization of individual endurance and potential.

Evolving Through the Phases

As you explore the first phases of cultivation, Earth level, the teaching will direct you in a simple approach to Qigong through practices that help you to discover, gather, and circulate Qi. At this level it is important to know when you need assistance from acupuncture and natural healing methods or even medical treatment. In the middle phases, the HeartMind level, the teaching will assist you in learning to purify, direct, and conserve Qi. It is important as well, at this level, to resolve and release emotional pain, investigate forgiveness of those who have transgressed against you, and adjust habitual attitudes that are not serving you. In the middle phases, it may become evident to you that you would benefit from the assistance of counseling or social and emotional support from like-minded students. In these phases a teacher can provide important guidance, but you must still be the practitioner. Very little of what is promised by the Qi can be done for you by someone else.

In the later phases, the Heaven or Spirit level, the evolution of personal cultivation will help you to access the part of yourself that knows more about your own place in the universe and your own pace of healing than anyone else can possibly know. There is no way that someone outside of yourself could, or would want to, compete with the quality of your personal connection with your highest self and universal

Ancient

source. The most enlightened teachers inspire us through their practice and actions and encourage us to apply the principles from the Ten Phases of Cultivation. In the Spirit Phases of Cultivation, our teachers become our peers.

In the contemporary sense there is really no limit to who can learn and practice Qigong and Tai Chi. There is too much need in the world for such powerful tools to be locked up behind barriers that were erected in completely different political and historical times. The Ten Phases of Cultivation is just one carefully distilled way of looking at the map of Qi cultivation practice.

The Phases as the Foundation of All Forms of Qigong, Tai Chi, and Yoga

Our fascination with these possibilities, our longing to continuously improve ourselves and maximize our potential and even to bring peace to our own little corner of the world leads us to ask, "How can I learn to do these things? How can I gain access to the promise of the Qi with all its benefits and gifts?"

The answer? Cultivate Qi! Master Qi! With sincere intent, you can evolve through these phases of Qi cultivation and mastery that have been recognized for thousands of years. In your personal practice, through exposure to wise instructors and in communication with your fellow practitioners, you will consistently evolve through these phases in perfect timing. There is no rush; this is not a race. Relax into it.

Most important is that every kind and style of Qigong—including Tai Chi and Yoga—shares a basis in essential principles. Many of these principles are applied in the Ten Phases of Cultivation and Mastery. However, in every unique school or system these phases and the essential principles are clothed in the accouterments of that particular approach. Each has its particular practices, movements, and philosophies. The good news is that this multitude of forms and traditions is rooted in a common foundation of principles that are inherent in the phases of cultivation contained in the chapters that follow.

For example, the Daoist forms reflect the phases as a process to behold and embrace nature's deepest secrets and refine within oneself a profound elixir, which perpetuates health, attains longevity, and supports access to transcendental states. This awareness of one's infinite nature is called Immortality, which means awareness of one's eternal nature. In the Buddhist forms, the essential phases of cultivation are embedded in the framework of the tradition of liberation from suffering and access to pure mind—called Nirvana or Pure Land. Medical Qigong employs the language of traditional Chinese medicine, including Yin and Yang, the Five Elements, and the organs and channels for Qi flow with the goal of healing. In the martial arts, the phases are revealed in methods for subduing the assailant by using Qi power and wisdom rather

Mastery

than physical strength and fury. The enemy is more often one's own confused inner self than it is someone attacking from outside. For that reason Tai Chi is often called Shadow Boxing.

My personal mission—in my practice, in my teaching, and in this book—has been to distill the essence of these wondrous traditions. My hope is to inspire you by revealing the essential framework—the prime technology—to empower your Qi cultivation practice. Numerous students I have worked with have remarked that they finally felt at home with ancient Asian wisdom and had a kind of awakening "Ah-ha" when they began to work their way into this phased framework of cultivation practice.

This phased system of cultivation principles is very practical. It has the great benefit of allowing you to immediately enjoy the simple gifts of Qigong in the earliest phases, while the more esoteric and transcendental aspects of the system fall into place during the later phases. If you already have a cultivation practice, consider applying the phased system to your favored lineage or teaching. Whatever your particular favorite form, style, or school of Qigong, Tai Chi, Yoga, or meditation, the Ten Phases of Cultivation can assist in deepening your practice.

The Phases and the Ancients

Patanjali, the great second-century Yoga philosopher from India, has written that healing and access to highly refined states of body, mind, and spirit must occur in stages.[1]

> *Mastery through practice in discipline*
> *gives access to the light of wisdom.*
> *The practice*
> *is achieved in phases.*

—PATANJALI, *YOGA SUTRAS*, SECOND CENTURY C.E.

The phased framework is present in the Qigong tradition as well. During the Tang dynasty, one of the great renaissance eras in every aspect of Chinese culture, there were many breakthroughs in Qi cultivation. Two particularly famous figures from this era—Sima Chengzhen, also known as the Master of the White Clouds of Tian Tai Mountain, and Sun Simiao, renowned as one of the greatest of all Chinese physicians—wrote prolifically on Qigong. These Qi cultivation luminaries have provided guidance and inspiration to me in my practice and to many who have come before me over the centuries in China. Master Sima wrote fifteen books, among which are the *Discourses on the Essential Meaning of the Absorption of Qi* and *Discourse on Sitting in Oblivion*.[2] Master Sun (pronounced "soon") wrote twenty-two books, including *Prescriptions Worth a Thousand Ounces of Gold, Handbook of Methods for Nourishing Life,* and *Visualization of Spirit and Refinement of Qi*.[3]

Scholars and historians of Qi cultivation agree that the Tang dynasty brought tremendous organization to both medicine and Qigong. Sima Chengzhen is renowned for helping to organize the Qi cultivation arts into a more structured and phased system. Master Sun, called the Emperor of Physicians and also True Person Sun, believed heartily that true health was to be gained through the most refined phases. This was not just a transformation of the body but rather a transformation of all three levels or domains of the self—body, mind, and spirit. Livia Kohn, in her work *Early Chinese Mysticism*,[4] clarifies that Daoist Qi cultivation has a threefold structure. "Practitioners move from refining the body to restructuring the mind, and ultimately to attain oneness." We will be exploring such a three-level structure in the Ten Phases of Cultivation and Mastery.

With the guidance of Masters Sun and Sima, through the wisdom of my own teachers, and through sincere personal exploration it has become apparent that the ten phases of Qi cultivation have a poetic yet practical structure that can empower Qi cultivators in deepening their practice. While most of the Chinese classics remain largely untranslated and there is no one system used in teaching in China, this phased, threefold approach is a reflection of time-honored traditions.

As you know, the Three Treasures provide a framework for an enormous range of philosophical concepts and practical applications in Chinese tradition, Chinese medicine, Tai Chi, and Qigong: "The Three gives birth to the Ten Thousand Things." The Three Treasures provide the framework for the Ten Phases of Cultivation and Mastery as well.

The following chapters will explore in rich detail the Earth and HeartMind phases and provide practical insights for your Qi cultivation. The Heaven phases are much more difficult to discuss, as the highest levels of cultivation are both mysterious and very personal. For this reason the discussion of these phases will be fairly brief. However, Phase Ten—Transmit Qi, The Phase of Compassionate Expression—provides a practical compendium on how to apply your cultivation practice as service to others.

The three domains of Qigong—Earth, HeartMind, Heaven—provide the foundation of this comprehensive framework for learning and practicing Qigong. For clarity we will explore this teaching and learning system briefly before we meet our master teachers and travel to our training center deep in the sacred mountains of China for comprehensive training in Qi cultivation.

Elixir

The Three Treasures and the Ten Phases

Treasure	Qigong Domain	Aspect	Elixir	Resource	Phase
Earth	Earth	Body	Body Medicine	Jing	1–3
Life	HeartMind	Mind	HeartMind Medicine	Qi	4–6
Heaven	Heaven	Spirit	Spirit Medicine	Shen	7–10

Earth Domain: Making Body Medicine

Typically when people commence with Qigong, their practice is focused primarily on the body—relieving pain, healing disease, and maximizing energy and productivity. In the Earth Domain of practice, no special knowledge is required. The focus of mind intent is simply to get out of the way of what occurs naturally. Qi will naturally gather into your system and circulate if you relax, focus your awareness, and move your body gently. Rather than being directed and specific, mastery of Qigong in the first three phases of cultivation is based primarily in gaining the ability to use the Three Intentful Corrections to access the Qigong state with simple practices to discover, gather, and circulate Qi. In the framework of the Three Treasures, Earth Domain Qigong is primarily associated with strengthening the Jing and healing the body.

Earlier we discussed the metaphors used to describe the Three Treasures. Earth Domain Qigong is associated with the image of the caterpillar crawling on the ground, which illustrates the level before transformation. As a caterpillar we live with a small view of the world and are not aware that we can fly. In Discover Qi we get a glimpse of the possibilities. In Gather Qi we nourish our potential healing by purposefully gathering resources from nature. In Circulate Qi we collaborate with the body's natural capacity to fuel the function of tissues, organs, and glands, which facilitates healing and pain relief at the same time it builds potential to enter the HeartMind Domain of Qigong. The sign of success in Earth Qigong is healthy and vital longevity.

HeartMind Domain: Medicine for Heart and Mind

When you evolve beyond the Earth Domain, your practice takes on new meaning. You enter the HeartMind Domain of cultivation. You have already learned how to discover, gather, and circulate the Qi. Now you are going to purify, direct, and conserve Qi; you are called to a greater degree of focus—increased mind intention (*Yi*). To achieve mastery in the HeartMind Domain it is not sufficient to merely perform the practice. Cultivation of HeartMind Qigong means that you are becoming conscious and alert in the process of purposefully redesigning, re-creating, or rebirthing yourself.

HeartMind Qigong is associated with the cocoon. The caterpillar enters the cocoon to melt down its former self and be transformed—it is reborn and takes flight. There will be an equivalent in your own practice and experience—a transformation including the dissolving of your old self, with its habits, attitudes, and conditioning. This level of cultivation moves toward Inner Alchemy, the process of transforming yourself purposefully using Qigong. Implementing shifts in personal behavior, thinking, and communication potentiates your transformation in the HeartMind phases of Qigong. Breathe and relax. As much as this may seem like an immense challenge, even terrifying, you are really looking at the possibility of giving yourself the gift of becoming more true to your nature.

The focus of HeartMind Qigong is to strengthen and heal the nervous system, thoughts, emotions, attitudes, and deeply held beliefs. Qigong is the power tool that can Purify Qi by detoxifying extra or blocked Qi from the Qi Matrix. Practitioners of HeartMind Qigong suffer less from stress as the nervous system is purposefully cleared of habitual reactiveness and resistance.

In Direct Qi you evolve your level of concentration and mind clarity. In this phase the intention is to overcome your busy mind and distraction through your practice. If your capacity to access this level of inner quiet is stalled, if the mind will not be managed, it may indicate that you will want to complement Qigong with additional strategies and support. Conserve Qi is only possible if the HeartMind is relaxed and focused enough to set limits on wasting Qi. Habits, compulsions, extreme emotions, and life conditioning that cause tension are addressed in this phase, which allows for the accumulation of inner potential and Qi. This is the gateway to the Heaven Phases.

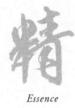

Essence

The sign of success in HeartMind Qigong is the ability to sustain calm in the midst of life's stresses, to say no to activities that drain inner resources, and to maintain a sense of cheerfulness through all conditions and outcomes. Honest self-assessment is an aspect of HeartMind Qigong.

Heaven Domain: Spirit Medicine

When you break free of the cocoon of HeartMind Qigong you are liberated to flutter, like a magnificent butterfly, into the ultimate phases of cultivation and mastery, Inner Alchemy. "Ultimate" is a key concept in Qigong. The Chinese words *Tai Chi* actually translate as "supreme ultimate." Very high level Tai Chi is neither martial skill nor health improvement; it is a form of spiritual Qigong. In this domain of Qigong you will have gained access to the most compelling level of mastery—a direct and conscious relationship with energy, universal intelligence, and spiritual light. Your cultivation evolves beyond concerns of the body and the Earth Domain and matures through the mental, emotional, and situational concerns of the HeartMind.

Practitioners of Heaven (Spirit) Qigong experience expansiveness and no resistance; they are open like sky, it is said. The organ channels and the Central Tai Chi Channel that connects the three Dan Tian are all so clear that Heaven and Earth are supremely present within and unburdened by issues of personality. In this state, practitioners cultivate *Jin Dan*, also known as the Golden Elixir. This is the ultimate spiritual medicine. Spirit Domain Qigong is largely focused on opening up to being and expressing your highest self in a context where you have realized that each separate being is woven into the fabric of boundless, unified totality.

In HeartMind practice your Qi has been purified, directed to maximize function, and conserved to accumulate inner potential. Now, in these most advanced phases of cultivation, the portion of this accumulated inner wealth that is not being used, moment-to-moment, to heal and maintain the body can be stored and then transformed into pure Spirit—Shen Qi.

Store Qi purposefully guides this accumulated Qi into storage in the organs, channels, and bones. In the Transform Qi phase, this stored resource is transmuted through the firing process of Inner Alchemy into a sustainable capacity to express the universal self. Finally, as you Dissolve in Qi, your universal self radiates the boundless and timeless qualities of your eternal nature, even if it is being expressed through your individual body and personality here and now. You merge with the One, Dao.

The Tenth Phase of Compassionate Service is both simple and challenging. Pure and abundant Qi spontaneously overflows, transmitting beneficial influence to affect others in a healing or inspiring way. You will learn how to help others by triggering the transmission of the Qi of the universe rather than spending the Qi that your body needs for personal health and endurance.

People who are successfully cultivating in the Heaven Domain express unconditional love, inspired acceptance of what spontaneously arises, and personal radiance. Spirit Qigong cultivates spiritual light which is unconstrained and flowing ever outward. Masters of this level of Qigong are not only content in all conditions, but palpably soothing and inspiring to others.

Our Training in the Phases of Cultivation

In the following chapters we will look at some of the richest of the Chinese Qigong traditions. This body of information comes from ancient roots and has been refined over many dynasties. We will travel deep into the Chinese countryside to ancient sacred mountains—to the site of a traditional Qigong and Tai Chi training center. The mountains, the center, our teachers, and our experiences will create a profound and memorable adventure of healing and transformation that is intended to inspire and empower your practice.

Sacred Mountains Qi Cultivation Training Center

Imagine that we have traveled deep into China across agricultural plains, rivers, and valleys. We have passed through many small villages where it is obvious that all of the sustenance is cultivated and harvested in the surrounding countryside. The residents of the villages interact through barter and direct exchange. Depending on the area we are in, home after home has some form of grain—rice, wheat, or corn—drying in the sun or hanging from the doors, windows, and rafters. In many such villages there is not even one store. Let that fact sink in—village after village where there are no stores at all. As we pass through these communities, especially in the early mornings, there are people out practicing Qigong and Tai Chi—in the streets, near the rivers, and in the courtyards of the houses.

Then suddenly, after miles and miles of flat farmland, the plains abruptly end and imposing mountains sharply etch the horizon. With the unexpected shift, following the miles of heated plains in their golden harvest tones, to the cool green of tree-covered mountains there is a sudden drop in temperature. Clouds are draped around the peaks and tumbling through the valleys. The images of mountains that you have seen in Chinese paintings suddenly become real. These mountains are that mystical domain of Daoist observatories and Buddhist temples. The Chinese people have historically climbed into these mountains for serenity and spiritual renewal—to get closer to Heaven. Qigong was born in mountains like these ages ago.

Mountain

Our bus follows a river that is rushing out of the rocky gorges, climbing upward. At the end of the road we begin on foot across a bridge. The river makes a musical sound as the water spills over the rocks. It is as if we have crossed a threshold and left the world behind. We begin the ascent to the training center. We will be climbing up into one of the high valleys, on a staircase of granite. Our guide and translator is named Intentful HeartMind (Yi Xin). It is typical for those who are deeply involved with Qi cultivation to take names that either express their personal goal or their status in Qi cultivation.

Yi Xin informs us that these steps were carved into the granite mountain so long ago that no one knows who did it or how. He says that the facility that we will be visiting, which was first built thousands of years ago and was destroyed several times throughout the dynasties, is experiencing a renaissance as a Qigong and Tai Chi training center. Our load is light as a group of Yi Xin's associates have agreed to carry the single bag that we each have brought on two-man shoulder carriages that can also carry a person seated. If you feel the hike is more than you could handle, take a ride up in one of these.

We are literally walking up through the clouds. After several hours of climbing, many stops, and numerous dramatic vistas, the steps open up into a wide area where small, neatly arranged gardens lie outside of a beautiful secluded monastery. As we approach the entrance, we are greeted by our teachers Eternal Spring (Yong Chun) and Jade Unity (Yu Yi).

These teachers will provide the metaphors for how we might think of the principles of Qi cultivation we are about to learn. Stories and metaphors are traditionally used to bring Qigong and Tai Chi teaching to life.

In the oldest systems of cultivation, from the eras in history previous to the written language, it was traditional to teach using songs or scriptures that for centuries had been passed along orally from teacher to student. In my training as a doctor of Chinese medicine, I learned from one of these songs called the Jade Dragon Song. This is the song of the Ten Phases of Cultivation and Mastery.

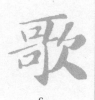

Song

Song of the Ten Phases of Cultivation and Mastery of Qi

In seeking to live vitally in accord with the true nature of the world,
I first become aware of the essential universal resource—Qi.
I find, observe, and sense Qi within myself,
in my surroundings, in all beings, and everywhere in the universe.
When this profound resource is gathered and absorbed,
its increased presence activates the circulation of Qi
in my channels, reservoirs, and fields.
I purify and cleanse the Qi
by dispelling extra, impure, and spent resources.
I direct the pure and fresh Qi in the internal pathways
to the organs, glands, limbs, and senses.
The activity of pure and ample Qi
empowers my capacity to fulfill my destiny,
my work, and my creativity.
To sustain and even multiply my vitality
I conserve, protect, and accumulate the Qi
through moment-to-moment life choices.
Qi that is spent is lost, that which I conserve
accumulates and may be stored.
Through cultivation, Qi that is stored
can be transformed within me,
transmuting inner resources,
through Inner Alchemy,
into the Golden Elixir.
When it is transformed the Qi is refined into pure Spirit [Shen]
which elevates my awareness of profound unity
with my limitless universal nature.
When I am unified with the universal
I am undifferentiated,
one with all possibilities, beings, and things.
United with all that is and all that could possibly be,
I dissolve into the boundless field of the One.
One with the Universe, I am the Universe.
One with all beings and possibilities
I am moved to serve those around me through Qi transmission,
knowing that they are none other than myself.

Qigong Method

Spontaneous Qigong

HISTORICAL REFLECTION Spontaneous Qigong is a paradox. Initially it might seem inconsequential and simplistic, but it turns out to be one of the most extraordinary of all Qigong methods for many reasons. There is no detailed method to learn; it is completely spontaneous and intuitive. It is the best Qigong method for dealing with shaking out or detoxifying Qi stagnation or emotional patterns that are trapped inside. Workshops in spontaneous practice are fun. The benefits are immediate and obvious. This practice causes an immediate and strong Qi sensation because it brings about coherence in the physiological and emotional aspects of oneself. Music to support the release of emotions makes Spontaneous Qigong even more effective.

Research has shown that after a traumatic event, animals shake and tremble until they have cleared the nervous system of the trauma. This is a very healthy and healing activity. Humans typically do not have such a tool; they hold trauma in the body—specifically in the nervous system. Spontaneous Qigong is equivalent to shaking out trauma, so you may find that the practice will engage or release emotions. In some forms of Qigong the practice of spontaneous trembling or shaking is recommended often.

Spontaneous Qigong was most likely developed forty thousand to sixty thousand years ago by ancient pretribal humans. The ancient names for Spontaneous Qigong—Primordial (Wuji) practice, Dancing Before Heaven, and Dancing in Chaos—all suggest that the method is used to reconnect with the eternal aspect of the self. To do this we must shake off our conditioning. As well as a warm-up, Spontaneous Qigong is a very powerful healing tool with a multitude of applications. Yet there is nothing to learn or remember.

INSTRUCTION Despite its ancient tradition and important benefits, the practice itself is very simple. Find a comfortable place to stand where you have some room to move about. Allow yourself to drift for a moment in the aligning and opening postures. Take time to align the Central Tai Chi Channel and the Elixir Fields, explained in Chapter 3. Now bend your knees slightly and begin to bounce by lifting and dropping your heels. Do some variations on this activity—shift your weight so the right side is bouncing and the left is just along for the ride. Then bounce the left and let the right side relax. Next add flopping your hands at the wrists or snapping your fingers vigorously or, better, snapping all of your fingers past your thumbs. The key is to wiggle the body and limbs vigorously in any way that is comfortable. Allow your head and neck to move about, lift and drop your shoulders, even jump up and down. Do this for a few moments with deep, relaxed breathing.

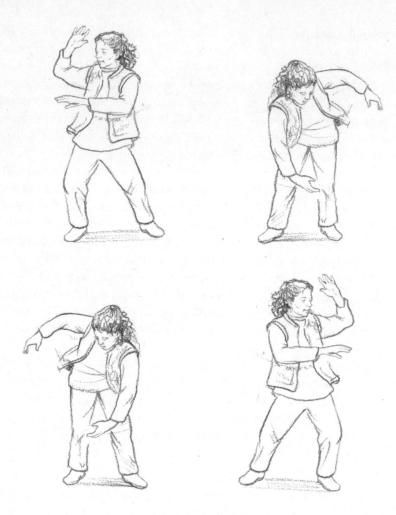

Spontaneous Qigong

Stop and turn your attention inward and feel the sensation. In your own mind answer the question, what do I feel and where do I feel it? There is no right answer; just sense the inner environment. Now, do the practice again.

After bouncing, wiggling, and snapping your fingers for a while use some of the sounds we have used with other postures—"ahh" or "ohh." Take in deep breaths and let out sounds that make you feel exhilarated—growls, shouts, laughter, or long, soft sighs. Which causes you the most relief? Do somewhere between five and ten sounding breaths with continued body activity.

As you wiggle, shake, and bounce think about shaking out that which does not serve you, that which causes tension and pain. Think about pulling in fresh Qi to replace that which is dispelled. After a while you may want to sit or lie down and just focus on the breath and feel the sensations and emotions within you. This is very similar to powerful therapies that have been developed by Wilhelm Reich, based on a Qi-like energy called orgone. The work of Alexander Lowen, called bioenergetics; Stanislov Groff's holotropic breathing; and rebirthing—all use the breath and body interaction to release trauma and open up inner flow.

Spontaneous Qigong consists of movements that come to you intuitively. Some will be from your own vocabulary of movement while others will occur to you from moment to moment. On some days, once you have warmed up to this practice you will find yourself vigorously shaking off tension and stress. Occasionally you will be lucky enough to get deep enough to release some old trauma with tears and laughter. On other days you will simply find yourself purring like a cat because you are, for some reason, in the comfort zone and feeling right with the nature of the world.

Phase I:
Discover Qi

If one cannot obtain medicines
one can live still to several hundred years of age,
if one fully grasps the principles
of Cultivating Qi and practices daily.
Indeed, humans exist within the Qi
and Qi exists within humans.
From Heaven and Earth to the myriad things,
Qi is pervasive.
There is nothing that does not rely on Qi for life.

—MASTER GE HONG, *THE BOOK OF THE MASTER WHO*
EMBRACES SIMPLICITY, FOURTH CENTURY C.E.

"Recall something important in your life that you did not notice at first. Now, remember when you became aware of it." Though a small woman, our teacher Eternal Spring speaks with authority and presence. She continues: "When I was first learning about Qi [Chi] cultivation from my own favorite teacher as a young student he told me, 'When you find the Qi it will amaze you. When you cultivate Qi you will discover something new every day. Some of what you discover will be realizations about nature and your surroundings. And some of what you discover will be revelations of the inner realm and your own true nature. It will be simple and practical, so just relax and have some fun.'

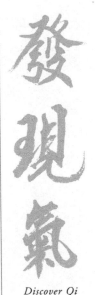

Discover Qi

95

"I knew right away what he was saying because of one of my most interesting experiences as an even younger child. When I was very small, a few years before the time that my teacher told me this, there was a woman's garden that I passed daily. One day I noticed that a vibrant green plant, about two feet tall, had appeared in the corner of the garden near the path. It was not there before—it was like a little surprise. In the spring things grow, so I took it for granted. I always thought the woman who grew this garden was very kind. My parents called her an immortal because she was very old and she was always happy and smiling. Her garden was extremely productive. She was constantly giving away food.

"Over a short period, the plant grew to equal my height. Its stalk was thick. I was standing there looking at it when the old woman came over to me and said this plant would be my teacher. I didn't understand, but the woman was smiling and the plant certainly had caught my attention. Over time the plant grew to twice my height, with an immense yellow bloom on it that was bigger than my head—a huge sunflower. I was amazed and kept wondering what it would teach me. Eventually the autumn arrived and one day the big plant was gone, just as suddenly as it came. I was kind of shocked. I was standing there feeling sad when the old woman came to me smiling and gave me a little bag of sunflowers seeds.

"She said, 'The seeds were like the lessons of a great teacher; they continue to teach long after the teacher is gone.' She said that to understand what this meant I should plant the seeds throughout the village before the first snow. Together we planted one of the seeds near where the big plant had been, so I knew how deep to place them. And so I did as she said. I placed several along the path where I walked every day, several by my school, and several near my home—twelve seeds in all. She said that someday I should tell others what my teacher taught me.

"The seeds sprouted in the spring. I was thrilled to have been involved in this miracle. They all grew into large plants, each with a flower on it as big as my head. I knew that each one contained hundreds of seeds. I wondered how one original seed could produce so many seeds, that then produced so many plants with so many more seeds. That original sunflower was not there at first and then it was there to capture my attention. It taught me so very much. That sunflower is still teaching. It helps me to teach you. From that flower I learned a great deal about the essential nature of life and life force and seasons, and about the productivity that happens spontaneously in nature.

"When my Qigong [Chi Kung] teacher said that the Qi would teach me something new every day I already knew what he meant because of the old immortal gardener and my teacher the sunflower. When you discover the Qi, watch it, and cultivate it, it will teach you and you too will learn something every day. Just like sunflowers that come from one seed and create hundreds of seeds that then create hundreds of sunflowers that create thousands of seeds—through your expanded awareness and your practice your Qi will multiply."

Eternal

Discovering the Qi

The first phase of cultivation and mastery is to establish a direct awareness of the Qi. Your consciousness is the observer and your own body, mind, and being are the laboratory. We can use the same methods now that the ancient Daoists discovered in their "observatories" millennia ago. Some Qigong teachers suggest that it takes a long time and a great deal of practice to discover Qi. I disagree. Between 80 and 90 percent of the people I have worked with feel the Qi the first day—many within a few moments.

Through the preliminary methods and the warm-ups from the previous chapters, you have likely begun to perceive the sensations of Qi as tingling, as warmth, as a sense of fullness or of flowing within.

Spring

The gateway to the wonder of Qigong swings open by first discovering or finding a direct physical perception of the Qi. This same perception is the basis for how you will eventually want to experience Qi in all your cultivation practice. It can lead to higher levels of cultivation and improved skills for self-healing, refining intuition, and helping others. This level of Qi awareness is not immediate for many people and so you may begin to discover Qi another way—through exploring the world around you with a new awareness.

Much of nature provides focal points for the study of Qi. The swallows return to the old mission in San Juan Capistrano, California, every year. The monarch butterflies return to the eucalyptus forest behind my house between Thanksgiving and the spring equinox. The tides are higher during the full moon. On the day of the full moon the sun sets in the west at the same time as the full moon rises in the east. These are all revelations of the order of the universe that the Chinese have determined is managed through the pervasive and essential force known as Qi. By becoming aware of these phenomena in nature, your experience of Qi will expand rapidly.

A pinch of seeds in the ground in my garden will give me pounds of carrots so sweet and delicious that I will brush them off and eat them while kneeling between the rows. Wide-eyed babies smile at everything. Just a glance from a certain person turns you on. These are all expressions of the power of Qi. With very little practice you will begin to get a feel for this. Over time you can evolve in your capacity to find Qi by simply watching. You can easily observe the power of Qi in a person's walk, gestures, and expressions. The differences between the expressions of vital people and depressed people, relaxed people and tense people, productive people and lethargic people are a striking reflection of the differences in their Qi.

In each of your Qigong practice sessions, and even from moment to moment throughout the day, you will learn to find and tune in to the Qi. When you begin this activity, it will be like finding an inspiring new channel on the radio or television, a channel that will change your life over time. Your practice is like carefully tuning to this channel for the absolute clearest, most dazzling reception. As you move through greater levels of Qi awareness and progress in the phases of cultivation you will find yourself transforming. Like the beautiful monarch butterfly, you will experience rebirth, uncover your latent essence, and become new.

Even if you are not as well and vital as you would like to be, your living system is spontaneously processing life resources—Qi—all the time with no special attention or purposeful activity. Qi is always in and around you, pouring its potential through you. You will begin to perceive your inner Qi by simply practicing shifting your attention with care and intention to note what is automatically occurring within and around you.

While many forms of Qigong include specific breath methods or movement forms, the essential foundation of Qigong is to practice attaining a certain state of increased awareness. In fact the breath and the movement in Qigong are intended to create a maximum awareness of Qi. Yes, healing and increased potential are important effects of Qigong. But it is this enhanced awareness of Qi that is the essence of Qigong itself.

You don't have to do much of anything to attain increased awareness of Qi. Think of your Qi cultivation as working smarter, not harder, by tapping into the natural power of the universe. Eventually, through cultivation, you may attain a capacity to sustain conscious awareness of the Qi for more than a few moments. This is one of the more profound goals in Qi cultivation.

By beginning to purposefully discover and sense Qi, within yourself and throughout the world, you are initiating the process of Gong—cultivation. This is the beginning of enhancing the extent to which you are processing and refining Qi. By simply attending to the natural properties, capacities, and tendencies of Qi, you will become aware of and improve the function of the Qi within you. It automatically optimizes the dynamic nature of your interaction with the world when you deepen your connection with the *one essential* that connects all things. You enter into an extraordinary, consciously directed relationship with your own internal wealth of invisible resources—and with the invisible forces in the environment around you. People will see this in you and call it good luck, good genes, intuition, and endurance.

How to Find the Qi

As you perfect your ability to find the Qi, you will be able to access it just by focusing your attention—and intention—on this subtle resource within you, within others, in your surroundings, or in nature. But because Qi has been circulating within you, beyond your awareness, for your whole life, some special techniques may be necessary to help bring about a shift in your perception.

Radio and television messages are pervasive in the atmosphere, around you all the time. However, you only perceive these frequencies and the information they carry when you turn on a receiver and choose a channel. In Qigong you choose the channel that has the messages you feel will enhance your well-being and optimize your potential. You are not aware of your heartbeat even though it has been beating faithfully since before your birth. But if you run around the block and then cover your ears, you can hear your heart beating. With some practice you can become aware of your heart, without the exertion, just by tuning in. Finding the Qi can be a lot like this.

The first and simplest way to find the Qi is to notice vitality in yourself and others. How do you feel? If you are tired often, depressed, or in pain, according to Chinese medicine your Qi is either deficient or blocked. Do you use stimulants or medications? Reliance on caffeine or pain medication is a sign that your Qi is in jeopardy. Also notice what excites you or moves you. When you cry in a movie or leap out of your seat at a sports event, it is evidence of the Qi.

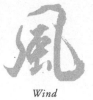

Wind

Observing the signs of the Qi is the foundation of diagnosis in Chinese medicine. As a doctor using traditional diagnostic methods I have learned to discern the status of the Qi by simply observing. Enthusiasm and humor are evidence of the Qi; exhaustion, depression, or complaining are indications of the Qi as well. When I walk out to the waiting area of the clinic, shake the patient's hand, and look into his or her eyes, the assessment of Qi status is already started. Then as I follow the patient to the treatment room I am observing body language and the walk—both provide clues to the Qi. Then I might say, "How may I serve you?" While the patient is answering the question I am listening to the sound of the voice. In the treatment room, I examine the color of the tongue. In Qi diagnosis, it is not actually necessary for the health complaint to be mentioned. The case can be fully assessed by noting the evidence of the Qi.

Are you hot before everyone else on a warm day or do you stick your feet out from under the covers? Are you the first person to put on a sweater at an evening event in early autumn? Tired at three in the afternoon? Quick to anger? Sensitive to criticism? Bloated after eating? Restless at two in the morning? These signs and hundreds of others are expressions of the activity, deficiency, or imbalance of the Qi.

The depressed person and the person wearing sunglasses on a cloudy day are expressing different qualities of the Qi of the liver. The overweight person, the emaciated person, and the person who exhibits compulsive activities are all expressing qualities of the Qi of the spleen. Being wakeful at night, talking back to the television, and laughing at inappropriate moments are qualities of the Qi of the heart. All of those little details including nail biting, addiction to sugar, and the tendency to speak softly or loudly or hum habitually are all expressions of Qi.

You can find expressions of Qi in nature as well. The wind is invisible but the flowing motion of the leaves and branches is evidence of the dynamic presence of invisible forces. Qi is particularly evident just before a storm, in the lightning, and then afterward as flowers leap forth following spring rain. How does that dry, wrinkled corn seed from last harvest become a bright green stalk and then produce six new ears of sweet, juicy corn? Qi. Why do trees and people grow upward against the force of gravity? Qi.

No matter how sophisticated science becomes there will always be an essential, pervasive element or force behind what we do and do not understand, behind what we can and cannot explain. It is the Qi. Simply being more aware of people and the environment is a study of Qi.

The Characteristics of Qi Sensation

Through your practice you will learn to feel the Qi within your own body. It is a sensation that is unique to each person. Here are a few of the sensations that are typical:

能
力

Ability, Skill

- tingling in the hands, feet, cheeks
- feeling fluffy internally, like clouds moving inside
- a sense of flowing or circulating
- feeling radiant or luminescent
- feeling that the surface of the body is porous
- spreading warmth in either the limbs or torso
- the feeling of being tipsy on wine
- energy moving in the belly
- release of tension in shoulders or neck
- decrease of pain
- sensation of a magnetic field between the hands
- sensation of heat coming from the hands as they pass over the face or body parts
- the urge to cry or the release of tears
- a sense of reconnecting with a lost part of oneself
- a sense of the transcendental or spiritual
- a feeling of coming home
- a feeling of ecstasy or bliss

There is no correct way to experience the Qi sensation. If you are fully awake and attentive in the experience you will probably ask "What is that sensation?" Most of us have these experiences but then fail to take the time to investigate them. As I discussed in a previous book, *The Healer Within*, this sensation is caused by the physiological mechanisms of self-repair. An amazing array of these powerful physiological self-healing mechanisms is triggered by Qigong and Tai Chi (Taiji) practice. But what activates the physiology? What causes the heart to beat, the blood vessels to expand, the cells to release water into the tissue spaces, the production of neurotransmitters, the activity of the immune cells, the flow of nutrients into the cells? What is the life-sustaining force, the internal cause or essence that drives the physiological activity and creates functional coherence? From the Chinese perspective, what we are feeling is Qi or the effect of Qi. The physiological sensation is a secondary effect of the primary cause—Qi. Qi is the underlying feature that sustains life, creates health, and generates the inner elixir—you can even feel it.

Because of the energetic nature of Qi you can feel the field of Qi around your body. You can also feel the Qi in a room full of people, in an old temple, and almost everywhere in nature. In the exercise that follows you will explore the sensation of the Qi between your hands and within your body.

Qigong Method to Discover Qi

Forming the Ball of Qi

HISTORICAL REFLECTION There are many Qigong practices that help to attune our aware-ness so that we can find the subtle energy of the Qi. This practice is a foundation method for personal cultivation and for building Qi skill for the healing methods from the tenth phase, Transmit Qi. This method is used in a great many systems of Qigong. It is considered a standing meditation (*Zhan Zhuang*). Many such methods are called *Yi Quan*, which means "mind skill" or "mind boxing," as we must box with the mind to get it to quiet. Standing meditation is a common form of cultivation. We will use this particular form, which has roots in the mists of prehistory, to feel the Qi.

When I first learned this method from Chang Yi Hsiang, I was fascinated to feel that sense of a magnetic field between my hands. In the Qigong classes we found and exer-cised our Qi as if it were a kind of muscle, then we would apply the Qi skills in the clinic. Many of my favorite teachers in China have confirmed that this practice is a foundation in Qi cultivation training. While this is actually a rather advanced practice, it is so fun-damental that it is frequently taught early so that students can be working with it over time. It is not important that you feel the Qi immediately. It will come to you in time.

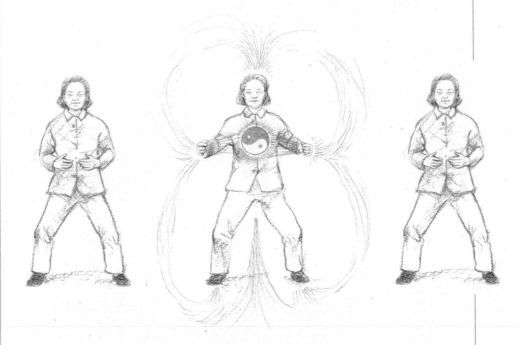

Forming the Ball of Qi

INSTRUCTION   Start from the preliminary Align posture. Align your Central Tai Chi Channel and the Elixir Fields as described earlier. Note that your feet are on a solid surface (Yin), and your head is in the open space of the air (Yang). Understand that in the terms of the Chinese worldview this creates a powerful potential. Yin and Yang have a natural urge to connect, and energy flows between them as in the negative and positive poles of a battery. The spaciousness of the sky and the solidity of earth meet in you, creating the conditions for a powerful charge of life force.

Initiate the opening posture. As you settle bring your hands together with the fingers or the palms facing each other. Deepen your breath and relax. The two energies, Heaven and Earth, are circulating within you, yet they are not confined within you. Your hands have a natural potential to transmit the Qi. Slowly bring your hands together and then apart. You can work and play with this energy potential and actually feel a field of energy between your hands. Many feel it as a kind of fluffy sensation like that of a cotton ball; others report a magnetic sensation. In later phases of Qigong you will use this Qi ball to help others. Some people have this Qi sensation with very little practice. Others will have more of a sense of the Qi internally, as described on page 100.

Mind Focus Affirmation

Discovering Qi, I connect deeply with nature and become aware of a powerful new way of perceiving and being.

Phase 2: Gather Qi

Gathering medicine
    means focusing consciousness within.
Quiet the mind,
    calm the emotions,
    cycle from movement to stillness,
    to complete the elixir.

—Li Dao Qun, *The Book of Balance and Harmony,*
THIRTEENTH CENTURY

To practice Forming the Ball of Qi (Chi), we go out into the courtyard of the training center. The energy on the mountain is pristine and vitalizing. It is obvious why the ancients built their observatories for internal and external exploration in such remarkable environments. Just being here creates a kind of automatic sense of healing and enlightenment.

The clouds are hanging low today. As they come off the plain, they wash over the mountains, huge waves of fluffy mist. It becomes clear why the Chinese are so fascinated with clouds. On the one hand they are simply beautiful and mysterious. On the other, we know that water (Yin) and sun (Yang) interact to form clouds. In the body, through Qigong (Chi Kung) the Yin and Yang interact to produce an inner mist—like clouds within our being.

When we return to the teaching hall for the lesson on gathering Qi, our teacher Jade Unity leaps enthusiastically to his feet to demonstrate. First, standing calmly, he

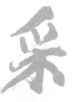

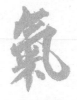

Gather Qi

aligns himself with Heaven and Earth. Then he does vigorous deep breathing, with strong exhalations, using a movement similar to the Warrior's Breath. Next he does a very graceful form where the movements are combined with walking and beautiful flowing gestures of the hands. At one point, one of our group members who has practiced Tai Chi (Taiji) whispers out loud, "Hands Passing Like Clouds." Finally, Jade Unity returns to a few moments of standing meditation as in Forming the Ball of Qi. His Qigong is very beautiful as he moves from one graceful gesture to the next.

Then settling into a cross-legged sitting posture he speaks to us gently:

"Have you noticed how little effort plants put forth to absorb water? It happens automatically. That's because they are naturally open to it. How easily the porous earth absorbs the rain? That is because the conditions are favorable. How hard is it for the color black to absorb light? Or for the color white to reflect? That is because it is their nature.

"It is the same with gathering Qi. We always have the potential to gather Qi, it happens naturally; it is our nature. There is one problem, however. Plants and soil, black and white do not have the capacity to become tense and distracted, but humans do. We can actually reduce our capacity to gather Qi by creating inner tension, which causes resistance in the natural gathering capacity of the system. This can cause fatigue, illness, and even death. Without the gathering of Qi, a primary problem of deficiency occurs which can lead to many severe secondary problems. Gathering Qi is like taking in nourishment. Food and water nourish and fuel the biological operations in the body. But it is Qi that allows our cells to use the nutrients and fluids. Without Qi the biology fails. So, the first lesson in gathering Qi is to open the natural gathering system with intentful adjustment of posture, breath, and mind.

"The second lesson is the matter of timing. Old Master of Pure Brightness, one of my favorite teachers, used to say, 'Do not wait to water the garden until after the plants have withered, do not plant seeds after you are starving, and do not wait to dig a well until you are nearly dying of thirst.' The timely gathering of Qi is like watering the garden in time, planting seeds before you are hungry, and digging a well while there is still ample water in the spring. Qigong is the method that we can use to nourish the system every day so that there is no risk of getting depleted and damaging the organs.

"Let me tell you a story that Master of Pure Brightness always told us. She said, 'If you wait to put the oil in the lamp until after the fuel is gone the wick will burn up, soot will damage the glass, and the light will become deficient. This is a huge waste of your energy. Instead of having trouble-free light, you now have to spend time and energy to do repair. Do your Qi cultivation on time, schedule practice so that you always fill your lamp before it is empty. This way it will always send out clear brightness, unfiltered radiance, with no extra effort on your part.'

"It is the same with the Qi. If people live a tense, worried existence, and do not neutralize inner turmoil, stagnation, or blockages with Qi cultivation practice, they are trying to live without refueling their lamp on time. They burn up their body and

Jade

their ability to see [think, learn] clearly becomes severely diminished by the soot that accumulates on the lamp. Then it is too late to simply add fuel. Now they need a full overhaul before they can get the light back on and clear the self so that the light can radiate."

Gathering the Qi

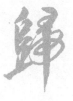

Unity, Origin

The human life force system automatically gathers Qi through air, food, earth magnetism, and the celestial influences of stars, planets, and boundless space. Through all activity and all rest the human absorbs, circulates, and processes Qi. Even before you were born, spontaneous interaction with Qi was the basis of your life. The channels of the Qi Matrix are natural passageways for the circulation of the Earth Qi and the Heaven Qi to enter, depart, and circulate through the human body. When these passages are open and operating optimally, health and vitality are an automatic consequence.

Naturally, the human system spends Qi as well, to process nutrients, accomplish tasks in work and play, and to sustain life. In cases where health and creativity are deficient, the natural capacity to gather Qi may be damaged or compromised due to a lack of information, absence of inspiration, or a wide array of direct causes including overwork, overindulgence, trauma, and injury. Our automatic birthright of access to ample, harmonious Qi can become dysfunctional; consequently a depletion or stagnation of Qi can occur. Over time this can lead to inefficiency, disease, pain, depression, and even, finally, to the loss of life.

By some marvelous instinct the Chinese in very ancient times figured out that by simply and intentfully turning one's attention to the Qigong practice of gathering Qi, the internal storehouse of energetic resource could be more efficiently replenished. In cases where Qi balance and integrity have been lost, the Chinese realized that through Qigong, nutritious food, herbs, rest, etc., we can gather Qi and thereby restore our health, vitality, and flexibility. While gathering Qi can occur spontaneously, the process can be accelerated or enhanced by all forms of Qigong and Tai Chi practice.

Gather Qi is a major key to all of the following phases of Qi cultivation. You must gather, collect, absorb, and accumulate the Qi that is to be cultivated. The Qi masters throughout many dynasties wrote extensively on absorbing Qi from food and herbs as well as from the natural surroundings through Qigong.

In the process of gathering the Qi, your goal is to add to the quantity and quality of Qi that is active throughout your system. A diet of vital foods, the use of herbs, plenty of water, rest, and pleasure are all sources from which to gather Qi. All forms and methods of Qigong help the body to open to acquiring Qi. There are two primary entry pathways for Qi in Qigong: the breath and the channels and points of the Qi Matrix.

Gathering Qi Through Breath

In China, India, and other ancient cultures, breathing practices are known to be profound methods for gathering vitality from nature. *The Spirit Immortal's Wondrous Record on Ingesting Breath*, a classic Qigong text written before 500 C.E., includes thirty-three Qigong movement practices with particular emphasis on the importance of the breath.

Most Qigong practices are based on the idea that the breath will regulate spontaneously through the practice over time. Special breath-holding techniques are not typically a part of Qigong. However, there are some practices that include special breath-holding forms. The following instruction is an excellent example:

> When you fall ill, first regulate the breath,
>   ingest the Qi, and fix your attention on the afflicted area.
> Practice holding the breath,
>   and by means of conscious attention
>   visualize the breath concentrating in the afflicted part.
> Visualize the Qi attacking the illness.
> When you can no longer comfortably hold the breath,
>   exhale very slowly.

—THE IMMORTAL MASTER'S TREATISE ON THE ABSORPTION OF PRIMORDIAL ENERGY

Try the following practice for three to four breaths. Breathe in fully, hold your breath for a count of one, one thousand; two, one thousand; three, one thousand. Then release through your nose very (very, *very*) slowly. Perhaps right away, perhaps after some practice, you will feel a warm, melting feeling inside—almost as if you've had a glass of wine. The effect is subtle at first; however, after some practice the effect of methods like this can become very dramatic. If you turn your attention to just this practice and nothing else, you will quickly enter a genuine Qigong state.

The inhalation is seen as the component of the breath where the gathering occurs. On the exhalation, as you may have felt from the exercise above, the Qi circulates. Interestingly, clues about using the breath to absorb Qi are found in the Chinese language. The character for breath in Chinese is *Qi Xi* (pronounced "chee she"), literally "to inhale Qi." It doesn't mean "inhale air with Qi in it," it means "inhale Qi."

Clearly, inhaling is a prime means of gathering Qi. There are hundreds of breath practices. One very traditional one is based on the gathering of Earth Qi (associated with the number six) and gathering Heaven Qi (associated with the number nine).

You can try this traditional breath practice of the Celestial Masters' stream of Daoism. On each of six breaths, focus on the Qi of the Earth. Then, on each of nine breaths, focus on the Qi of Heaven. In the alternative approach, divide the inhalation into six shorter puffs to absorb Earth Qi. With the single long, slow exhalation, circulate the Earth Qi throughout the Qi Matrix. If you are attentive you will feel the effect. Then to absorb Heaven Qi, divide the inhalation into nine shorter puffs. On the long, slow exhalation, feel the Qi of Heaven circulating in the Qi Matrix.

Gathering Through the Qi Matrix

The second major entry path for universal energy into the individual human system is through the body's energy gateways, often called acupuncture points. There are more than one thousand of these Qi gateways that connect the internal Qi Matrix of the human body to the external Qi system of the environment and the universe. These points intersect the surface of the body, along the course of the energy channels, pathways, or passages. These points act naturally as nodes of passage between the external world and the inner self; they allow you to gather fresh Qi and disperse expended or waste Qi. The Qi Matrix operates optimally when the body and the HeartMind are free from the effects of stress.

Celestial, Divine

However, with the intentful focusing of one's attention through Qigong, the extent to which the gathering of Qi into the matrix occurs is increased. Even if the practice does not include movement as in Tai Chi or other moving Qigong forms, the simple act of turning one's focus to the Qi and relaxing will initiate the Qigong gathering effect.

Inner tension constrains the Qi and life's details and distractions cause the Qi to scatter. Turning your attention, with intention and relaxation, to the natural capacity of the living system to absorb Qi enhances the absorption through these points, channels, and reservoirs of the Qi Matrix.

There are a few very key gateways, many important secondary ones, and a huge number of additional points. The top of the head (which is the soft spot in the newborn) is called the Point of Celestial Convergence (Bai Hui). This is a major entry point for the Qi of Heaven. The points that create our connection with the ground, Gushing Spring (Yong Quan, at the ball of the foot), along with Gathering Yin (Hui Yin, the point in the muscle group between the legs where they join the body), make up the major entry gateways for the Qi of Earth. Palace of Reward (Lao Gong) is the key point of Qi entry and exit on the palm of the hand. It is located approximately where your middle finger curls back to touch the center of the palm of your hand.

Celestial Convergence and Gathering Yin are directly related. They form the top and bottom of the Central Tai Chi Channel—the most powerful channel in the Qi Matrix. The HeartMind at the level of the physical heart in the chest is the meeting and merging point of Heaven and Earth. The hand point and the foot point are also related, forming a major channel of connection within the matrix. Many believe that the foot channel and the hand channel also meet and merge in the HeartMind. While the Central Tai Chi Channel represents Heaven and Earth, the hand relates to fire and the foot to water. These points and the related channels are the foundation of the Qi Matrix.

Also associated with the Qi Matrix are the trillions of pores of the human skin. Recall that even in Western cultures we say the skin breathes. One of the most frequently cited impressions from those who relax deeply and enter the Qigong state is that the skin is porous, that the boundary between the inner and outer self becomes ambiguous.

The idea that the surface of the self is at the surface of the skin is an illusion. We are only body-sized in substance; as multidimensional beings we have numerous additional sizes. First, there is our energy field around the body including the magnetic field. Then there is our mind field, which is of undetermined size. Finally, there is our portion of the universal informational or consciousness field that is boundless. This dynamic, diverse, and pervasive matrix of energies and influences creates an amazing system, within which the substance of the human body exists. Gathering fresh Qi and dispersing used Qi through this matrix is a major foundation of Qigong. The quality of the Qi may also be improved through the gathering process, although we will focus more closely on refining the Qi to a higher state of purity and potency in later phases.

We can use a simple metaphor taken from Chinese medicine and philosophy to express how gathering can dispel spent Qi with fresh Qi. Imagine filling a clear drinking glass with the turbid waters from an active stream. The water is murky with silt. The glass represents the body—the vessel of your life. The clouded stream corresponds to the thoughts and activities in your busy, creative life. If you are unwell or in pain, imbalanced Qi—which includes your symptoms, disturbing thoughts, and distressing inner dialogue as well as perhaps exhaustion or depression—shows itself as the cloudy water in your body vessel. Now visualize pouring a pitcher of pure, clean water from above into the glass of murky water. Keep filling the glass until it overflows with the crystal water from a higher source. The fresh water pouring in forces the turbid water out of the vessel, and soon the water in the vessel is completely clear. Health and optimal function are restored. Now, imagine that the pitcher filled with the clear water (Qi) is an endless source that just keeps pouring, like the natural process of Qi gathering that happens spontaneously in your body when you are in a state of openness.

Chinese medicine is based on this idea: the natural influx of vitality removes turbidity and sustains the pure. Gathering Qi is a primary method for achieving this. To be sure to maintain and maximize this natural process the Chinese invented Qigong.

Qigong Method to Gather Qi

Gathering Qi from Heaven and Earth

HISTORICAL REFLECTION This very poetic as well as moderately vigorous practice is one of the most ancient Qigong methods, invented long before China's written history. Gathering Yin from Earth and Yang from Heaven were likely practiced by shamans in magic rituals.

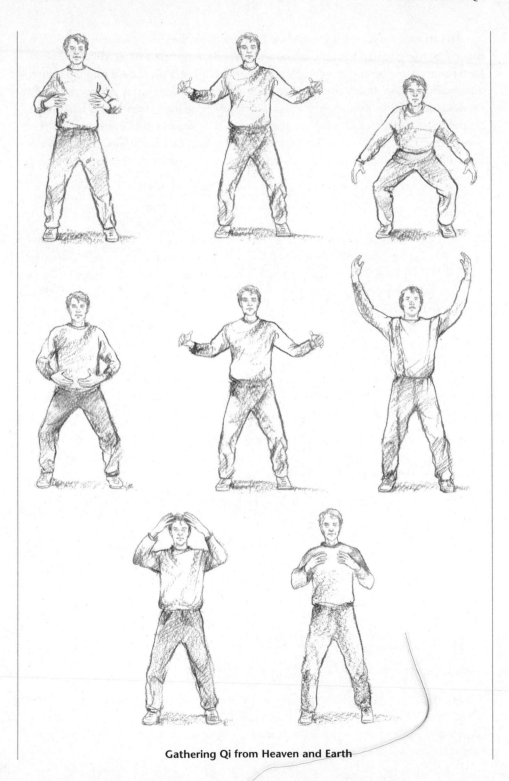

Gathering Qi from Heaven and Earth

All forms of Tai Chi, long and short, use a movement similar to this to close the form. I learned it as a Qigong warm-up for Tai Chi from my first teacher in the sixties. There is nothing more essential in Qigong and Tai Chi than gathering, merging, and balancing Yin and Yang. And there is no physical cultivation more obviously focused on the collecting and harmonizing of the energies of Heaven and Earth than this one. I've used this gathering method often in special areas in China—at the Great Wall, in sacred mountains, at the White Cloud Temple, and at the Shaolin Temple—to gather the Qi of a place.

INSTRUCTION Beginning from the opening posture, open your arms and sink down to gather Yin. It is important to be careful of your back and knees—go down only as far as is comfortable. Gather the resource of Earth in your arms and rise up carrying the Yin upward. When your hands come in front of your heart begin to open your arms again, this time reaching up toward Heaven. Gather the resources of Heaven and carry them downward until your hands are again in front of the heart. Repeat these two movements as many times as you wish. Notice that you are bringing first Yin and then Yang to the HeartMind center.

The breath can be directed a number of ways, including simply breathing naturally. As you advance you can experiment with other breathing methods. Try exhaling on the downward movement as you gather Yin, inhaling on the upward movement as you gather Yang. Then reverse it and inhale as you gather Yin. You can experiment with other breathing methods that feel right for you. The point is to feel free to innovate. However you do it, this practice is a powerful Yin-Yang mixer.

Mind Focus Affirmation

Gathering Qi, I access and purposefully draw upon the forces of nature for healing and empowerment.

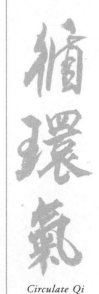

Phase 3: Circulate Qi

The human body needs movement
to balance right and left,
to distribute and assimilate the Qi,
to circulate the blood and fluids,
to prevent disease and aging,
and to extend life.

—HUA TOU, RENOWNED PHYSICIAN, 100 C.E.

Following our practice of Gathering Qi (Chi) from Heaven and Earth, several of our group decide to go for a hike in the mountains. We are with our guide, Intentful HeartMind (Yi Xin). The well-marked trail winds among cliffs and valleys. Along some sections of the trail there is a spectacular scene every ten to twenty steps. The trees seem to grow right out of the rock. Chinese pilgrims visiting the mountain's sacred sites are walking here—many very slowly in deep states of introspection. We cross a rustic stone bridge over a small creek of clear water, and stop to notice that it makes a cheerful laughing sound.

A bit farther up the path Yi Xin stops our group. "Now I will take you to a secret place. Sometimes one of the residents of the training center will spend a few days, a couple of weeks, or even a season in the small cave that we will visit. There is no one there now. The most famous master of Qi cultivation from our mountain used this cave for a period of several years more than one thousand years ago." We all promise to tell no one except those sworn to tell no one about this place. He waited, looking

Circulate Qi

right into the eyes of each member of our small group, as we gave a bow or nod of agreement to keep the secret. "No one has ever spoken while in this place. Pay attention to what you feel or learn here. I promise you will be astounded. Watch the stream of laughing water to your right and think about your life."

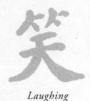

Laughing

After waiting for several groups of visitors to pass out of sight, Yi Xin pulls a large branch aside and we quietly slip onto a hidden trail, beside the rushing stream. We walk silently. After about two hundred feet we have left the forest and stepped onto a wide ledge with a beautiful view of the surrounding mountains. Then we are confronted by an awesome sight—looking to the right, back toward where we have just passed, the stream suddenly plummets in a dramatic, beautiful fall along a sheer cliff with at least a thousand-foot drop. We are standing on a naturally formed ledge, a terrace hanging on the vertical face of the massive stone mountain. Behind us, in a granite wall, is a shallow cave that could easily provide shelter from the weather. We each sit down to reflect in silence and to gaze—entranced—at the laughing stream's free fall, the wide open blue sky, and the clouds churning below us. Close your eyes and make the Three Intentful Corrections—join us for a few moments of quiet practice.

The immensity of nature allows the mind to understand how narrow our conditioned priorities may be. Water flowing then dropping in sudden free fall implies the value of surrender rather than resistance when reaching the dramatic changes in life. Inner awareness says, "Why try so hard? Look at what nature accomplishes by just allowing herself to be. What would happen if we were to trust what life offers?" At this point each of us begins to tingle slightly. Why? It's simple. When you open the channels by relaxing in trust, the circulation of Qi and consciousness multiplies radically. Later, walking in silence back to the training center, we know we are deeply inspired and on some level changed by having been in this place.

In the training hall the whole group is reunited. Everyone has by now had a handful of unique experiences. We are beginning to realize how removed we are from our homes and our usual lives. But while we have definitely traveled a great physical distance, the distance we have come in our ways of being and ways of experiencing is even greater.

Eternal Spring offers a brief demonstration, beginning with the opening and aligning of the Central Tai Chi Channel. As she goes through the methods we've learned so far, Forming the Ball of Qi and Gathering Qi from Heaven and Earth, we notice that her external activity seems secondary to her extreme level of inner focus. As she adds several new movements that signal the next phase of cultivation, that tingling that we felt at the ledge by the waterfall starts up again. Just watching someone do the methods activates the Qigong (Chi Kung) state. Our teacher takes her seat on a small stool.

"What makes the Qi circulate?" she asks. In a moment she answers: "Allowing it. You may have said, 'I am going to learn how to make the Qi circulate.' I would urge you to reconsider. The easiest and best way to circulate Qi is to become aware of what Qi does naturally and then arrange yourself so that you allow it to do what it is prepared and empowered by all of nature to do. Through your practice, get your conditioned internal tension out of the way of the natural gift of nature.

"Visualize a stream or river after many seasons of moderate flow. Logs and branches have collected among the rocks. Clumps of debris have accumulated and created numerous small dams that hinder flow. Puddles of stagnant water have formed. This is not an unusual scene from nature, and it is quite beautiful in a way. However, the perfect state of Qi circulation would be a completely unobstructed pathway for flow.

"Now, in this story about your own inner circulation, imagine that you become aware of how to open to the natural field of universal potential that is all around you using intention, breath, and movement. The act of opening causes a tremendous rush of fresh water into the river, as if a huge rain of pure water has fallen higher in the mountains of yourself. The volume and pace of this rush of pure, fresh water releases a powerful natural force that washes away collected debris, log jams, and stagnant puddles. All of these inner blockages and constraints are the conditioning and stresses that cause our inner resources to become less capable of expressing their natural self-healing capacity. Following this dramatic flush the riverbed is clear, all the accumulated obstructions are washed away.

"To use another metaphor, over thousands of years we have learned how to arrange our fields (externally our gardens, internally our Elixir Field) so that irrigation with life-giving water can happen automatically. Your Qi Matrix is like these fields. You open to the Qi and because of the careful arrangement of the fields and rows (Dan Tian and Qi channels) the resource is circulated to give life and create a bountiful inner harvest. But the gardener must, through careful tending and cultivation, ensure that all of the rows are open. You can imagine that when you come to a row that is not receiving water due to some twigs or weeds that have accumulated in the channel, you use your hoe to remove the blockage, and the water flows again. It is the same in Qigong. You use the practice and your intention to adjust yourself in relationship to the Qi of nature so that it automatically flows in your channels."

The Third Phase of Qi Cultivation and Mastery—Circulate Qi—is all about flow—the circulation of nourishing, healing, and empowering natural resources. It is taught in the Chinese traditions of healthy longevity and spiritual Inner Alchemy, that the fundamental state in nature is resistlessness. Water, the classic image for flow, operates spontaneously, even overcoming obstacles, by simply flowing around, over, or through.

Lao Zi says, "Water nourishes all things, naturally, with no effort." Qi has a natural capacity to circulate like water. Inner resources are delivered to their destinations in an effective and timely way. When no resistance is encountered, Qi flow is ample and harmonious and nothing restrains its natural tendency to circulate. All of the body functions are nourished without effort. The promise of circulation is that the potential of the human being may be enhanced, not by forcing it, but by simply allowing it. Remove resistance and energy flows.

Just as your energy system is constantly and spontaneously gathering Qi from nature, it is also constantly and spontaneously circulating this life-sustaining resource. The first promise of the Qi and the traditional Chinese view of the world is that life force, the essential source of life, is present and dynamic everywhere, always. The flow

Flow

or circulation of Qi through living beings and in all things is irrevocable. There is no way that Qi will not spontaneously and naturally circulate to its usual destinations and fuel its naturally destined processes—if the Qi is not constrained, blocked, tangled, spent, or wasted. This is the essence of Qigong.

Simply by virtue of your presence in the world, you have access to Qi. From the moment of your conception, with no effort from you, your Qi circulates; it nourishes your growth from just two cells, to fetus, to newborn, to child, and on to youth, adult, and elder. Most interruptions in Qi circulation that cause disease, discomfort, or dysfunction arise from behaviors, habits, accidents, and traumas in life.

The main reasons why Qi circulation becomes restrained is due to inner factors that we can consciously choose to change—factors such as fear, worry, compulsive behaviors, inappropriate dietary practices, smoking, or overworking. Only frank trauma—accidents, the effects of violence, etc.—cause restrictions to the circulation of the Qi that are not preventable through managing our choices.

As a starting place in Qigong, we can celebrate this miracle of universal Qi circulation by simply turning our attention to the Qigong state. This is Natural Flow Qigong. Qi will increase its circulation spontaneously as soon as we have removed the first and most disastrous block—constant, insidious, low-grade internal tension.

Circulation of Qi and Blood

Two classic sayings in the Chinese tradition of medicine and philosophy are "Qi and blood are like a brother and sister" and "Qi is commander of the blood." In a practical sense, this statement from Chinese medicine declares that the functional capacity of life and healing is founded in the circulation of the Qi, which delivers the blood. When Qi is efficiently circulating to particular parts of the body, the blood is circulating there as well. The promise is that enhancing Qi will enhance function and therefore cause healing. Physiologically we know that these benefits are due in part to the oxygen and nutrition carried in the blood. In China and in the Qigong worldview these physiological mechanisms are an expression of the vital capacity of the Qi itself.

That said, the mere presence of Qi is not enough to create optimal vitality and mental clarity. In fact, when Qi is present but not circulating efficiently, illness may develop. The classic ancient writings of Master Sun state that, "Water that does not flow breeds disease and door hinges that don't get used will be eaten through and destroyed by worms." The stagnant water refers to stagnant or blocked Qi and unused hinges are the body's joints, which may become dysfunctional when the Qi is not circulating effectively, particularly through the gentle movement aspect of Qigong or Tai Chi (Taiji).

One highly respected modern-day Qi master, Yan Xin, stresses the continued wisdom of Master Sun's philosophy. "It is not sufficient to do Quiescent Sitting Qigong alone," he says. "Meditation practice with no dynamic movement can cause the Qi to become stagnant. The benefits of the moving forms of Qigong practice complement and balance the benefits of cultivation in stillness. Qigong with only inner cultivation can result in an enlightened person falling into ill health. The greater and most preferred outcome is to be an enlightened person who achieves and maintains supreme health. Practices that move the body and activate the circulation of Qi, blood, and the body's internal fluids will typically be a prominent component of the cultivation practices of a highly successful Qi master. This is why people are spontaneously motivated into dynamic movements as they deepen their Qigong practice."

We can cause the Qi to move by relaxing. Through Qigong training over time you can learn to go into a kind of comprehensive relaxation that maximizes Qi flow. Movement can also facilitate circulation, particularly when combined with focused intention, to achieve deep relaxation. You have already experienced some of this more vigorous movement in the warm-up practices. The easiest way to accelerate circulation of the Qi, particularly for those who are early in the evolution of their Qi cultivation, is to move the body while in a state of relaxation achieved through, among other things, full, relaxed breathing. This simple approach engages the Three Intentful Corrections (body, breath, and mind), the classic formula for attaining the Qigong state.

The shift from a constrained Qi Matrix with accompanying health deficiencies to a clear open path to the flow of the inner resource can be achieved simply through the practice of Qigong. When we do our practice, even at the most introductory level, in a deep state of sincere intention, it fosters the rush of fresh Qi through the channels.

Two Ways to Circulate Qi

There are two ways to purposefully enhance the natural circulation of Qi. The first method stresses *allowing* rather than *doing*—the internal approach of Quiescent Qigong (*Jing Gong*). The second method is more active—the external approach involving movement that characterizes Dynamic Qigong (*Dong Gong*).

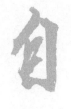

Spontaneous

In both approaches, the foundation of the practice is to relax and allow the mind to shift intentfully toward resistlessness. There are numerous Qigong metaphors for accessing this state. Frequently, the leader of a Qigong practice in a park or hospital in China will say, "Turn your attention, with focused mind intent, to the prebirth state of being. Before birth, what is there to cause stress, what is there to resist? Unborn you float comfortably in the ocean of the womb with nothing to remember, nothing to accomplish." Embryo breathing and fetus mind help to access the prenatal state in which the prebirth or Original Qi (Yuan Qi) circulates freely.

An equally poetic but more practical statement used by many of the contemporary master teachers in China is "Enter into and sustain the state of cheerful indifference." The purpose of this state is, essentially, to be happy about nothing in particular. When you tap natural internal joy that is not based on particular expectations, you achieve a state of maximum trust in the world and its processes. In the state of trust, inner tension and the resistance that compromises Qi circulation is eliminated and flow is enhanced.

In both approaches to circulating Qi the goal is to neutralize inner resistance to natural flow.

Allow Flow Methods: Quiescent Qigong

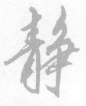

Quiescent

Quiescent Qigong is usually meditation that can be done either standing, sitting, or lying down. Natural Flow Qigong, introduced in Chapter 2, is also a form of quiescent practice. The goal is to relax deeply and clear the consciousness, mind, and nervous system of any effort, concern, or any other form of thought or action that would create stress or contraction anywhere in the substance (body) or the field (energy and consciousness) of the self.

To remove internal resistance is the only thing necessary to free the Qi to circulate to its maximum capacity. In this state, the Qi is naturally unencumbered and will circulate to its natural destinations and foster natural function and accelerate healing. Stagnation and accumulation do not immediately disappear. Those areas where the body is injured, traumatized, or contracted will require perseverance and continual improvement in your practice of Qigong and Tai Chi. In some cases much more vigorous Qigong is required to break through these blockages. Tools such as massage, herbs, acupuncture, emotional release, and forgiveness of others are frequently necessary to potentiate one's capacity to use the "allowing" methods for enhancing Qi circulation.

Beyond a few moments it is extremely challenging for most people to remain still. To advance in the quiescent, allowing methods requires a major personal transformation that can take a large portion of a lifetime to achieve. Most practitioners who elect to pursue cultivation and refinement of the self toward a higher level of health or being will eventually commit to some form of quiescent practice.

Activate Flow Methods: Dynamic Qigong

Another approach to circulating Qi is to use an array of less subtle, more active methods. These methods accelerate the circulation of Qi to cause either a temporary or permanent dissolving of the barriers to inner flow. The primary goal, as usual, is to relax. In addition, certain body postures, movements, either mild or vigorous breath practices, and self-massage techniques are used.

Focused intention and deep relaxation—the Qigong state—can transform calisthenics, swimming, and even walking into Dynamic Qi cultivation methods. The breath is frequently used purposefully to move the Qi, alone or in conjunction with the body movements. The gathering occurs on the inhalation. On the exhalation the Qi of Heaven and Earth are circulated.

The thousands of Qigong forms and the dozens of Tai Chi variations are all dynamic methods. They are all constructed around the theme of maximizing the gathering and circulating of Qi. Some are gentle, some are vigorous—they are all dynamic. They can be very simple, as in Spontaneous Qigong, or quite complex, as in the 108 movements of Tai Chi or the 64 movements of Wild Goose Qigong.

Qigong Method to Circulate Qi

Inner Rivers Flowing

HISTORICAL REFLECTION This beautiful, graceful gesture causes and represents the flow of Qi. It is a whole Qigong form by itself. The Qi of Heaven and Earth meet in the HeartMind center. Inner Rivers Flowing represents circulating that mix of Heaven and Earth Qi into the arms and hands and then down into the legs and feet. The upper movement, representing circulation in the arms, is the classic push gesture from Tai Chi. Circulating the Qi in the rivers of the lower limbs is an ancient gesture that was likely practiced long before written history.

I learned this practice from Dr. Cai at the Xi Yuan Hospital Qigong Training Center in Beijing. He has traveled throughout China to meet with numerous old masters and to study many different styles and traditions of Qigong. Dr. Cai taught Inner Rivers Flowing as a part of a longer medical Qigong form for deep healing.

INSTRUCTION Begin by aligning and opening. Then, with palms facing each other at the level of the heart, inhale and turn to your right. Press and shift your weight forward gently and exhale. It is not so much that you are pushing something, rather, in a deep state of relaxation you are encouraging flow, signified by the movement forward. Imagine, or feel if you can, the Qi flowing into your arms as you exhale and shift your weight forward. Now turn your palms to face you and shift your weight back. It is as if you are gathering in fresh Qi from around you as you inhale. When your hands reach the heart and you are ready to breathe out, turn your palms downward and begin to bend down. Your weight remains on the rear leg and you lift the toe of the front leg as you run your hands down along the front of the leg as if you are encouraging the flow in the channels of the leg.

At the end of the exhalation and being careful not to bend too far, turn the palms up and return to the upright position as if you are encouraging flow upward now. Breathe in. When your hands reach the heart, repeat. You can do several of these movements and then return to face the front as you do a final pull upward along the legs. Then turn to the left and do the practice to the other side. Exhale, push forward, and shift the weight forward, then inhale, turn the palms toward you, and return breathing in. Then exhale pressing down and inhale rising up. Repeat several times to this side and return to center. There are a number of variations to this practice. I encourage you to explore variations for fun.

Rivers or channels of life force travel out along the arms and down the legs, and these rivers return from the limbs back to the torso. As you do this practice feel that you are accelerating the natural flow in these channels. Understand that movement and breath accelerate flow. Realize that by clearing your mind and simply relaxing into this practice, you are reducing constraint and resistance in the channels, which also

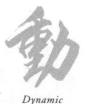

Dynamic

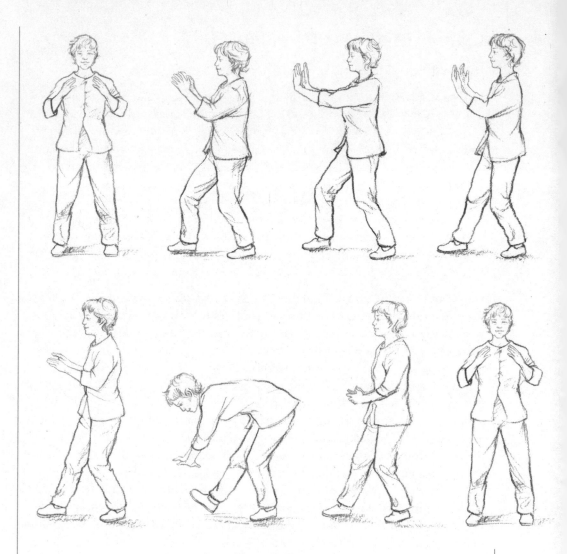

Inner Rivers Flowing

accelerates flow. So, by regulating the body movement, the breath, and the mind in this practice there is a major increase in flow and circulation.

Mind Focus Affirmation

Circulating Qi, I deliver potent restorative resources to strengthen and fuel my organs, glands, and tissues.

Phase 4: Purify Qi

Those adept at Dao Yin and respiration
can nurture the vitality within
and dispel illness.
Those who fully grasp the principles of cultivating health
and practice morning and evening
to purify and stimulate blood and Qi
can indeed attain longevity and freedom from illness.

—MASTER GE HONG, *THE BOOK OF THE MASTER WHO
EMBRACES SIMPLICITY*, FOURTH CENTURY C.E.

Purify Qi

A number of us are up very early to watch the sunrise. The terrace at the entrance of the training center faces east and south, affording a perfect view of the sun and moon rising over rows and rows of mountain ranges, often covered with banks of clouds. The sunrise this morning is exquisite. The sun, *Tai Yang* (literally, "absolute Yang"), rises from a cloud ocean that appears to continue far beyond the horizon.

To the right, south, is the trail of granite steps that we arrived on several days ago. To the left, a smaller, more natural trail leads from the temple complex along the face of the granite mountain. We notice a solitary figure, an older man, moving briskly along the trail among cragged rock and pines that have been sculpted by time and the elements. It is obvious that he is moving toward a clear and level place higher up along the trail.

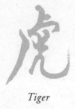

Tiger

The elder, likely a mountain hermit or one of the senior residents of the temple, steps out onto a natural terrace, at the very edge of the mountain's abrupt slope. After standing for a moment facing east, he turns to the four directions, reaching out, collecting, and bathing himself in the invisible resources of nature. He is bathing in and absorbing the powerful healing elixir of nature.

He begins to stretch his body vigorously, in a variety of directions and dynamics. Next he slowly moves about the leveled place, first swirling like the clouds themselves and then like a large graceful bird. Then standing and holding the ball of Qi (Chi), as we have learned to do so recently, he turns to the east with a gesture that looks as if he is placing the rising sun into the morning sky. He turns to the west and places the moon, as if it were setting. Gathering the invisible energies of Earth and Heaven he rises and sinks with his arms churning in the Gathering Heaven and Earth practice. He drifts momentarily into stillness, holding the sun or perhaps the moon in his arms.

Then in a sudden burst of vigorous activity he leaps about kicking and flying like a much younger man. He appears to have been visited by the nature of the tiger—moving stealthily, then the monkey—moving cheerfully. Next, he becomes the butterfly—moving lightly—the turtle—moving very slowly—the phoenix—sweepingly—and the dragon—with flying kicks. The movements are mesmerizing. At some points he expresses powerful vigorous activity; at other points he seems to be taking the forces of nature inside with very little external movement. We turn to each other, exclaiming without speaking, amazed.

Finally, the elder moves to the edge of the clearing and sits cross-legged with the astounding morning glowing before him. Through his eyes he drinks in the elixir of the moment. We too, in a kind of timeless freedom from the personalities that we left back home, drink in that special healing of night becoming day, when the Tai Yang first throws its heavenly light upon the earthly world. Just as he is likely closing his eyes to plunge into the practice of profound stillness, we are called to our morning practices. Before this journey we had been thinking of Qigong (Chi Kung) and Tai Chi (Taiji) as wonderful self-healing exercises. Now, with just three days at the mountain training center and already a number of deeply inspiring experiences, we realize that cultivating Qi is much more.

After practice and breakfast our teacher Eternal Spring leads a brief review of the Earth methods—Find Qi, Gather Qi, and Circulate Qi. Again it is obvious that the essence of Qigong lies not so much in "what" she is doing but "how" she is doing it. After the closing movement, she stands quietly for several minutes, and we are all pulled into deep contemplation. Finally she takes her seat and begins:

"When we make medicines in the clinic, we use pure ingredients. Pure water and pure mountain-grown herbs. It is the same when we make the inner medicine, the ingredients must be pure: the Qi, the blood, and the fluids.

"How to Purify Qi is central to cultivation practice. Purify Qi is the first of the three phases in the HeartMind level of cultivation. The body dispels by-products of metabolism including waste, spent cells, and toxins through blood, lymph, bile, urine, sweat, and even tears using the kidney, bladder, liver, large intestine, lungs, and skin. Similarly, the Qi Matrix dispels extra, spent, or toxic Qi through the centers, channels, and points as well as through the breath and the pores in the skin. In Chinese medicine we speak of the body and mind having the ability to separate the pure from the impure, the clear from the turbid, or the righteous from the imbalanced. In Qigong, this process, whether spontaneous and innate or enhanced by the intent of the HeartMind, is often simply referred to as fresh Qi replacing exhausted Qi. We can accelerate the rate that the body purifies Qi through Qigong and Tai Chi.

"Take some time while you are here to sit by Dragon Well. Listen to it for a while as the water spills from the spring. The spring has been called Dragon Well for so long no one can remember when it was named. People come from all over China to drink this water. It is called Elixir Water; it is medicine all by itself. It is renowned because it is blessed by the influence of many centuries of Qi cultivators here at the center. This water is already an elixir when it comes from the ground because it has been purified by this sacred mountain. We use this water for everything so its influence is within and around us all the time—in our tea, our medicines, our food, as well as our laundry and our bathing. [Many of us had already been commenting on the fact that the water tasted exceptional, particularly after days of bottled or boiled water in the hotels in Beijing and Shanghai.]

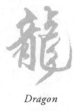

Dragon

"You may find here a useful inner picture for what happens when we purify the Qi. The countless vessels and passageways for the Qi and fluids in the body are like the countless passageways for water and Qi in the mountain. The Earth influences of stone, density, and compression plus the openness of Heaven that surrounds and penetrates the mountain create this pure water. The Earth influence of organs, tissues, inner dynamics of fluids in the presence of Heaven, which surrounds and penetrates the body, create pure Qi.

"When you use the breath, the movements, and the mind to Purify the Qi the essential process for separating the pure from the impure is inherent within you, as it is in the mountain. Do your practice knowing that the nature of the mountain is inherent within you, as the natural capacity to purify—creating pure elixir Qi within."

Purifying the Qi

By now you understand that merely being alive nurtures a wide range of important Qi interactions. This is particularly true in gathering and circulating Qi within Earth level Qigong. Now, in the HeartMind level, the focus shifts. Greater intention and will are useful and even required. Earlier it was enough to simply turn your attention to cultivation and use the Three Intentful Corrections to absorb and circulate Qi. Purposeful focus plays a much more significant role in the HeartMind phases.

In the Purify Qi phase our inherent nature causes the human system to dispel extra and unneeded Qi that may be wasted, spent, excessive, or toxic. Through this innate purifying of Qi you have survived and even thrived in your life—at least until your health was perhaps compromised at some point. For most people survival is satisfactory, but Qi lovers seek greater vitality and a refined state of being. To purposefully purify the Qi promises a higher level of function. One must purposefully purify the Qi.

The most effective way to purify Qi is with increased intention and will. This is the natural domain of the HeartMind in Qigong. In the incredible eloquence of the Chinese language the character for HeartMind, *Xin*, is the foundation character for both intention (*Yi*) and will (*Zhi*). *Yi* actually means "voice of the HeartMind." To gain greater purity and refinement of your internal resources and to increase your healing capacity and personal power, you must purposefully engage HeartMind Qigong.

HeartMind Qigong: Gateway to Inner Peace

Just as the body filters the Qi and fluids, so the HeartMind can be trained to filter thoughts, feelings, emotions, attitudes, and philosophies. Interestingly, the Chinese language characters for all of these concepts include *Xin*, HeartMind. Thought in Chinese basically means to *examine* the HeartMind. Attitude means to *express* the HeartMind. The characters for emotions and feelings, *Qing Gan*, have the character for the HeartMind in them twice.

So does this mean that we purify the Qi through the mind? Probably not. It is my interpretation that the heart is the key. Heaven and Earth merge in the middle Dan Tian, not in the head, to create the human experience. The HeartMind is the merging of the body and the nonbody aspects of our being. Thoughts, feelings, emotions, attitudes, intention, and will are all rooted in the HeartMind. To pass through to any deeper level of Qi cultivation, you will have to go through the gateway of the HeartMind.

In the ancient traditions the teachings of the great masters point to the Gateway of Mystery or the Mysterious Pass. When you approach HeartMind Qigong you are at an important gate. When you achieve success at HeartMind Qigong you have passed through that gate. At that point you will have access to the possibility of success at Heaven Qigong. As you will see, the phases of cultivation at the HeartMind level require a kind of focus that was not required in the earlier Earth-level phases.

Ancient Chinese medical philosophy honors the mind/body connection. The HeartMind is evidence of the Chinese recognition of what we in the West have recently come to call the BodyMind. Fortunately there has been a rise in interest in caring for and healing the mental/emotional self here in the West. The cultivation of the HeartMind through Qigong is likely to become a primary tool in this mind/body renaissance.

Cleansing and Renewing the Qi

In healthy newborns a kind of natural Qigong happens spontaneously, due simply to the nature of life. Then, through life, an array of factors challenge this natural, inner Qi cultivation process: accidents, emotional trauma, extreme environmental impacts, infections, stress, poor diet, and other factors can jeopardize the body and spirit, creating dysfunction, disharmony, or pain. To regain inner harmony or health the disturbed Qi must be purified, cleansed, or refined out of the system.

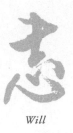

Will

To return to a state of efficiency, where the automatic capacity to cleanse and purify Qi can operate optimally, requires conscious Qi cultivation. The HeartMind level of Qigong is distinguished from the earlier Earth-level practices by the presence of greater consciousness and focus in the engagement of intention and will. This does not mean that it is useless to use Earth Qigong practices. Earth Qigong is profoundly useful. However, if your objective is to maximize your potential and attain true peace of mind, then cultivating the HeartMind influence in Qigong is relevant.

You already know that Qi can sometimes become sick, toxic, or disturbed. Through many causes, Qi that is less than pure and fresh can stagnate within, leading to deficiency and disharmony. Toxic Qi, pathogenic Qi, turbid Qi, impure Qi, excess fire Qi, excess water Qi, aggressive Qi, disturbed emotional Qi, and evil Qi are all forms of extra Qi or Qi by-products. These can become lodged in the internal matrix of the organs, energy centers, channels, and energy points. Inharmonious Qi can also have an influence on the external aspects of the matrix: your magnetic field and what some call your aura.

Strategies for Purifying Qi include acupuncture, herbal formulas, massage, and Qigong. One of the great gifts of Qigong is that you can take action personally, without a practitioner, to purify your own internal Qi. As we have seen, one method for Purifying Qi is to gather fresh Qi, which displaces extra or unneeded Qi with the deluge of fresh, a new natural resource. In acupuncture and herbal medicine, as well as in medical Qigong, there are variations on the theme of purifying, cleansing, and refining the Qi system that have specific meanings. Techniques called dredging and purging are used in herbal medicine; dispersing and draining are applicable to acupuncture.

However, Qigong self-healing practices can help to resolve the diverse forms of Qi disharmony as well. If it becomes important to complement the healing and cleansing effect, Qigong practice can be combined with the other aspects of Chinese medicine or combined with therapeutic strategies from Western medicine in an integrated health-care program. If a more aggressive Qigong approach is required to manage difficult cases or speed up recovery, a trained practitioner of medical Qigong can recommend specific Qigong practices targeted to a person's particular deficiency or stagnation of Qi. If it is warranted, a medical Qigong therapy practitioner can administer Qigong healing methods in conjunction with your personal Qigong practice. Some general Qi healing methods are detailed in the Tenth Phase of Cultivation and Mastery, Transmit Qi, where your cultivation practice is directed at serving others. Most people can do their own Qigong practice and get excellent results in purifying the Qi. Through relatively simple and consistent practice over time, remarkable and natural Qi cleansing effects can be achieved, evidenced by more energy, better sleep, less anxiety, clearer mind, greater productivity, less pain, and greater flexibility. Because your Qi Matrix is inherently designed to absorb the fresh and dispel the extra, the most important thing is to enter a deep intentful state—to fully activate the natural process of Qi renewal.

The purposeful focus of the HeartMind in purifying Qi multiplies the natural, inherent capacity just as using a leverage makes it easier to accomplish a difficult task. Tension patterns, residue of trauma, and other restraints lodged in the Qi Matrix caused by factors such as busyness, worry, overeating, and overworking, along with a multitude of other major and minor torments cannot be overcome without engaging the HeartMind.

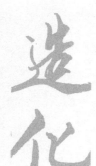

Blessing

Since the HeartMind is the secret gate through which you may wish to pass, thoughts, feelings, emotions, and attitudes, as well as intention and will, become major focus areas in your practice. In China and in many ancient traditions, retiring to a cave in the mountains or going to the desert or monastery and leaving the material world behind were primary ways to pass through this secret gate. That is why it is often called the Mysterious Pass. Bodhidharma, who brought Buddhism to China and was the founder of the Shaolin Temple school of Qi cultivation, sat facing the wall of a cave in deep meditation for nine years.

In modern times, however, most people find it difficult to clear the HeartMind with years of solitary meditation. Yet the need for inner peace remains. It is completely appropriate to use psychotherapy, counseling, and group support as complementary tools for clearing the HeartMind as a part of these phases of cultivation. The point is simply this: if you are distracted, busy-minded, or constantly listening to self-judgment or worry, the fourth, fifth, and sixth phases of Qi cultivation will not be accessible. If Qigong practice does not seem to be clearing the HeartMind, you may want to move into the cave. Or, more likely in contemporary times, you may want to explore a sincere process of emotional, attitudinal, and self-esteem healing.

Kinds of Qi Purification

There are numerous ways to purify, cleanse, and refine the Qi by intentfully maximizing the natural purifying mechanism. Active or dynamic methods employ movement, breath, and sound to accelerate Qi activity. Methods for mind focus are more quiescent and internal.

Dynamic Focus

The most common way to cleanse the Qi is through dynamic focus that includes movement, breath, and sounds.

Movement

Body movement pumps the Qi as well as the internal fluids that are recognized as being the conductive medium of Qi flow, allowing for the automatic purging and dredging that displaces and dispels extra or unneeded Qi. Spontaneous Qigong is particularly useful as a way of shaking out and dispelling spent or stagnant Qi and replenishing the system with fresh Qi. It is common for students to comment that Spontaneous Qigong causes an immediate sense of emotional relief.

Breath

In the West we discovered that oxygen is gathered and carbon dioxide is eliminated through the breath. The ancient Chinese scientists found that Qi is absorbed through the breath and that extra, used, or unneeded Qi is expelled with the breath. One of the warm-up practices, Warrior's Breath, is based on the idea that dynamic movements stir up the Qi and dredge the extra and unneeded Qi, which is then dispelled with deep and vigorous exhalations. The breath and movement cause the release of unneeded Qi through the channels, points, and pores, as well as the breath itself. This is often called a cleansing breath.

Sound

Adding sound to the exhalations, as it is traditionally taught in Qigong, vibrates the organs. This circulates healthy organ Qi and releases the Qi of the emotions associated with them. The most common use of sound in Qigong takes a traditional form known as the Six Healing Sounds, Six Power Sounds, or the Six Secret Healing Words. There is a healing sound for each of the organs associated with the five elements or phases. The Triple Heater, or 3 Burner, represents the pelvic, abdominal, and chest cavities along with the organs located there. Because there are two organs associated with fire, there are two sounds for fire. This method uses sound to vibrate and purge the energy reservoirs, organs, and channels to discharge extra or unneeded Qi and infuse the Qi Matrix with fresh Qi.

What in the West we often call a sigh of relief is also a traditional Qigong practice, to exhale making a sound. Try it a few times. Use one of the sounds in the chart on page 126. In my own teaching we use "Ahh" in brief or beginning classes because the Six Sounds require some time and interest on the part of the learner. We follow the adage "Simplicity Enhances Qi; Complexity Depletes Qi." New students are inspired by the effect of the use of sound in a very simple context. Later, when they demonstrate their interest in going deeper, we teach the Six Healing Sounds.

The Six Healing Sounds		
Traditional Element	**Organ**	**Sound**
Wood	Liver	Xu (Shuu)
Fire	Heart	Ha (Haaa)
Earth	Spleen	Hu (Whoo)
Metal	Lungs	Ah (Ahhh)
Water	Kidney	Chui (Chruee)
Fire	3 Burner	Xi (Shee)

Begin by breathing in deeply. Express a sighing sound to soothe the organ and the Qi associated with it. To expel extra Qi, express a louder, more forceful sound. Experiment with adding movement. It is particularly effective to use the shaking and wiggling of Spontaneous Qigong.

Quiescent Focus

The mind leads the Qi. This is a promise of the Qi that we will explore in detail in the next phase, Direct Qi, but it is important to realize now that you can utilize meditation, visualization, purposeful choice making, declarations, and blessings to purify Qi. You can combine meditation and visualization into very powerful imagery that can be used in either stillness or movement. For example, when you exhale visualize pressing outward with your hands. The inner image is one of clearing the space within and around you. In the relaxed state the mind-directed image can be combined with the breath. All work together to purify Qi. Gathering and circulating Qi are secondary effects to this practice. The Qigong practice at the end of this chapter is an example of such a practice.

When you make the choice to let go of a grudge or to forgive someone who has been unfair, that is also purifying Qi. You are removing a factor that has been depleting or stagnating your inner resources. You've probably noticed that a grudge or withheld forgiveness does not hurt the begrudged or the unforgiven. Instead the damage is done to the one who holds the grudge or withholds forgiveness. That is because the Qi is exhausted when these feelings remain unresolved.

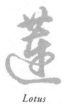

Lotus

Declarations and blessings are like chants or prayers that are used while you practice. Zhu Hui often suggested that clearing the HeartMind to enhance Shen makes what appear to be simple exercises into powerful Qigong practices. He suggested the following chant during his training for use in either still meditation or moving meditation. He often discussed it in conjunction with his teaching of one of his favorite Buddhist forms, Lotus Flower Qigong.

> *Extra Qi is pulled out into nature,*
> *Disturbed Qi is pulled down into the earth.*
> *In this my heart is purified.*
> *Who seeks Dao*
> *Will achieve Dao.*

This combination chant and declaration helps the practitioner to sustain the focus on purifying the Qi in the practice. While it is not mentioned, healing is implied as extra and disturbed Qi, representing everything from physical sickness to mental disharmony, is being dispelled. "Who seeks Dao will achieve Dao" is a Qigong promise that cultivation in a purposeful state will connect the practitioner with his or her true state of radiant health—the state of all in Dao. The mind focus affirmations following each of the Qigong methods are example declarations that enhance our cultivation.

Natural Flow Qigong

It is possible to accelerate the inherent process of Qi purification with Natural Flow Qigong. Use the Three Intentful Corrections—deepen the breath, adjust the posture, and clear the mind—to induce the Qigong state. Inner constriction and stagnation are reduced and a steady flow of fresh Qi is fostered, which allows for the displacement of extra Qi with pure new Qi. You may wish to refer to page 41 to review Natural Flow Qigong.

To Elevate, Flush, or Radiate

One particularly interesting method for purifying Qi is to use mind focus, intention, and visualization to place your concerns and distractions into the Central Tai Chi Channel and flush them out. Allow yourself to slip gently yet fully into the Qigong state by using the Three Intentful Corrections. Place the issue, attitude, worry, person, or relationship into the Tai Chi Channel. Acknowledge the inherent wisdom of the universal intelligence of the Qi. Notice what occurs. The issue may be pulled up or elevated to Heaven; it may be pulled down or flushed into the Earth as in Master Zhu's declaration; or it may be radiated and infused with Qi. The universal and benevolent field of energy and consciousness will naturally assist in clearing and purifying the Qi, if we will let it. From your place in that Qigong state simply observe whether elevation, flushing, or radiation is occurring. Allow yourself to feel gratitude for the assistance. In certain cases it will help to add in the benefits of breath, sound, and movement.

Spontaneous Qigong is a perfect tool to maximize elevating, flushing, or radiating to purify Qi. Simply visualizing may not be enough to activate the purifying, so add some intuitive body movement. If you find that you cannot hold the focus well enough to clear or purify certain issues, then it is reasonable and recommended to engage supportive assistance from any number of approaches. Practicing with a like-minded group that will support you in sustaining new behaviors can actualize Qi purification. Being in a group support process, with or without professional facilitation, can help to initiate or sustain the benefits of purifying the Qi as well.

Qigong Method to Purify Qi

Clearing the Small Universe

HISTORICAL REFLECTION This practice comes from the Shaolin Temple's traditional method called the Tendon and Muscle Transforming Practice (*Yi Jin Jing*). It was originated by Da Mo, also known as Bodhidharma, who created many health and martial Qigong forms for the monks. You may have seen these movements demonstrated by Qigong masters who are preparing to demonstrate some special skill such as walking on sword blades or absorbing brutal punches with no obvious negative effect. In addition to purifying Qi, this portion of the Tendon and Muscle Transforming Practice has a beneficial effect on all of the connective tissue, including the tendons.

I have learned dozens of different variations of Yi Jin Jing from numerous teachers in the United States and China. Some teach it as a martial practice; some teach it as a healing practice. It has a wide range of application and can be used easily to circulate Qi as well as to purify Qi.

The Small Universe is your personal Qi Matrix. In Qigong and Tai Chi it is a central concept that each individual is a reflection of the cosmos—a small universe. Yi Jin Jing is preliminary to Iron Shirt Qigong, in which the whole form is used in a very vigorous context to build the connective tissue into an impenetrable suit of body armor. In the martial context it protects against attack. In health care it protects against disease.

INSTRUCTION Start with the hands at the level of the heart. Breathe in and turn the palms to face out to the right and left. Exhale and push the palms away from the center as if you are pushing something very heavy. The palm is open and the fingers are reaching upward forcefully. This is not a relaxed movement. Perform it as if you are clearing away mountains of unwanted material or breaking free from between a rock and a hard place. Now relax completely, breathe in, and return your hands to the area in front of the heart. Then press upward, exhaling forcefully with your palms open to the sky. It is as if you are lifting the weight of the world from your shoulders. Stretch up and sink your pelvis and tailbone downward. Then inhale and return your hands

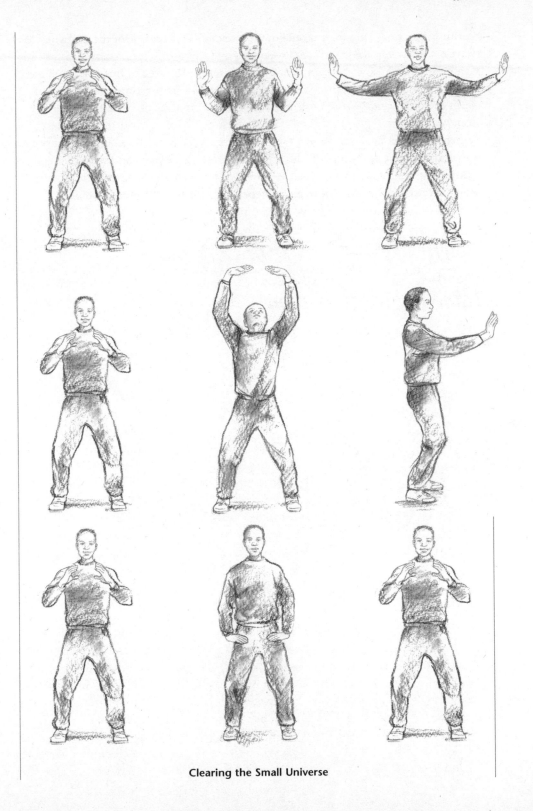

Clearing the Small Universe

to center, relaxing. Rest for a moment. Now, exhale and press forward as if you are moving something heavy. You are purposefully and forcefully clearing the space before you. Relax and breathe in. Bring your hands back to the area in front of the heart. Finally, exhale and press downward. Visualize that you are pressing down or holding down the rising tide of stressful situations. Relax and return your hands to the area in front of the heart.

Clearing the Small Universe is a powerful method to purify the Qi. The forced breath dispels extra Qi through the exhalations. The vigorous hand movements are clearing the area around you as well as opening the Qi channels. As you push, particularly if you allow your pelvis to sink, it opens the torso. As you push right and left, it opens the center of the body. When you push down, the spine lifts up, also opening the torso. This clearing and opening accelerates the flow of internal water, which is conducive for fresh new Qi, which comes rushing in.

Mind Focus Affirmation

Purifying Qi, I restore inner harmony by cleansing and dispelling spent, toxic, and unneeded Qi, and by opening to the inflow of fresh, natural life force and power.

Phase 5:
Direct Qi

> *To nourish health and life*
> *by distributing the Qi,*
> *adjust the posture*
> *to facilitate flow.*
> *Direct the Qi throughout the body*
> *to dredge the channels,*
> *moisten the flesh, and*
> *regulate the organs.*

—RECORDS OF DAOIST ESSENCE PRESERVATION
GATHERING OF SPIRIT IMMORTALS ON WESTERN
MOUNTAIN

Direct Qi

When we gather back at the training hall we are surprised to find a guest instructor, one of Jade Unity's favorite teachers. "This is my honored teacher Mrs. Zhang," he tells us. "She has a large following in southern China. You will see why she is known as the Pearl River Master. Before we begin with the practice Master Zhang will demonstrate her short Tai Chi [Taiji] Sword form. As a young woman she took many awards as a sword champion. Pretend you are alone, no one is paying attention to you, use these practices to neutralize any inner tension, allow your new self to be revealed, allow your perfect self to be expressed."

The Pearl River Master appears, as is usual with those who cultivate Qi (Chi), quite young and nimble—although it is very likely she could be in her middle to late seventies. In the Tai Chi form she is fluid, as if the whole sequence is one movement. There are between thirty and forty separate postures but just as she reaches the completion of one of the gestures, she gently shifts forward or drifts back into the next one. We begin to get a message from the hypnotic movements. The suggestion of her gestures is that she is using the sword to slay her own inner demons and cut away Qi that is not serving her. The sword is inner spirit and truth killing off doubt, fear, and ongoing anxiety.

It becomes apparent from the movements, and even more from an inner sense, that she has now turned her intention to us. Just watching her, our breath shifts to become fuller, slower. Deep within something changes—a door opens, a cord is cut, we begin to feel as if we are slowly filling with warm, fragrant tea. We are aware of not caring too much about who we have been or who we might become.

As she concludes, we are all in awe. She bows and we applaud, enraptured by her obvious skill and filled with the sense that she has done us an important favor. As she asks that we stand and spread out for practice, we each notice that we still have that very comfortable feeling inside. Jade Unity says gently, "Allow yourself to become new." Pearl River Master nods to our teachers to commence playing a large drum and a deep sounding gong. The rhythm is soothing and mysterious; the resonating gong is a calling reminder of something deep within.

Teach

Pearl River Master begins the instruction: "Your teacher suggested that you relax. No one is paying attention to you. Use your breath to open your channels and your Qi gates, open your consciousness, open the gates in your crown to the influences of Heaven, open the gates in your lower body to the influences of Earth. You may have noticed that in my sword form I was freeing us from past traumas; allow that to benefit you in our practice here today.

"Spontaneous Qigong is not a form—it is formless. You may just go ahead on your own or you can take some clues from the words that I will speak. Whenever you feel that you understand the idea, stop listening to me and listen to the beat of the drum and the occasional sound of the gong. The point is to neutralize inner resistance to natural Qi flow, dispel extra and useless Qi, direct the Qi into the places where it is the most deficient, and break through where stagnation has created blockage. This is intended to reveal or release the inherently more healthy and more radiant self that is latent within you.

"Begin to shift your weight from right to left, or forward and backward from the ball of the foot to the heel. Move your arms. Pretend you are a bird or gather Qi from Heaven and bathe yourself. Remember that this practice doesn't look like anything— no one is watching you; we are not doing a form. If you have a kind of dancing that makes you feel free, employ that. If you feel like you need to cut some internal bonds, use your body to do that. If you become aware that it would help to make some sounds, please do. Sighs, shouts, and cries are excellent ways to shake loose the inner tension that constrains the Qi. Don't pay attention to the person next to you."

That warm feeling inside, that sense that something has been altered, the sound of the drum, and every once in a while the sound of the gong have conspired to create a great sense of freedom. There is no form; there is nothing to learn. The only goal is to circulate, purify, and direct the Qi, and to uncover and reveal the inherent self. In the background you can hear the voice of Pearl River Master but you have taken her advice and stopped listening. You are deep in Spontaneous Qigong (Chi Kung).

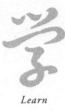

Learn

The relaxation and openness of this practice allow you to recognize the perennial tightness of your shoulders and chest. How might you shake this loose? What if you start to rotate your arms like windmills with the idea of throwing off Qi that has gotten stuck around your throat and heart? It feels right, so you try it. Somewhere almost out of range of your awareness the sound of the gong reminds you to go deeper. You start to whirl your arms like a windmill. It feels liberating so you go faster and faster. After a very short time you feel the chest opening and the sound of your exhalations getting louder. In your mind's eye you see an image of dark-colored Qi whirling off the tips of your fingers.

After a few moments more you are exhausted to the point of slowing down and then stopping. Standing in place you decide to use the Qigong closing and stand for a while with your hands over the Earth Dan Tian in the aligning posture. Notice a strong sense of openness in the area around the chest, heart, and throat. The sound of the drum and gong begin to enter back into your awareness. The Pearl River Master's voice also enters your awareness: "Please, conclude now; bring yourself toward a comfortable conclusion." After briefly readjusting you open your eyes. Looking around, notice that several of the group are lying down or sitting cross-legged on the floor. Others are still standing. Everyone is facing in a different direction. It is obvious that each person has had a unique and spontaneous experience.

We all applaud Pearl River Master. She bows, then steps back to take a seat. Jade Unity steps forward: "This combination of circulating, purifying, and directing the Qi is very effective. Please take the time on the breaks to share your experiences with each other.

"One of my favorite teachers had several traditional word pictures that helped me to learn how to direct the Qi. Have you noticed what happens with a Chinese fan? Air that is invisible can be accelerated and directed using the fan. It is the same with Qi. Your intention and your actions are like a fan. With your practice you can concentrate and direct the Qi, which is naturally available everywhere, to a particular destination. Directing the Qi is like using a magnifying lens to concentrate the sunlight to a pinpoint of intense heat. The light, like Qigong, is already present but is not intensified. Holding the magnifying lens in the proper place allows for a resource that is naturally available to be concentrated for increased effect.

"With both the fan and the magnifier, it is important to notice—you must use intention and will. The fan is still a fan lying closed in a drawer. The magnifying lens is still a lens closed up in its case. They are the tools that can be used to concentrate natural resources to create benefit. However, the tools only become useful when you use them. With your intention and skill, Directing Qi can become a powerful tool for you."

Directing the Qi

By its very nature Qi is constantly directed to its appropriate destinations and interactions with body structures, organs, glands, tissues, cells through the Qi Matrix of points, channels, passages, Qi reservoirs, and centers. In the healthy state where there is little tension and where Qi is neither deficient nor blocked, the need to consciously direct Qi is minimal.

However, if your health is challenged and your goal is to heal and restore vitality, or if your goal is to attain extraordinary personal capacity, intuitive insight, and healthy longevity, then it becomes appropriate to attend more specifically to cultivating a conscious ability to direct Qi. When pain and disease caused by deficiency or disharmony create the need for healing, specifically directing Qi is more powerful than simply circulating Qi. This level of focus requires agreement of the HeartMind—the brain, mind, nervous system, and psychological components of your body/mind/spirit complex. If you spend much of your practice time making lists or trying to figure out solutions to the millions of problems in life, you probably have not found the subtle skill needed to direct Qi.

If the HeartMind Domain of Qigong is the bridge between the beginning Earth phases and the highly advanced Heaven phases, then Direct Qi is the bridge within the bridge. Earlier it was possible simply to relax and the Qi would self-cultivate; however, from here on in the Ten Phases of Cultivation and Mastery require much more focused use of HeartMind skill, in the form of will and intention. Directing the Qi requires the ability to remain attuned to a particular focus. This can only occur when the HeartMind is clear and attuned to resist distraction and neutralize inner resistance. The low-grade tension that exists throughout the body, caused by the conditioning of life, is the adversary of your ability to sustain your focus and successfully direct the Qi.

HeartMind Is the Commander of the Qi

In medicine and philosophy, "the mind is the leader of the Qi." In general terms this means the heart in its integrated relationship with the mind leads the Qi, because in Chinese there is only Xin—HeartMind. This same sentiment is also stated, "Qi follows intention." Whether it is by placing the hands on points or centers of life energy or using mind intention, Direct Qi requires a greater degree of focus and intention and the development of a higher level of skill than that needed for the earlier phases of cultivation. The level of mind focus and clarity that is necessary to Direct Qi is greater than just simple relaxation.

It is necessary to train the HeartMind to sustain a single focus for an extended period of time as in meditation. This is why Direct Qi is the bridge between initial more simplistic Qigong and more mature and experienced cultivation. In less advanced Qigong practices the discipline required is to *do* the practice—move your body, deepen your breath, relax, and clear your mind. Direct Qi demands more than this. It requires that you *be* in a whole different way. People who have attained this level of Qi cultivation skill are unique. Whether the realm is business, sports, education, or otherwise, people who have advanced to this level of skill are intuitive and insightful as well as compassionate. It is impossible to master this phase while distracted by the complex world of personality, the social scene, or the compulsive accumulation of material things.

Practice

Intention and Will

No matter what methods are used to direct Qi, sustained calm focus of the HeartMind will maximize the effect. This means you must listen to the voice of the heart. In your meditation, use visualization and the focused intention of the HeartMind to guide and propel the Qi. No matter what methods you use to direct Qi, *Yi* (focused intention) and *Zhi* (will) enhance the effect because only a focused mind can lead the Qi.

Breath

Use the breath to guide the Qi to specific destinations, particularly on the exhalation. The simplest practice is to gather and concentrate inner resources on the inhalation and direct those resources on the exhalation. On the exhalation, remembering that the clear and calm HeartMind can guide the Qi, focus on the part of body where you wish the Qigong effect to have its influence. You can even add a declaration or directive, "And now on the exhalation I send internal healing resources to my head (heart, or whatever area you are working with)." You can use the same sounds that we explored in the last chapter, with strong intention, to direct fresh Qi to and release tension from the organs that are associated with the sound.

Massage

One of the best ways to direct Qi is with massage, hand placement, or tracing the acupuncture energy channels. With massage or near-touch, use your HeartMind intent to direct the Qi to your hands and from the hands into the points, centers, or organs. Some of the practices at the end of this chapter are focused on this means of directing Qi. True, it is more fun to have a massage from someone else, but this kind of self-massage is free, spontaneous, and convenient; in other words, you don't have to set an appointment, go somewhere else, or pay to get it.

Movement

You probably have already figured out that body movement can be used to direct Qi. The body movements of Qigong and Tai Chi or even random wiggling get the Qi to flow into areas that are blocked or stagnant. Almost every Qigong movement can be used as a Direct Qi gesture by coordinating it with the intention and the breath.

Other Methods

Using acupuncture, herbs, oils, magnets, and hot coins (a useful folk remedy that is used in place of acupuncture) on the points can direct the Qi without the HeartMind intent. Herbs can be used externally in salves and poultices or internally as formulas to guide the Qi. Oils can also be applied externally. Magnets are used to attract or disperse Qi. And heated coins direct heat into the specific points where there is blocked Qi.

Direct Qi to Others: Transmit Qi

You can also direct the Qi to assist others. To direct Qi with out-flowing intention, meaning to direct the Qi to another or to cause the universal forces or resources to have a positive influence on others, is an entire realm of Qigong. We will explore this in detail in the tenth phase of Qi cultivation and mastery, Transmit Qi.

Qigong Methods to Direct Qi

HISTORICAL REFLECTION   Each of these three methods of directing Qi—Trace the Yin-Yang Channels, Direct Qi to the Organs, and Direct Qi in the Microcosmic Orbit— comes from a slightly different historic origin. Trace the Yin-Yang Channels is a common health improvement method based on the theory of energy flow. It has been used for thousands of years. The Yin energy of Earth comes up the front channels and the Yang energy of Heaven flows down the channels of the back. Trace the Yin-Yang Channels and Direct Qi to the Organs are both part of the Vitality Method, a contemporary form of medical Qigong designed for general use with all disorders and health conditions. It is intended to be modified for all populations including elders and the young, those who are sick and those who are well. It can be adapted for people who can stand or for those who must practice sitting or lying down. Direct Qi in the Microcosmic Orbit is more esoteric and subtle. Also known as the Small Heaven and the Small Universe Circuit, this practice reflects the traditional Chinese idea that the human system is a microcosmic representation of the whole universe. In all schools or traditions of Qi cultivation, Direct Qi in the Small Heaven is an early form of Inner Alchemy. It creates the foundation for the more advanced phases of the Heaven level of cultivation.

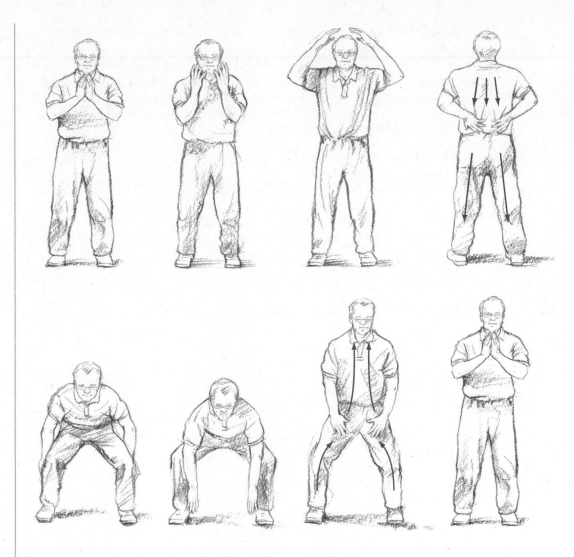

Trace the Yin-Yang Channels

Trace the Yin-Yang Channels

INSTRUCTION Start by rubbing your hands together to make some heat. Turn your palms toward your body, lift your chin, and starting at your neck, wash your face. You can either touch the body surface lightly or pass the hands slightly above the surface. Proceed upward over the top of your head and down your neck, shoulders, and back. Reach up and get as close to the kidneys as possible, then trace down over the sacrum and down the back of the legs. It is not important to bend over all the way—go as far as you comfortably can. These are the Yang channels—urinary bladder, gallbladder, and stomach. Then trace the Yin channels—liver, spleen, and kidney—up the insides of the legs, up along the torso, and to the neck and face again. You can stop to rub your palms together to make more heat. Repeat this as many times as you wish; try to do it at least three times. Allow yourself to enter a deep state of meditation; your mind is not taken up with details. You can coordinate the breath with the movement or just relax and breathe naturally.

Direct Qi to the Organs

INSTRUCTION Rub your palms together to make heat and build up the Qi. Place the right hand over the lower border of the right rib cage, the location of the liver and gallbladder. Place the left palm at the lower border of the left rib cage, the location of the pancreas and the spleen. Make a circular motion with the palms to further stimulate the Qi. Then be still. Feel the sensation of the energy flowing from your hands into the organs or from the organs into your hands. It can go either way as the natural tendency is for the body systems to seek harmony. You don't make this happen; it happens naturally. Simply place your hands, relax, and deepen your awareness of what is happening.

Now place one hand over the HeartMind center and one hand over the Earth center at the umbilical area, make some circles, and build up Qi. Then rest and allow yourself to feel. Allow the breath to be full, not urgent. Again, relax and allow the healing and harmonizing. Take a moment to feel gratitude for your organs. Send them a sincere smile. After centuries of observation the Qi masters assure us that our organs are happier if we thank them occasionally and send them some Qi.

Now place your hands on your back. Make some rapid strokes to build up heat. Place your palms flat against your back as high as it is comfortable. Send energy to the kidneys. Take a moment to send your gratitude for their service to you.

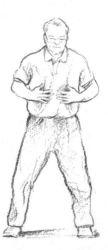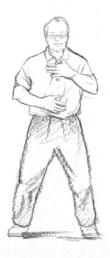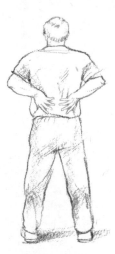

Direct Qi to the Organs

Direct Qi in the Microcosmic Orbit

INSTRUCTION The human system is a replica of the universe—Heaven. Two primary Qi channels, the front and back central channels, form what is called the Microcosmic Orbit or the Cycle of the Small Heaven. Each of the points or gates on the Microcosmic Orbit is related to a major inner function. This practice directs the energy from gate to gate. Typically the process starts at the Earth Elixir Field and progresses as the points are numbered in the illustration. Many believe that this method is associated with the Circulate the Light practice from *The Secret of the Golden Flower.* Start

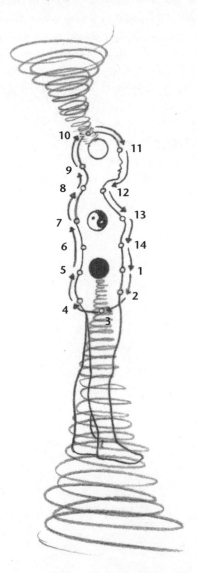

Direct Qi in the Microcosmic Orbit

with an inhalation and focus at the umbilical point. On the exhalation, imagine or feel the Qi moving downward to the second gate. Imagine that the point becomes warm (you may feel this). On the inhalation, allow the energy to flow through the gate and into the body. Then, on the exhalation, send the flow, the river of light, on to the next gate. Continue this transmission from gate to gate for fourteen breaths, which will bring you back to the first gate. On each inhalation pull energy in through the gate; on each exhalation send the energy on to the next gate.

After fourteen breaths, the gates should be open. Then continue. On the inhalation the Qi moves from the nose to the umbilical point in the Microcosmic Orbit and on the exhalation it passes down between the legs and rises along the back and over the top of the head, where you begin the next inhalation. When you can do this for the fourteen breaths and then do the full cycle for ten breaths or so without thinking or becoming distracted, it demonstrates that you are becoming an advanced practitioner who is definitely making progress in HeartMind Qigong.

Mind Focus Affirmation

Directing Qi, I transmit empowering resources to specific areas to accelerate healing and to restore balance and harmony.

Phase 6:
Conserve Qi

> *Longevity is related to sufficiency of Qi.*
> *If the Qi is strong, life is long.*
> *If you cultivate Qi*
>   *with senses protected to conserve essence,*
>   *and use tonic foods and herbs in proper timing,*
>   *you can conserve and increase the production of Qi.*
> *Your life will be long and vital*
>   *and you will never experience the challenges of old age.*
>
> —WONG CHONG, *ESSAY ON BALANCE*, 400 B.C.E.

During our visit, we have learned that there are many hermitages and small temples located throughout the mountains. Some are inhabited by monks, others by retired physicians and scholars seeking through personal retreat the roots and origins of Chinese medicine and philosophy. During our free time, a small group of us have started out looking for the adventure of meeting one of these mountain hermits. Earlier our guide Intentful HeartMind invited us to meet an elder physician who has retired to the mountain after a successful career in medicine.

After about forty-five minutes of easy walking on trails where we pass groups of Chinese travelers, Intentful HeartMind stops and tells us more about the doctor we will encounter. "Dr. Chen is very interesting," he begins. "He studied with old masters who practiced classical medicine from long before the Cultural Revolution. His approach to medicine was always very closely associated with the traditions of Daoism

Conserve Qi

141

and Qi cultivation. He now focuses mostly on his own cultivation practice although he does see patients who come from afar and residents of the cultivation communities here on the mountain. His treatments are unique because he typically only needs to treat the person once. Following that treatment, with the use of herbs and Qigong [Chi Kung] practices that he recommends, most people are so inspired by what they have learned that they practice Qigong vigilantly and recover their health. He is very humble and will not tell you that part of the story."

Intentful HeartMind pulls back a branch and we enter another hidden trail. This one climbs sharply up into a mountain valley. There is a very small creek to our left. After a while we step out into an open area where a small hermitage dwelling stands surrounded by gardens. An elderly gentleman looks up from his gardening and waves. He greets Yi Xin enthusiastically, and we are invited to take seats on large logs turned on end as stools. He serves tea.

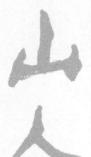

Hermit

Nature crafted the place perfectly for a hermitage. The area is just large enough for a very small house with small garden beds all around. The little valley faces due south so that it is warmed during winter days. In the summer the sun rises late and sets early, and the mountain keeps the temperatures cool. The valley is not large enough to capture much rainwater but by coincidence of nature there is a small spring that arises from the ground nearby. Rows and rows of mountain ranges spread in a wide panorama before us. When the conditions are just perfect, the sea of clouds would likely come right up to Dr. Chen's front door.

Intentful HeartMind says to us, "Several days ago, I told Dr. Chen that you are very enthusiastic about learning of his studies and his reasons for living here. He has agreed to discuss that with you. He likes to inform people about the richness of Chinese medicine. I think you will be amazed by his story."

Our teacher nods to Dr. Chen who begins to speak with an easy smile:

"You may be wondering why a successful doctor is living in the mountains so far from his home. Of course you can see that this place is very beautiful. I have learned that one's life does not go as it seems it could. As a very young man in the later 1930s I had traditional training from a monk at a Daoist temple near my home who felt strongly that I should be a physician. I learned Qigong and a secret kind of Tai Chi [Taiji] and many unusual medical methods. China then entered a very complex and distressing period. Much later, following the Cultural Revolution, when I was allowed to continue my practice as a doctor, it became important to practice medicine in the style of the 1970s. It was, I must admit, a very stressful period between 1943 and 1970. For many reasons it became useful to have forgotten the Daoist medicine methods. But I did not really forget.

"During that same period I was diagnosed with liver cancer—a frightening experience. I did have some very trying times and I suspect that both the difficult time plus some pent-up inner tensions could have aggravated my condition. We were beginning to use Western medical treatments with the Chinese medicine of that period, but I was not responding to the chemotherapy. I decided to reestablish my connection with some monks from these mountains and discreetly took up a search for a Qigong form that was consistent with my earlier training.

"I made the acquaintance of an elder monk who was involved in the lineage of the secret Tai Chi I had learned many years earlier. He taught me a Qigong form that is based on reversing time that comes directly from the master who created the original Tai Chi, Zhang San Feng. Master Zhang had a background in the tradition of Inner Alchemy, and a strong feeling for the value of moving meditation. The form called Primordial Qigong [Wuji Qigong] reverses time to reconnect the practitioner with the past and with their prebirth state to alter the course of the future. I practiced this Qigong faithfully and took some herbal formulas and, over some time, completely recovered from the cancer.

"The new medical synthesis of the 1970s created a standard form of medicine. The new methods, partly based on the ancient traditions, were usually quite effective and many people were served. When I needed to, I could use some of the Daoist methods from my earlier training, because nobody but I really knew the difference anyway. I got excellent clinical results and over the years I felt comfortable passing on a number of the ancient insights to a few senior students. I waited patiently to reach my retirement so that I could take up my personal cultivation in earnest.

"Some years back my beloved wife passed away. Our children were all grown. I was called by my inner sense to return to this mountain to continue with my personal cultivation practice and to go back to using the methods from my earliest training. I now teach people the Primordial Qigong that helped to neutralize my cancer and study the ancient principles of time reversal and Inner Alchemy."

Dr. Chen pauses briefly and then asks, "Would you like to see the Wuji form?" He takes a stance on a little rise. A circle has been worn on the ground where he has apparently practiced this form many times. "Notice that, in the form, each set is done in a way that represents the seasons. On one level it progresses forward in time from spring to summer and so on. Within each set there is a movement against the seasons, which turns back time." As he begins his practice, it is obvious that he quickly settles into a kind of deep meditative state. His eyes are half closed; the movements are slow and fluid. It appears that he is gathering resources, turning them this way and that in his hands as if preparing a special inner medicine. The practice combines a deep Qigong meditation while moving the body gently. As he had said, the sets move with the seasons to the right. Simultaneously there is a powerful and consistent contrary movement against the seasons—to the left there is a turning back of time. It is exciting to see an approach to Inner Alchemy that is so simple and yet so profound. The four rounds, one for each direction and season, took only twelve to fifteen minutes. Dr. Chen had clearly collected and processed a significant dose of subtle energy and inner elixir—he seemed to glow as he bowed in conclusion and returned to his seat at the table.

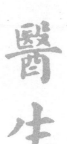

Physician

Back at the training center Jade Unity resumed our training. "More than any aspect of cultivation Conserve Qi is focused on our lifestyle. With most of the phases of cultivation the practice of Qigong creates the outcome. In cultivation to Conserve Qi, the focus is more on intention and will creating action in our lives and the capacity to be foresightful and proactive to sustain our Qi for a long healthy life."

Jade Unity recounted a story to illustrate Conserve Qi. The story went something like this: "In ancient times, there were two of our ancestors who each had some grain. They could cook and eat the grain for nourishment or plant it to grow more grain. The first man wanted others to see him as well off, so he cooked his grain and spent his time appearing to be a person who could afford leisure. The second man refused the temptation to eat his grain. He busied himself with two jobs, to prepare the soil to plant the grain and to forage food for his nourishment so he could save the seeds.

"The man of abundance and leisure invited the industrious man to share a meal. They talked late into the night each expressing his different views. The one who was saving his grain talked of his plans to plant and the other boasted about his life of luxury. In time the one who had conserved his seed had planted, cultivated, and harvested enough grain to have plenty to eat and enough left over to plant again. He was healthy and well nourished. The man who had consumed his seed was now hungry and his energy was waning. Eventually, the man who conserved his seed became the leader of the region and the other man became one of his followers.

"This is one of the legends of the beginning of the Han people, the original tribe that gave birth to the Chinese civilization. Qi cultivation teachers for thousands of years have used this story to emphasize one of the most important phases of Qi cultivation—Conserve Qi. To master the most advanced level of Qigong—Inner Alchemy—a high level of intention must be cultivated and a store of Qi must be accumulated. Conserve Qi, the final HeartMind Phase, is the threshold to the Heaven phases of cultivation—Store Qi and Transform Qi—and the ultimate phase of cultivation and mastery, Dissolve in Qi. The Heaven phases of cultivation do not occur spontaneously. Conscious cultivation in Heaven Qigong cannot happen without advancing in HeartMind Qigong. These are advanced practices. To accumulate resources and inner potential, so that the inner elixir can be achieved, Qi must be replenished, conserved, accumulated, and protected. Conserve Qi is more than a Qigong practice; it is also a way of engaging in life."

Conserving the Qi

The Qi masters, through millennia of exploration, practice, and refinement, discovered one of the most important insights of Qi cultivation. You can become aware of and cultivate Qi, yet not actually accumulate Qi. A maximal store or reservoir of this essential life-sustaining and healing resource can only come through conservation and protection. Nature, in combination with our inherent state of health at birth, causes the human system to collect and circulate Qi automatically. However, every action, internal function, and emotion uses or spends our life force as well. Work, play, digestion and metabolism, sexual activity, stress, emotional challenge, extreme weather, pollution, and many other factors compromise the Qi. To put it another way, simply living one's life can spend a person's needed reserves of Qi or even deplete his or her vitality.

This constant, natural spending of your inner resources suggests that Qi conservation should not be isolated to thirty or fifty minutes of practice in the morning or after work. The ideal in Qigong is to maximize the inherent capacity to replenish, conserve, and accumulate the inner reserve of Qi while natural Qi expenditures are occurring. We can improve our inherent capacity or reservoir of Qi throughout our day by using mindfulness in decisions and behaviors that help to conserve Qi.

There is a maxim in Chinese Qi management tradition: "From moment to moment Conserve Qi and replenish spent or lost Qi to accumulate Qi wealth—otherwise you must live with the consequences of a diminishing store of vital life-enhancing resource." As we saw in Jade Unity's story, the metaphor of grain storage is a useful one. To sustain the security and prosperity of the community it is vital, in addition to cultivating nourishment, to replenish, conserve, and accumulate a portion of the resource to be stored. For the internal community of organs, glands, tissues, and cells it is vital to replenish, conserve, and accumulate Qi.

Control, discipline, focus, and intention at the Conserve Qi phase are highly refined, way beyond what anyone simply using Qigong practices for better health would naturally attain. For many, however, once they have tasted the Qi they want it all, it becomes a kind of positive addiction; it is legal, as Qi costs nothing and is always available to everyone. The consequence of such an addiction is, at the very least, health improvement. At the most, you may become a sage. What do you give up to attain these higher levels of Qi mastery? Fear, worry, guilt, anger, revenge, negative addictions to food, alcohol, or self-judgment, and other useless habits.

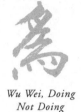

Wu Wei, Doing Not Doing

Inner Accounting of Your Qi Wealth

The ability to modify or curtail the negative habits or addictions that deplete Qi does not come easy. Such behaviors are frequently lifelong and are even, unfortunately, rewarded by popular culture. Large portions of low-nutrient foods, lots of stress, and constant work without sufficient rest are signs of success in the minds of many people. The necessary quality of focus and concentration in your HeartMind cultivation must be very high for you to transform to your new, more healthy, more efficient self. Your Qi is your wealth, the inner treasure in your life.

Your Ancestral Qi (*Yuan Qi*) and the Original Essence (*Yuan Jing*) from your parents and other prebirth influences make up the initial principal in your inner wealth account and called your prenatal resources. The Qi acquired from nature—breath, food, peace of mind, pleasure, inspiration—are the daily contributions to your Qi assets; these are called postnatal resources. The highest level of Qigong practice yields high interest, it is like an up market of Qi wealth or a year in which the grain harvest is extra robust. Only minimal to moderate returns can be expected to accumulate when the conservation of your asssets is neglected.

The down market occurs when stresses accumulate to compromise the Qi account. Often life is undirected and driven by external pressures—social trends and the compulsion to accumulate thrills or material wealth. These attractive external distractions often cause people to ignore the cultivation of inner resources. Unfortunately, in this context, there is typically no reserve and every stress on the system depletes the assets in the account all the more. This translates into less vitality, less productivity, lower life expectancy.

In the Conserve Qi phase, your practice becomes the foundation for your purposeful choice making in a mindful way of being. Posture adjustment, gentle movement, breath focus, mind focus, and self-treatment with acupressure and massage, the classic components of Qigong, are tools to help you *Gong* your Qi. However, in HeartMind Qigong, these methods are not enough to foster the highest levels of healing and transformation. These highest levels of cultivation require that we aim our Gong at behavior, personality, and character. Doing Qigong methods is still very valuable, but at the sixth phase of cultivation the greatest power tools are focused determination, resoluteness, and discipline—the force of will. Will is a profound expression of the HeartMind. *Xin*, the character for HeartMind, is also the foundation of the Chinese character *Zhi*, will. This level of Qigong provides the leverage to move one's practice into the highest domain of cultivation and mastery, Spirit Qigong.

No: The Conserve Qi Power Word

In a way the most powerful tool at the level of preserving, protecting, and accumulating Qi is the word *no*. To say yes to the more advanced benefits of Qigong, it becomes critical to be able to say no to the things that cause a deficit in the Qi quotient—leaking of Qi into fear, worry, depression, and extremes in food, addictions, work, sex, and so on.

Interestingly, while Conserve Qi is an advanced level of practice, people who are simply dieting or who have quit smoking are also somewhat involved in this level of Qigong. They too are in the process of saying no to something that depletes or compromises their Qi. However, there is a major difference. A person who vigilantly practices Qigong methods (as in phases one through five) and also declines to engage in activities, attitudes, and emotions that cause the loss of Qi (phase six), has a maximized approach to all of life. This person is not just saying no to one depleting habit—he or she is transforming the whole of his or her life by saying yes to bringing the practice of Qigong to a moment-to-moment level. Therefore, compared to the dieter

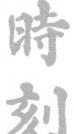

Moment

or the former smoker, the Qigong practitioner's Qi cultivation is all the more powerful because it is a whole-life devotion to personal improvement in many areas. Succeeding at dieting, recovering from drugs, or quitting smoking are, however, wise life choices that definitely engage the HeartMind. Such changes empower people to engage in Qigong at a fairly high level, whenever they choose to explore the Qi.

You know that to accumulate Qi you must conserve, retain, build up, preserve, and protect. The causes for the loss, damage, or depletion of Qi are the same as the causes of disease studied by physicians of traditional Chinese medicine. The remedy in cultivation is easy to discuss but challenging to actualize. The most advanced phases of Qigong can take a significant amount of practice and time to master (or even explore). Learning how and when to use *no* is a major breakthrough for most people.

Managing the Emotions: Fear, Worry, Guilt, Anger, and Grief

In advanced Qigong, your cultivation leads to important realizations about emotions, habit patterns, and attitudes. Xin, HeartMind, is implied in emotions and feelings. Qi cultivation in the advanced phases requires attending to the feeling aspect of oneself. You may have noticed that worry doesn't change anything, aggression does not lead to peace, fear does not enhance the ability to respond to crisis, and guilt does not increase personal power. These emotions and attitudes, learned and conditioned into us, neutralize our ability to conserve and accumulate Qi. Advanced Qigong cultivation reveals that the remedy for the depletion of energy is to cultivate tolerance, forgiveness, communication, trust, surrender, and acceptance. These virtues activate the capacity to conserve rather than spend Qi.

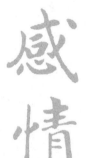

Emotion

The challenge is that most of us have been conditioned to act upon or express emotions in certain ways and to accept those actions and expressions in others. Children tend to mirror those behaviors they learn from their family members and teachers. Some emotions or inner patterns of response are infused into them by physical or emotional trauma. Personal discipline, focus, and intention is required to alter these deeply ingrained habits. In many cases additional professional support or trauma release can facilitate and even accelerate progress in Qigong.

The ability to express emotions and feelings at the appropriate time is a powerful method for conserving and protecting Qi. Expressing sadness when tragedy strikes or fear in the face of extreme violence are automatic and reasonable responses. Restraining sadness or fear will actually spend more Qi than expressing it would. According to Chinese medicine and Qigong philosophy, chronic anger, fear, and other emotions drain and stagnate Qi, which make it impossible to build up a strong reserve. The more spontaneous Qigong methods, which do not require constant concentration on the details of the form, can foster a major release of emotions that may be accompanied with weeping or laughing.

When the HeartMind is stagnant, deficient, or unfocused, the necessary capacity to evolve to the domains of HeartMind and Spirit Qigong can be severely compromised. The internal chatter of the busy mind usually is driven by unresolved emotions stored in the nervous system and Qi field. At this point there could be real value in seeking facilitation through some form of mind/body treatment that helps to accelerate emotional clearing or Qigong healing that addresses emotional stagnation and disharmony. If, after some assistance to clear the HeartMind, your practice becomes successful in aspects of meditation and internal focus that were formerly difficult to accomplish, it is a sign that the evolution of your practice is no longer stuck.

The great Qi masters eventually clear their Qi field of emotional pain and gain the ability to remain steady in the midst of all that arises. They do so by making it a priority to say no to habitual responses that drain Qi and yes to new responses that conserve Qi. Purposefully cultivating your ability to sustain a practice of Qi conservation makes it possible to adjust your alignment to the universe, optimize your relationship to the natural flow of Qi, express spiritual light, and rest in clear-minded acceptance of the present. These skills build powerful Qi wealth.

Managing Excesses in Lifestyle

To work, play, eat, learn, and be sexual are associated with both building and spending Qi. The Qigong challenge is to spend less and conserve inner resources. Overwork, overplay, overeating, underresting, habitual use of drugs or alcohol, prolonged use of medications, an overabundance of stress-inducing information or entertainment, and excessive sexual activity or sexual distraction are all major causes of Qi depletion.

It is Qi that makes sex so wonderful and such a powerful flash point for life and procreativity. Qi makes our work inspiring. Appropriate food intake is nourishing, a source of Qi. Play and creativity can be so energizing that they can neutralize stress and connect us with two powerful sources of energy—inspiration and fun. In excess, however, even these positive activities can become serious drains on our Qi.

The most challenging factor in Conserve Qi is that many of these lifestyle excesses are regular features in most people's lives. In fact, these excesses are even expected and glamorized. Overwork is nearly a way of life in many professions. Alcohol is vigorously promoted in the media; the media nearly always depict successful people having fun. Is fun really limited to the rich and famous? Sex and violence are prevalent in all forms of entertainment. Given the amazing potential of Qi, this glamorization of Qi-depleting excesses is a significant compromise to human potential in the twenty-first century. It may even be that problems such as hunger, violence, and poverty could be resolved if the people of our world would purposefully conserve Qi.

Corporations are suffering from billions of dollars of losses in work absenteeism and stress injury claims. It was recently reported that one major corporation spends $52 million on ulcer drugs alone. Strange new diseases of fatigue, exhaustion, and pain, with no certain cause, are becoming commonplace. Preventive training in Conserve Qi methods could reduce these losses considerably.

Health, longevity, social or personal enlightenment, and peace among cultures are certainly not the top focus of exhausted people who are driven by the more commonplace excesses of our culture. Any sort of widespread human enlightenment is constantly neutralized by our cultural fascination with the worst of lifestyle habits, which have become the basis for our consumer society. The wisdom of Lao Zi and Confucius proclaimed, "It may be impossible to fix the ills of culture, but it is never inappropriate to cultivate Qi to repair the shortcomings in oneself."

Those who practice Conserve Qi by managing their energy and activities become part of the solution to the challenges of living in the modern world. To conserve Qi, it is not enough to do Qigong practices. To say yes to a richer, more harmonious, more inspired life, some people must change jobs, refuse to take on new projects, set limits and boundaries in their relationships, or change their diets by refusing old favorites. Knowing when and how to communicate clearly about personal boundaries is powerful Qigong, as is the ability to pass on foods, drinks, and activities that deplete Qi.

Managing Extreme External Influences

When it is cold, you can either choose to put on a coat, or be cold and suffer the consequences. You can decide to stay in on extremely windy days or to avoid exposure to bright sun, or you can live with the consequences of exposure to these forces. The climate has the potential to enhance the Qi or, in excess, deplete or damage the Qi. You know that watching the sun set over the mountains in nature stimulates and inspires the Qi. The same sun at midday in the summer, if you are unprotected, can deplete energy in the short term and cause exhaustion and dizziness. In the longer term it can cause much worse problems, including cancer, which severely depletes Qi. Besides the natural climates there is a wide assortment of external influences, including exposure to stressors and toxins in food, water, air, and the environment, that have the potential to damage and deplete the Qi as well.

The key point regarding Conserve Qi and these external factors is *choice*. You have to take that coat, wear that hat, use that umbrella, take care to shield yourself from excessive sun, build a fire, make hot tea, take a vacation.

If it is too grueling to drive to your work through heavy traffic, you are the only person who can find yourself a new job. If it is obvious to you that certain foods cause you sudden fatigue, it will be you who must make the choice to avoid that food.

If you find yourself saying that you don't honestly think you can change your behavior or the behavior of others in regard to weather, work, food, and other external stressors, then definitely accelerate your Qigong practice. This can neutralize the negative effects of many stressors. However, if you accelerate Qigong and become more skilled at conserving Qi through your choices, this will create a radical multiplication of your personal potential and Qi wealth.

Sexual Qigong

Sexual

The fact that humans produce powerful sexual resources—the sperm and the egg—is in itself amazing. That these resources then merge to create a brand-new human being that grows from two cells into vibrant men and women is no less than astounding. Because the amount of Qi required to do this is immense, the sexual aspect of the Conserve Qi Phase is pivotal in Qi cultivation. Ancient Chinese Daoist monk scientists, those revolutionary Qi specialists, have always been fascinated with the amount of Qi involved in every level of sexuality.

Qi masters agree that management of the powerful resources inherent in the sexual context is among the great secrets of cultivation and mastery. The ancient literature on cultivation is full of references to sexual Gong and the fact that it is at least as important as exercise, breath practices, and meditation. To conserve those resources protects a radical internal treasure called *Jing*. Jing, and the Qi associated with it, is considered in Chinese medicine and Qigong to be a major component of your Yin, the root that holds and secures inner Yang, vitality. Yang is our aliveness. If there is only deficient Yin for the aliveness to root in, there will be deficient aliveness.

Dharma, Calling

The balance and harmony of Yin and Yang is the foundation of vitality and longevity. The depletion of Jing through stress or frequent sexual expenditures depletes Yin, which depletes the potential of the Yang components of life. Think for just a moment of living with a deficiency of energy, alertness of mind, and physical stamina—all Yang. The Chinese observed this carefully for several thousands of years and determined that more than any other single factor, it is through sexual activity that we stand to lose or gain the most in cultivation. Thus the emphasis on sexuality in the cultivation and mastery of Qi is not so much about sex itself, but rather on energy management and the optimization of personal potential. In advanced Qigong men enjoy sexual satisfaction and participate sexually with their wives and lovers, while conserving semen (Jing filled with Qi) by reserving ejaculation. Women conserve and protect their essential resources by retreating from demanding and stressful activities for a few days a month at menstruation. Both men and women benefit from cultivating the capacity to communicate and establish personal boundaries that conserve Qi. Conserve Qi is the most advanced phase of HeartMind Qigong, and conservation through sexual cultivation practice is an advanced aspect of the Conserve Qi phase. Sexual cultivation is a component of Inner Alchemy (*Nei Dan*) and a key gateway to the Qigong of the Heaven or Spirit Domain.

Qigong Reflects Important Differences Between the Feminine and the Masculine

Just as Yin and Yang are very different, so are women and men. This polar yet complementary state is what makes attraction, love, and sex so wonderful. So, too, the recommended methods for the Conserve Qi phase, regarding sexuality, are different for men and women as well.

The Feminine: Yin

Women's capacity to cultivate the powerful inner resources associated with sexuality requires practices that conserve Qi by creating a period of stress-free, relaxed, low-demand time each month. The word *period* has two meanings: one is "span of time," the other is "a stop." Ancient cultures typically had an inherent framework for protecting women during the menstrual period in which the egg and a significant amount of blood is lost. This is particularly true of those cultures that have roots in ancient eras when matriarchal social structures were in place. China, being such a culture, has a rich foundation of wisdom associated with conserving feminine inner resources.

As we have discussed, in Chinese medical theory the blood—which is called the Red Dragon in the sexual context—and Qi are associated. During the menstrual period blood maximally infused with the female Jing, a major inner resource, flows out of the body. The dispelled blood and Jing—including one or several mature eggs—represent a significant loss of Qi. So, the greatest loss of Qi and potential for the woman, sexually, is concentrated at the monthly period. This is particularly true when she continues like a warrior at work or with family responsibilities during this time. However, the woman actually gains Qi from the sexual encounter itself.

The excitement of inner resources during sexual activity—intercourse and otherwise—can be a major form of cultivation activity, particularly if it is engaged in purposefully. The ideal practice for women, particularly during the period, is to harvest the Jing, to retain it as an energy resource, before it is released from the body. This is part of how women can contribute their feminine energy and creativity to a situation, to their family, and to the community. For women, conserving protects personal health, which becomes a feminine asset that they can then contribute to the world.

Beyond declaring the menstrual period as a time of decreased activity and stress and using sexual interaction as a cultivation opportunity, feminine sexual Gong can be quite provocative. One such practice includes inserting smooth pieces of jade the size and shape of an egg into the vagina (called the Jade Palace) and doing an array of muscle contractions to enhance sexual potential. Similar muscle contractions are used by men as well and are common in Yoga. In the West, similar contractions are called the Keigel exercise. In Taming the Red Dragon (also called the Deer Practice), a technique to curtail ovulation, the practitioner rubs her breasts gently in a circular fashion for more than three hundred cycles. There is quite a bit of debate about whether it is wise or natural to curtail ovulation. For more information on this subject, readers can check out a number of dynamic groups devoted to female cultivation. There is a listing of Qigong organizations in the references at the back of this book. Alternatively, readers can contact the National Qigong Association.

Generally, the goal in sexual Qigong for women is to stimulate and sustain youthfulness and foster a long and healthy life. According to Chinese medicine Jing regulates your sexual hormones. If Jing is low, sexual hormones can't regulate themselves, no matter what a person's age is. Qigong helps to retain the Jing, which contributes to the store of inner medicine. Given that women do not lose as much Qi in the sexual act as men, there is less literature about female sexual Qigong. The most important point is that normal sexual interaction and orgasm with a loving partner is a very powerful way to build Qi.

The Masculine: Yang

For men the challenge of mastering the sexual aspect of the Conserve Qi phase of cultivation is a major undertaking. The writings of Master Sun Simiao, one of China's most famous physicians, are heavily laced with wisdom on all phases of Qi cultivation, including the sexual aspect of the Conserve Qi phase.

> *When a man is in his youth,*
> *he does not usually understand Dao.*
> *If he does hear of Dao, he is not likely to believe fully or practice it.*
> *However, when he reaches vulnerable old age,*
> *he will realize the significance of Dao.*
> *Then it is too late,*
> *for he has lost most of the vitality necessary*
> *to cultivate Dao.*

—SUN SIMIAO, *PRESCRIPTIONS WORTH A THOUSAND OUNCES OF GOLD*,
SEVENTH CENTURY

In the vitality of youth, the human body produces so much semen, the male aspect of Jing that is spent in sexual ejaculation, that it is practically overflowing. Young men frequently have "wet dreams," engage in repeated masturbation, and can have sexual interactions with numerous ejaculations in the period of just a few hours. This is an overt demonstration of the robust amount of inner resources that are available in the youthful human system driving this high level of semen production. However, by the age of forty or fifty the capacity to replenish spent semen is significantly altered. Many men feel drained after having sexual encounters that include ejaculation.

The cultural myth in the West is that strong men can have loads of sex with no consequence. What the Chinese figured out through their centuries of attentive observation is very different. In fact, most men, if they are honest, will admit that their capacity falls off significantly after the age of fifty. The Chinese insight: the earlier in life that men begin to conserve sexual resources, the longer they will have dynamic sex and the greater their general vitality and longevity will be. This practice of conservation leads to actual increases in personal energy and stamina.

In the Chinese view, the immense amount of Qi required to produce an ample reserve of semen after ejaculation can actually be conserved to produce the inner elixir (Nei Dan). Through sexual cultivation, particularly through the withholding of ejaculation, a person can conserve sexual resources and produce inner elixir to increase health and even cure disease. Traditionally, for many diseases Chinese doctors recommend sexual interaction without orgasm as a healing practice.

How is it possible, you may be wondering, to have sex without ejaculation? You may also be thinking that such sex may not be very desirable and that the women are being deprived. Prepare to be astounded again by the incredible breakthrough thinking of the ancient Chinese scientists of long life and vitality. It actually turns out, for those who pursue this aspect of Qi cultivation, that it is a huge win for both of the lovers. Men in their fifties and sixties (and even older) can have frequent sexual encounters with their partners and numerous, very inspiring climaxes by having ejaculation only rarely.

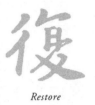

Restore

The language is very important here. Most men see the whole sex act as a run for the finish line of orgasm. Look more closely—there are multiple components of the sexual encounter. For both of the partners there are actually a number of possible climaxes, which are like peaks or rushes. These prejaculative rushes, multiple climaxes, are often at least as wonderful and more lasting than the final orgasm. Finally, there is orgasm, with the ejaculation of semen and sperm by the male. Most people have never even thought of this, but men can have all of the sexual experience, with foreplay and numerous climaxes plus the complete satisfaction of their partners, and still reserve the ejaculation to conserve Jing and Qi—two critical internal treasures.

In the sexual cultivation aspect of the Conserve Qi phase you gain the capacity to say no to ejaculation while saying yes to all the wonderful components of sexual activity. This is an ultimate form of HeartMind Qigong. It requires a significant amount of internal focus, practice, self-understanding, and communication with your lover. One bit of encouragement: once you have cultivated this capacity you will find that you pass a threshold in the love-making process where you can continue vigorous intercourse with almost no sense that you will lose it. This sort of Qigong will have far-reaching effects in your relationship and in your personal vitality.

Some may make the argument that this type of sexual activity is not as much fun. Have you ever wondered how emperors and tribal chiefs who had harems, with many consorts or concubines, were able to have so many sexual encounters? They are having a lot of sex and lots of climaxes, but they are only having occasional ejaculations.

Would you rather have sex occasionally and feel wasted or have sex frequently and not feel wasted but replenished? Unlimited sex with no depletion is very attractive, isn't it? What about the idea that this approach may be less desirable for women? As a doctor of Chinese medicine one of the most frequent complaints that I hear from women is that their lovers ejaculate and then fall asleep, frequently without providing satisfaction.

Women whose husbands or lovers have discovered these Chinese sexual arts typically are very happy. Sex lasts longer and it involves more subtle interaction and a lot more communication, the very things that women seek in a relationship. Men who don't ejaculate at every loving encounter stay awake and continue to be affectionate even after the woman is satisfied. In other words, women in relationships with men who practice sexual Qigong are enthusiastic proponents.

For men, engaging in frequent sexual interaction, particularly with a loving partner, is excellent for cultivating Qi and sustained health. Master Sun also said, "If you make love one hundred times without emission you will easily attain longevity." In *The Secrets of the Jade Chamber*, a classic book on the "bedroom arts," the Yellow Emperor gets some advice from Su Nu, his female advisor on sexual Qigong: "Love once without losing semen, it will strengthen your body. Twice improves vision and hearing. Three times without emission, diseases disappear. Four times, you will have peace of your soul." She continues through five, six, seven, and eight, and then says, "At nine times with no emission you will access longevity. At ten times, you attain immortality."

There are special and unusual practices in addition to this basic method of cultivation. Several writers on Qi cultivation have claimed that having the ejaculation but retaining the semen internally by applying pressure to the *Hui Yin* point between the scrotum and the anus is a Conserve Qi method with merit. You might try this a time or two as it is an amazing technique to experience, but this is not suggested as a regular practice. It has caused urinary tract complications in a number of men that I have communicated with. Like the Deer Exercise for women, there is much debate on the use of this method and I urge caution.

As in the sexual practices for women, the most important point is this—normal sexual interaction with a loving partner is a powerful Qi cultivation method for men. However, frequent sex with ejaculation can be a cause for severe depletion. But sexual cultivation with the retention of the Jing is a major Conserve Qi practice that actually helps to create a profound inner elixir.

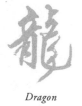

Dragon

The Simple Rule

Our rule in this book has been to keep it simple when possible. Chang Yi Hsiang proposed this sexual guideline for women: "The most important method for women is to act on the fact that they are especially vulnerable for losing Qi to stress and overwork during their menstrual period. The sexual cultivation focus should be to sustain a happy sense of peace. They should also carefully develop mild Qigong practices for this period as intense Qigong can be counterproductive. This plus loving sexual activity is powerful sexual Qigong for women. For postmenopausal women, please understand that the best strategy is to conserve at all times—not just a few days a month. The challenge for the woman is to be able to communicate about her commitment to be conservative during the menstrual period with her loved ones and associates."

What about the simple rule for men? Tang Yi Fan, the chief of rehabilitation medicine at the Hangzhou Medical University, has a very practical approach to Qigong. "There are many exaggerations that have developed around the mystery of sexual Qigong. If you eliminate all of that, it is very simple. Men can lose a large amount of Qi in the emission of semen and a major amount of Qi is required to replenish the natural semen reserve. Paradoxically, significant enhancement of Qi occurs through sexual interaction. So the formula is easy: have a lot of sex but do not lose it. Probably the most powerful single form of Qigong is having sex in a calm (Yin) yet excited (Yang) state. This creates harmony of Yin and Yang in a very dynamic way."

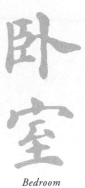

Bedroom

Successful cultivation of sexual Qigong requires that the frequency of ejaculation be calculated carefully and that climax only include ejaculation at a rate that allows for a net gain of Qi wealth over time. Dr. Tang stated a formula for how to calculate when ejaculation does not compromise Qi wealth. "Everyone is different, so the formulas in the ancient books do not take into account variations; they are more like averages. Simply become aware of how long it takes you to feel fully vital after an ejaculation, then never have ejaculation without allowing that time span to elapse. It is important to communicate your plan to your spouse or lover.

"A younger man may replenish after two days. So the formula for him might be to go ahead and have sex every day but only ejaculate on the third or fourth day. This allows for two days where the Jing and Qi are free to focus on inner healing. For an older man who is aware that he feels fully replenished only after a week or so, he might have sex every few days but conserve emission for two to three weeks. The sexual encounters that a man has after replenishing but before the next ejaculation are powerful sexual Qigong practice sessions. Healthy older men who intend to cultivate longevity could easily have sex once or several times a week or month, but might ejaculate only once or twice a year or even not at all. Remember to have lots of sex because it is very healthy; just don't lose the treasure."

Accumulate Qi to Cultivate Elixir

Careful choice making and the practice of Qi-conserving behaviors form the gateway to the highest levels of cultivation. In gaining the ability to master the Qi management arts you will learn to redesign yourself. You may drive the same car, live in the same house, and answer to the same name, but at an essential level you will actually be reborn. Conserve Qi is like a birth canal to what the Chinese refer to as becoming innocent like a baby who has just been born—with no cares. This is known as mastering HeartMind Qigong and qualifying to practice Heaven or Spirit Qigong in which you are reborn in a very special way. In the Heaven Phases you will give birth to the awareness of the eternal spirit child within you. This is your immortal self.

The threshold to Spirit Qigong is more about choices and behaviors than specific Qigong methods. To cultivate the Golden Elixir in the Heaven phases you must accumulate your inner resource. To accumulate Qi you must conserve Qi. Beyond a conscious Qigong practice, Qi cultivation at the higher levels requires the management of personal resources by cultivating a moment-to-moment capacity to choose to conserve and protect the Qi. As you conserve and protect, particularly in conjunction with purifying, you accumulate high-quality pure Qi. This accumulated resource becomes the primary ingredient in the practices in the storing and transforming phases to follow.

Qigong Method to Conserve Qi

Watching Clouds Pass

HISTORICAL REFLECTION Watching Clouds Pass is part of all classic Tai Chi traditions. In the martial application of Tai Chi Chuan (*Taiji Quan*), this movement of the hands and arms is a block for incoming punches. For health and enlightenment, your hands are like clouds. The movement goes by many names, such as Hands Like Clouds and Cloud Hands. When asked to name their favorite Tai Chi movement people almost always mention Watching Clouds Pass.

Imagine you and your best friend are lying on a grassy hillside on a perfect day watching big puffy clouds pass by. You say, "That one looks like a dragon flying." And your friend says, "That one looks like a pioneer wagon with four horses pulling it." You are each purely in the present. Past and future have collapsed into this moment. You have no place to go, nothing to make happen, nothing to keep track of—you are simply watching clouds pass.

The benefit of relaxing into the present is extraordinary. The Qi masters say that direct access to fresh Qi can only happen in the present. The past is gone and likely laden with regrets and unfulfilled aspirations. The future looms in an anxiety-producing unknown. When you have surrendered to the present, the channels open and the inner flow is free of restraint. Because it takes you out of busyness and complexity and into calm openness, Watching Clouds Pass is the perfect practice for conserving Qi.

INSTRUCTION Starting with the opening posture, breathe slowly and relax. Allow the right hand to make a circle. Do this a few times. Drop the right hand gently down the right side, pass the belly to the left, raise your hand up the left side until your hand is to the left of your face. Now, the palm of your hand passes in front of your face. Imagine that it is a cloud passing. Make this circle with the right hand a few times. The hand should be relaxed with the fingers gently curved and the wrist relaxed and flexible.

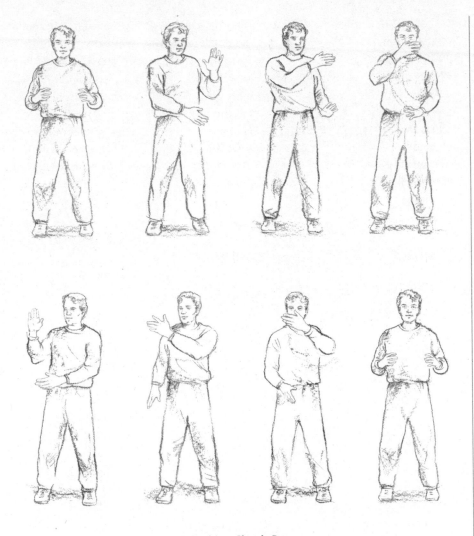

Watching Clouds Pass

Now do the same with the left hand, down the left, across the belly to the right, up the right to the right of the face and eyes, then passing like a cloud before your face. Do this a few times. Next you will coordinate these two. When the right hand cloud is passing from the left of your face to the right, the left hand is passing the belly to the right also, below. As the right hand then continues down on the right, the left hand is coming up. When the left hand cloud is passing from the right of your face to the left, the right hand is passing the belly to the left below. As the left hand now drops down on the left, the right hand is rising up the left getting ready to be your next cloud.

This gentle motion requires some alert mind focus to learn at first. We are conserving Qi, so don't bother getting tense. Look for someone to practice with and make this fun. Eventually, it becomes second nature and you can sink into the blissful perspective of watching clouds pass.

Mind Focus Affirmation

Conserving Qi, I protect my inner essence and accumulate the subtle ingredients for refining the inner elixir.

Phase 7: Store Qi

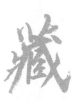

In the state of concentration,
when the light first arises,
make sure to hold onto it
and never let it go.
There will be nothing within
that would not be brilliantly illuminated
and the one hundred diseases will be driven out.

—TAI PING JING CHAO, *SELECTIONS FROM THE SCRIPTURE
OF GREAT PEACE*

It is a perfect misty morning in the Chinese mountains. Everyone along the trail is friendly and lighthearted. As our small group travels farther from the training center, the trail becomes steeper.

About an hour up the trail we round a bend to find a flat open space between the slope of the mountain and a small stream. We stop suddenly seeing a bareheaded man dressed in gray leaping about. We step back into the full cover of the shrubs to watch. Perhaps this is one of those hermit monks that we have been reading and hearing about. His dress is less well tended than the monks in the temple. He does not wear robes but his clothing is the same color gray as the traditional dress in the community of Buddhist monks. We have heard that there are some Buddhist monasteries here in the mountains and that many of the monks live purposefully isolated in nature.

Store Qi

He leaps and crouches, kicks and punches. He appears to be middle-aged but is as flexible as the younger students we have seen practicing at the training center. He seems to be acting out an epic story; in one moment he appears to be in battle and then in the next it seems that he has been transformed into a huge bird or perhaps a flying dragon. Then he slows down and performs a beautiful set of Tai Chi–like movements, clearly focusing on circulating and centering the energy that has been stirred up during the earlier part of the form. Every movement emerges from his center—even the footwork. Every extension of his arms and hands is like the waving of a large flag on a flexible pole deep within his torso.

Monk

His movements take him to the edge of the stream where he stands and begins to reach out and gather Qi (Chi) from the water, the mountains, and the sky. It is as if he is bathing in invisible healing resources from nature and storing them. He repeats the gathering and bathing movements fifteen times and then settles into a standing meditation. He stands absolutely still for about ten minutes and then closes his practice. What an incredible gift it is to witness this.

The next morning after our practice session it is clear that Eternal Spring is excited about the upcoming lessons:

"Now we explore the deepest practices. At the advanced phases of cultivation we actually become more Qi than substance and dissolve into oneness with universal resources. The ancients understood that the Earth level and the HeartMind level of Qigong [Chi Kung] prepare us to achieve an alliance with the natural activity of the universe. Once we have gained the capacity to manage our Qi through the earlier phases it becomes possible to act in complete accord with the universe.

"The Qi that is stored in water as it falls as a river or crashes as a wave, the Qi that is stored in wood that can become fire, and the immense potential of the Qi of the sun—we have the natural capacity to store all of these influences within us. One of my favorite master teachers taught us that through alchemy we become the universe and gain direct access to its power for healing and good works. When you store Qi you are filling yourself with the resources necessary to create the highest medicine—Heaven Elixir, the medicine of the spirit.

"To have automatic access to the energy of the sun and the universe, store Qi. Be like the tree that absorbs Qi and even gives Qi away in the form of seeds and fruit. But the tree is also storing Qi as wood. We know that this stored energy is its strength because of the retained strength of wood that is used to build houses or the fuel inherent in wood that creates fire.

"Plant your roots firmly, be patient, notice that your fruits appear and ripen without any effort, due to your relationship with the seasons that is completely natural and requires no effort. It is a rare person who will actually become like the tree, the water, or the sun. Most people are overexposed to the marketplace and the strains of life. The usual attitude in society is that if you want something to happen, you have to make it happen. The inner teachings of Chinese tradition declare that nothing happens that is not in accord with the highest organizing forces of cosmic design. This is why the most advanced levels of Qigong—Inner Alchemy—are such a mystery. It is only rare individuals who even find their way to this level of Qigong."

The Heaven Level

Most spiritual and religious traditions declare that "Heaven is at hand," which suggests that access to the heavenly domain is always possible. The Chinese Qi masters created special practices and ways of being to access and reveal Spirit. Now we are at the threshold of Dao.

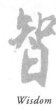

Wisdom

Thousands of years ago the Qi masters, cultivating in their observatories in the sacred mountains, found that the body stores Qi. Contemporary scientists are at long last realizing that this is not just a poetic idea. Contemporary research has found that energy is stored in the body in numerous forms—from body fat and oxygen to ions, electromagnetic energy, and even as invisible light. All of these forms of energy along with consciousness are aspects of the Qi.

In Qigong practice, Store Qi marks the transition from the HeartMind cultivation methods to Heaven cultivation methods. Celestial Qigong, Spiritual Qigong, Universal Qigong are all versions of Qi cultivation that focus on the Heaven phases—Store Qi, Transform Qi, and Dissolve in Qi. In addition, the tenth phase, Transmit Qi, is the most effective when the practitioner is operating at the Heaven level of complete openness.

You can learn about, explore, and practice the Heaven phases of cultivation, even if you are just beginning your Qigong practice. If you have only just begun to cultivate your garden, it is not inappropriate to experiment with unusual varieties of vegetable seeds. It may be disheartening to reach beyond your ability and discover just how much you have to learn. However, it could just as easily be inspiring. You may find yourself more enthusiastically focused on the Purify Qi practices, knowing that they will ultimately benefit your capacity to cultivate the Heaven phases.

You Are Already Perfect in Spirit

It is important to understand that we cannot improve Spirit—Spirit is already perfect. We can only reveal it. In alchemy, rough ingredients are transmuted into gold— through fire. In the Heaven or Spirit level of Qigong you reveal what is already within you buried among your own raw ingredients. Tending the fire can take many forms including caring for your inner fire (metabolic fire and elemental fire related to the heart). It can also be the willingness to bear the fire of experience. The Earth level activates the body potential that is already present, but that may have become deficient or blocked. The HeartMind level reveals the true nature by clearing the consciousness and nervous system of conditioned thinking and emotional disharmony. In the Spirit level there is nothing left to do but radiate your universal and eternal essence.

Storing the Qi

According to the Qi masters, Qi is stored in special areas throughout the body—the primary channels of circulation and storage include the Central Tai Chi Channel, the Twelve Organ Channels, and the Eight Extraordinary Channels. The organs themselves store Qi, as do the Dan Tian—Earth, HeartMind, and Heaven. The names of the Qi points of the lower Dan Tian suggest this—Ocean of Qi (*Qi Hai*) and Gateway of Original Qi (*Guan Yuan*). Another primary storage area is in the marrow. This includes not only the bones, but also the brain, spinal cord, and nerve trunks, believed by the ancients to be like biological batteries in which Qi may be stored.

In the knowledge base of ancient Chinese science, energy, light, and consciousness are all highly refined Yang. Qi is stored with Yin. Extreme Yang is paired, for balance and harmony, with extreme Yin. Yang also tends to link with and travel in the most prevalent Yin resource in the body, water. The main areas of focus for storing Qi are the marrow (hidden deep in the core of the bones, skull, and vertebral column), which is very Yin, and the Lower (Earth) Dan Tian where the highest concentration of lymph (water) in the body is found.

While it is true that the body stores energy naturally, it is also true that electing to seek a higher level of function by storing Qi purposefully requires advanced cultivation skill. It is much easier to gather Qi and circulate Qi; you simply use the Three Intentful Corrections. However, storing Qi requires more. You must have the ability to purify Qi and direct Qi. You must live a lifestyle that fosters conservation, allowing for the accumulation of purified Qi. And you must have the skill to get deeply enough and securely enough into the cultivation state to build the Qi in each of the Dan Tian and to direct the Qi into the storage areas.

Many Qi masters believe that the advanced practices cannot be taught. Store Qi, Transform Qi, and Dissolve in Qi are advanced stages of Qigong. Progress at this level of Qigong is largely due to personal internal discovery through practice.

Because of the nature of Heaven Qigong, storing Qi and transforming Qi can really only happen when you have mastered the HeartMind phases. To practice at the Heaven level, your universal nature must be present and awake; distraction, worry, judgment, desire, and an agenda with great expectations all sabotage the effect. Practice doesn't *create* your Spirit; cultivation *reveals* your Spirit. Inner Alchemy is the practice of accepting and surrendering to nature, or *Wu Wei*. In Wu Wei—translated as doing not doing, or nonaction—we have so fully cleared inner resistance and opened so fully to flow that the inner light of pure Spirit radiates spontaneously.

> *Hidden within is vitality and light.*
> *How does the Master express this truth?*
> *By allowing it to be so.*

—Lao Zi, *Dao De Jing*, #21

Even in the earliest levels of Qigong there is something to *do*. In Earth Qigong we cultivate through the Three Intentful Corrections. In HeartMind Qigong we cultivate through intention and will. In the later stages, the essence of cultivation takes us deeper into being. To access Heaven Qigong we must lift ourselves up through the HeartMind phases, where the hardest work of Qi cultivation will take place. In the Heaven phases there is even less to *do* because in Spirit you are already perfect. These phases are more devoted to accepting or surrendering to a highly refined version of yourself—radiating the hidden splendor that was always there.

The Practice

In the Heaven phases the practices for storing, transforming, and dissolving in Qi are more internal. We will explore specific methods, but it is very important to know that at the Spirit level there is much less external practice than in the earlier phases. Body and breath methods are very useful in the earlier phases. Simply moving about, eating wisely, and resting can cause the Qi to circulate and purify. In the Heaven phases the methods can be used as reminders, but it is really the way you react to situations in your life that shows the level of cultivation you have achieved.

If you use the methods described in this and the next two chapters but are stressed or habitually distracted, the truth is that you will not be able to make the transition to the Heaven level. It is a very rare person who has authentically progressed to Heaven Qigong without much sincere cultivation, so don't get busy judging yourself. There is no law that says you can't explore Heaven while you cultivate Earth.

Qigong Method to Store Qi

Bathing the Marrow

HISTORICAL REFLECTION This method has both ancient and historic roots. Long before any written record of Qigong, this simple yet deeply profound method was used in ancient China as well as other prehistoric cultures.

Root

In historic terms this method is a central aspect of the Bathing the Marrow practice that was reputed to be developed at the Shaolin Temple. Bodhidharma is credited with creating this form. However, several of the Daoist streams have also used Bathing the Marrow for many centuries. We know that one of the most famous Daoist observatories was located in the Song Mountains near the Shaolin Temple, so it is very likely true that the method has a Daoist and even pre-Daoist shamanic origin.

There are numerous versions or forms of the Bathing the Marrow method depending on whether it is a Buddhist version, a Daoist version, or a version modified for healing or building martial power. My favorite is called the Four Seasons Method of Absorbing and Storing the World. It is similar to the Native American Medicine Wheel;

Four Seasons Correspondences of Absorbing and Storing the World

Direction	Season	Time	Plant	Focus	Life	Organ
East	Spring	Morning/Dawn	Sprout	Beginning	Birth/Child	Liver
South	Summer	Noon/Bright	Bloom/Fruit	Work	Adult	Heart
West	Fall	Afternoon/Dusk	Harvest	Reward	Elder	Lung
North	Winter	Night/Dark	Seed	Rest	Rebirth	Kidney
Center	Whole Year	All Time	All Phases	All Focus	Every Age	Spleen

it draws on the four directions plus Heaven and Earth and stores the powers or forces of the seasons, and all of the natural qualities of plants—seed, sprout, fruit, and harvest—in the marrow of the bones. In this version you do the Bathing the Marrow practice to the four directions.

In contemporary science we now know that the marrow produces all blood cells and immune cells. The only exception is T-cells, which are produced in the thymus gland. The Chinese did not know this. But they knew that the marrow was so important they developed an entire Qigong methodology to enhance and refine it. Why? How? The earliest Chinese physicians were in awe of the deepest, most hidden, most mysterious part of the human system, the marrow, which is buried in and protected by bone. In Chinese tradition Mystery is good; it is the source of everything. The mysterious hidden marrow was understood as an important inner source.

When you face each of the directions and gather these qualities, store them in the bones, organs, and Dan Tian to be used as medicine—extra resource that you can call upon to prevent disease and be more vital in times when you need extra inner strength.

INSTRUCTION From the opening posture, open your arms, reach out into the universe; this is a good time to take a deep breath. Gather from the resources that surround us—air, water, mountains, plant life, space, influences of stars and planets, the prayers of loved ones, the best wishes of departed philosophers and saints, and universal love. Bathe yourself in those influences as your hands pass your head, your face, and your torso. Send these essences to be stored in the marrow of your bones. Do this as many times as seems reasonable.

Many people use this as a meditation for gratitude. Of course the point is always to relax deeply. With each gathering you acknowledge and celebrate an item on your gratitude list. As your hands are passing the body you are sending these positive influences in through the surface of the body to the channels of the Qi Matrix, the Elixir Fields, the organs, and, most importantly, into the marrow of the bones. To conclude the movement, bring your hands to rest over the Earth Elixir Field and just drift there for a few moments.

To do the Four Seasons Method of Absorbing and Storing the World continue with this practice facing the four directions. As you face the east focus on the sunrise,

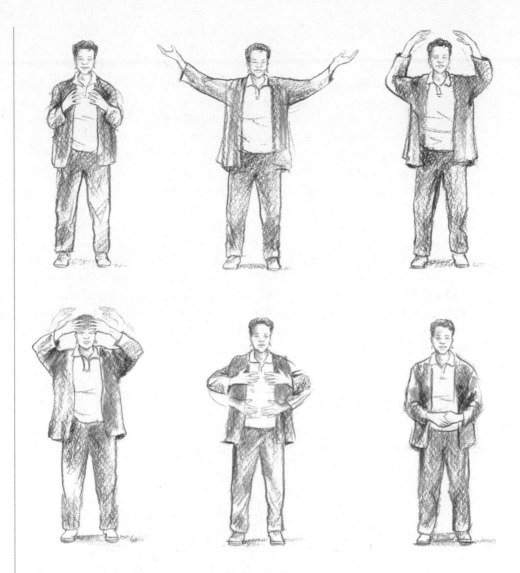

Bathing the Marrow

the powerful energy of the beginning of a relationship or a project, the strength of the sprout as it breaks out of the seed reaching up into Heaven and down into Earth. Send these energies and influences into the bones to be stored.

As you face the south focus on the immense force of the sun and what it causes in nature. The sweet juice pours into the fruit as it ripens, work gets done, the world is bright and full of light. This is the season of vigilance and accomplishment. Send that energy to be stored in the bones.

Face the west and relax as the heat of midday cools off, the harvest is assured, the fruit is ripe. This is the time of reward. Imagine relaxing after a hard day of work. This is where you get paid, where you recognize and celebrate your accomplishments; it is the season of the harvest and thanksgiving. Send these energies to be stored in the marrow of the bones.

To the north is the most profound season. It is the time of rest, redesign, and rebirth. What is going on in the seed that waits in the ground during winter? It seems like nothing, stillness. Stillness yes, but not nothing. The seed is busy, quietly absorbing celestial influences. This is the season when we make tea and write poems, the season when we stop and take some time out to get the bigger picture before the next beginning. Store these forces and influences in the marrow.

Notice that you are now ready to face the east again. Are you the same person who faced the east moments ago? The implication in Qigong is that these seasons are turning at every moment throughout the days, months, seasons, years, eras. The intention is to celebrate transition and change at the same time you gather the radical resources of nature and life and store them internally as ingredients for making the ultimate inner medicine. The ancients declared that you can reverse time and access your eternal nature by reversing the direction. Instead of turning from east to south (spring to summer), go the other direction, from east to north (spring to winter). In a deep state of meditation this turns time backward and gives you access to your prebirth self, when your body was flexible and your HeartMind clear and innocent.

Mind Focus Affirmation

Storing Qi, I create, maximize, and sustain an inner reserve of potential to optimize my health, life, and being.

12

Phase 8:
Transform Qi

*Our health is derived from the Yang
    of the prenatal inner world,
        constantly accumulated and refined over time.
    Through this cultivation we are transformed
        to reflect our eternal nature.*

—MASTER SHANG YANG, COMMENTARY ON THE CAN
    TONG QI, TWELFTH CENTURY C.E.

Every evening at about nine we hear three deep sounding gongs toll from the temple building near the center of the training complex. There are five minutes between these gong tolls. Tonight we decide to have a look. Following the cobblestone alleyway through the maze of buildings, we walk into the courtyard near the temple just as the gong is struck for the third time. Large red lamps cast a dim but rich and mysterious glow.

The sky is extraordinarily clear. Here, high in the mountains and far from civilization, the number of stars is astounding. The immense expanse of universal space above us causes a stirring of the Qi (Chi). We decide to take the opportunity to practice some of the Qigong (Chi Kung) that we have been learning.

Align—adjust your posture, deepen your breath, clear your mind.
Become aware of Heaven above—vast, open, boundless.
Become aware of Earth below—solid, dense, contained.

Transform Qi

Absorb Heaven into the upper Dan Tian.
Absorb Earth into the lower Dan Tian.
Open the Central Tai Chi Channel and allow Heaven and Earth to mix in the
    HeartMind.

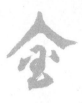

Golden Elixir

Just as we are about to begin the opening movement, we become aware that across the courtyard, in the dark, someone else is practicing. Perhaps it is one of the Qigong masters from the temple. He or she—we cannot tell which—is doing a beautiful form that has the grace of Tai Chi (Taiji) but appears much simpler. We sense the excitement as we realize that we could easily follow along for a private lesson in some secret Qigong form in silent agreement with this teacher we will probably never know.

The figure is barely visible in the soft glow of the lamps. Slowly we work our way closer, and continue to follow the movements of the teacher as well as possible. He or she seems to be encouraging us to continue and so we do. We sink down, gather Qi of Earth, and reach up to gather Qi of Heaven. Our hands pass in front of the heart as if to bathe away tension, followed by a movement that looks as if we are offering the calm heart outward to others. The lesson continues for quite a while. We experience a deep sense of gratitude for this moment. We realize that the practice is concluding as our teacher reaches out, gathering from the universe in the closing movement. He or she bows gently, nearly invisible in the dim glow of the red lamps, steps back into the shadows, and disappears.

The next day, after morning practice and breakfast, Jade Unity declares in his forceful yet soft voice:

"Transform Qi is where the most important cultivation of Spirit Qigong occurs—where Inner Alchemy takes place. Transform Qi is the alchemical firing. This is where the reversal of fire and water takes place, surpassing the usual. While it is usual for Yang fire and openness to be above and Yin water and density to be below, through the Transform Qi phase Yang fire of Heaven and Yin water of Earth do an amazing reversal. The Yang is now below and the Yin above, creating the conditions necessary for the practitioner to transcend the physical limitations and be fully aware of and expressive of the radiant soul. The practitioner, through Inner Alchemy in the ancient Chinese tradition, becomes immortal—meaning aware of, immersed in, and expressive of his or her eternal nature.

"Let me tell you the legend of Master Shen. Even as a child he was interested in gathering healing ingredients with his grandmother who taught him about the medicinal powers of herbs. He always asked to be told the stories of the legendary immortals—known in Chinese tradition as the Eight Immortals. He eventually became a physician and was a compassionate healer. His success was based on the fact that he understood that within all beings is not only the local, personal self but also the universal self. His acupuncture and herbal treatments were always directed by that knowledge. He always taught his patients to practice Qigong and Tai Chi.

"When Master Shen completed his household phase of life as a husband and father, he retreated to China's sacred mountains. He took up residence in a humble hermitage. He collected the freshest plants and herbs from the slopes and valleys. He found the purest spring for water. He established in his kitchen a carefully designed cooking fire and cooking vessel. He made powerful formulas and discovered 'secret' ingredients and special processes. Master Shen cultivated a refined state of mind, heart, and spirit. He eventually found the formula for the Golden Elixir of Immortality. They say that, like the Yellow Emperor and many of the great immortals, he ascended into heaven riding on the back of a dragon [the Chinese symbol of spirituality and eternal life].

"This is a metaphoric story about us all. Old Master Shen's story reveals our process of Inner Alchemy. When he moves to the mountains it represents our decision to cultivate and refine our nature by limiting distractions. The gathering of ingredients signifies becoming aware of what is necessary for our cultivation including nourishment, Qigong, and the ability to say no to activities and people that drain our Qi. The water is not only the water we drink but the Yin aspects of ourselves, like rest and meditation. The fire is our intention, focus, and will. The kitchen and the cooking vessel are the body and the inner cauldron, specifically the middle Dan Tian, where Yin and Yang merge in harmony, the HeartMind center. When Master Shen discovers secret ingredients and processes, it is the learning and practicing of the Ten Phases of Cultivation and Mastery. When Master Shen cultivates the HeartMind and Spirit, it is our realization of how to rise above the habits and conditioning of the body and mind. When he makes the Golden Elixir, it is our ability to sustain a centered and calm state in the midst of life's wild ride. When Master Shen ascends to heaven on the dragon, it represents our potential to awaken to our ultimate spiritual nature."

It is a tradition in China to use these metaphors. The large universe is related to our personal smaller universe, the body and the consciousness are a personal observatory likened to a research laboratory or institutional observatory, ingredients from the world are associated with inner ingredients, and pure gold is associated with our highest self. The history of this man named Shen, which means "Spirit," is representative of the story of each of our lives—in cultivation.

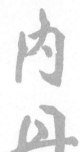

Inner Alchemy

Transforming the Qi

With purification, accumulation, and storage of Qi, the human system becomes a vessel filled with powerful universal resources. This is highly refined Qi. In terms of cultivation the body now becomes the alchemical vessel, the cauldron for making the Golden Elixir.

One of the most profound yet least understood promises of Qi is associated with the Three Treasures—Jing, Qi, and Shen—which are equivalent to Earth, Life, and

Heaven. This promise is stated in numerous proverbs and aphorisms from ancient writings. Here is one example:

> *Conserve Jing and transform it into Qi.*
> *Maximize and transform Qi to create Shen.*
> *Transform Shen to Dao.*
> *This is the supreme practice.*

—Traditional Chinese wisdom, from a multitude of texts over many dynasties

Qigong for healing and longevity, activated from the preliminary practices up through Conserve Qi, focuses on Jing and Qi. The Heaven phases focus on Shen and Dao. In the earlier phases, the medicine within is cultivated to heal and cleanse the body, mind, and emotions. In the Transform Qi phase this medicine is transformed into Spirit medicine. Ultimate Spirit is never sick, so this is not medicine *to heal* the soul. Rather, it is medicine that reveals the soul—our eternal self.

In this level of the practice, the veil between our forgetful local self and our super conscious universal self is pierced. Ancient and contemporary Qi masters agree that, as Zhu Hui said, "In Qigong we open ourselves to the outpouring of virtue and beneficence from Heaven and Earth."

Transformation of Qi into Spirit and the rebirth of the self into a new being is the essence of Qigong. Once transformation occurs you are liberated to dissolve in Qi. In the Chinese story of transformation and Inner Alchemy, the practitioner realizes over time the merit and worth of full immersion in the super state of pure universal awareness and openness. You cultivate awareness of your universal nature to heal the split between the local self and the universal self. Because the universal self is eternal, you gain immortality, the awareness of your eternal nature.

Transformation creates a self beyond the body that is born and exists as a transcendental or heavenly aspect of your being. Transforming the Qi not only refines, enhances, and heals the local self but also opens the gateway of conscious awareness of your Spirit self by transmuting Qi into Shen.

Master Ge Hong refers to this state of transformation, "You will never know exhaustion, fire will not burn you, water cannot drown you, no wild beasts will harm you, creatures will not attack you, and you will be free of fear of demons or poisonous insects, ghosts will not approach nor the blade strike." This is like becoming conscious of your unseen eternal self that can never be harmed, and then living henceforth from the point of view of that eternal self.

Transforming Qi Through Alchemical Firing

How can we achieve this sense of immortality? The ancients use the image of alchemical firing to explain it. Alchemy has an ancient history in China. In both China and Europe, alchemy was the predecessor to what we now call chemistry. In alchemy the transformation is created through heating or firing a secret set of ingredients to create a profound inner elixir. The more advanced the alchemy the more subtle the ingredients.

In the Heaven level of Qigong we use these secret ingredients to produce the Golden Elixir, which transforms our conditioned and habitual nature into a highly refined and enlightened self. Many ancient teachings give formulas for creating the Golden Elixir that gives the practitioner access to ultimate knowledge and truth. In alchemy the highest result is to make gold, to become aware of and act from one's pure eternal nature. In China we call the person who succeeds at Inner Alchemy an immortal. This is not a person who lives forever in their current physical body, but rather it is someone who lives and expresses his or her eternal nature. Actualizing one's boundless, universal self is immortality.

Legends about Inner Alchemy abound. In most the practitioner retreats to the mountains where the environment is conducive to elixir making. The practitioner gets closer to Heaven by going higher up. He or she has access to nature and quiet; pure water and air; clear views of the sun, moon, and stars; and freedom from the distractions of the complex world below. He or she carefully collects the elixir ingredients by eating a healing diet complete with herbs and tea. Through the fire of sincere and intentful cultivation these ingredients purify to reveal the true self of pure gold. Through our own experience of the inspiring beauty of nature, exploring our feelings, and shaking out and resolving emotional trauma we too can make this Golden Spiritual Elixir. Stored Qi is a primary ingredient in the transforming process.

The Transform Qi method below is one of many methods that are representative of Alchemy practice. There is an illusion that you can learn to make Spirit Elixir. My most revered teachers have shared that the elixir makes itself when you be a certain way. You cannot do the making of the Golden Elixir. You can only become more capable of understanding how it is naturally produced and then purposefully allow that to occur through "the way" that you be.

Spirit Gate

Qigong Method to Transform Qi

Immortal Dragon Cultivating Golden Elixir

HISTORICAL REFLECTION This practice depicts an immortal dragon cultivating the Golden Elixir by transforming stored Qi. The dragon is the Chinese symbol of universal wisdom and immortality. It is associated with primordial nature and the origin of the universe. This Qigong method comes from a form called Primordial Qigong (Wuji Qigong). It is said to have been developed by Zhang San Feng who created Tai Chi (Taiji), a Daoist Qi master. From the first time I experienced Primordial Qigong it impressed me as a profound elixir practice. I currently use this method and teach it frequently.

The Primordial Qigong form is easy to practice and yet it has many unusual qualities. One of these is that the form promises to reverse time. It does this by reversing

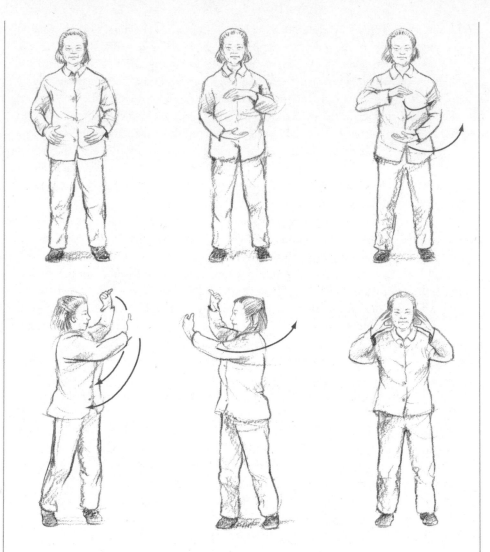

Immortal Dragon Cultivating Golden Elixir

your progression as you face the four directions. As you do the segments of the practice, you turn to the right, which is consistent with our usual perception of the passage of time—the clock, the seasons. However, in the primary movements of the form you turn to the left. Energetically, this reverses the passage of time and takes you back toward your prenatal or original state—the state of pure health and pure spirit.

This Immortal Dragon segment of Primordial Qigong is simple; you face only one direction. There are two familiar components to keep in mind as you are learning and practicing Transform Qi—the Microcosmic Orbit, which we discussed in Direct Qi, and reversal of Yin and Yang, which we discussed earlier in this chapter. As you are

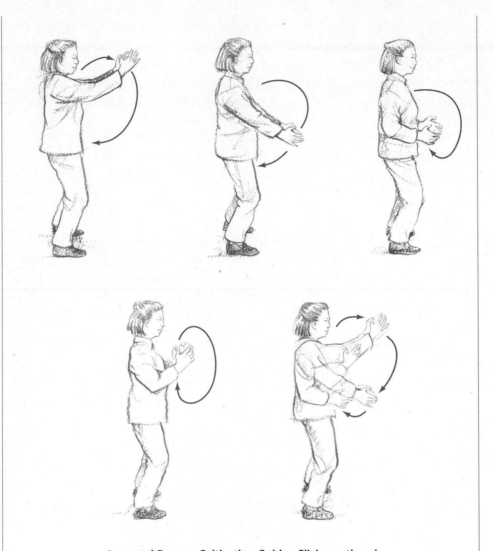

Immortal Dragon Cultivating Golden Elixir, continued

doing this practice link it to the Microcosmic Orbit as the illustration suggests. You will eventually get a feel for how this associates with reversal as well. In reversal what happens is that the fire represented by Yang, which characteristically rises and is positioned above, is purposefully directed below. The water represented by Yin, which characteristically descends and is positioned below, is purposefully directed to rise. In nature water and fire separate. In Alchemy they rise and fall into each other. This transcends nature. It creates the refined and purified steam—essence—of the Heaven Elixir. One clue to the effectiveness of your practice is reversing your responses to news, opportunities, challenges, expectations, and habits. Before alchemical reversal news matters; after, news is less important. Before reversal expectations run one's life; after, expectations carry less weight. This is not an easy assignment, but one that is well worth exploring.

INSTRUCTION   Align the Central Tai Chi Channel and the three Elixir Fields. Form the Qi Ball as in Discover Qi and begin turning it around. Carry it up to the right and to the left. After you have become comfortable with this movement, you can allow it to become more spontaneous and free flowing. Then come to the center, holding the Qi in front of your face like a crystal ball. If you get into a deep enough relaxation and a state that is free of projections, preferences, and expectations you can use this crystal ball to get intuitive insights. Ask the question that has been on your mind; do it without caring what the answer is. When you do this in the deep Qigong state you can hear the voice of your eternal nature.

Gently push the ball away, then lower it to the level of the umbilical area. Now bring it closer, raise it to the level of the heart, and sink into a meditation that can easily lead you into the next phase, Dissolve in Qi. This last gesture, as seen in the second set of movements, represents the cycle of the Microcosmic Orbit.

Mind Focus Affirmation

Transforming Qi, I am changed deeply, expressing my eternal nature and unlimited potential.

13

Phase 9:
Dissolve in Qi

Secrets within secrets,
Wonders within wonders,
Mysteries within mysteries—
The gateway to deepest knowing.

—LAO ZI, *DAO DE JING*, 500 B.C.E.

Our teachers have mentioned on several occasions that the best time to practice the most advanced forms of Qigong (Chi Kung) is deep in the night. The Yang and active nature of the daytime concludes at sunset and the sounds of civilization are quiet. In these mountains the silence is immense. The flow of celestial energies is strong and the stars are clear.

A small group of the students has decided to practice Qigong at night to experience this special time for elixir making. Our friend Yi Xin will lead us to a new place where we can see the Big Dipper. We have been sleeping only lightly in anticipation and at midnight we arise, dress in a few layers, and slip out into the cool night. The group is gathered at the entry terrace of the training center. The stars are so bright that we can see our shadows, even in the dark. Yi Xin suggests that we use the walk to the practice site as a form of stair-climbing Qigong—clearing the mind, moving the body smoothly and rhythmically. He suggests using Xi, Xi, Hu breathing (see page 48), as it builds Qi and stamina. We start off in a different direction than usual on a section of the granite staircase that climbs steeply upward. As we ascend we allow ourselves to slip into the Qigong state that Yi Xin recommended.

Dissolve in Qi

Stars

After quite a while the dome of the heavens opens before us as we step out onto a natural plateau. The sense of exposure to the immensity and the raw energy of the universe is awe inspiring. There are higher peaks to the northeast and northwest. Directly to the north, in the valley between the peaks, we can see the North Star and the bright Big Dipper wheeling around it. It is obvious that this spot has been used for centuries to view the heavens, particularly the northern sky. To the east and west the mountain peaks are lower, providing a perfect view for sun- and moonrise and sun- and moonset. Eight almost perfectly square stones are set in a circle. The three of our tiny group and Yi Xin take seats facing the North Star. Yi Xin speaks quietly:

"As you can see, the ancients used this site as a vantage point to study the heavens and draw upon the Qi [Chi] of the universe. This place is an astronomical observatory. From here the sun, the most profound resource for life, can be absorbed just as it arises or as it sets. On the day of a full moon, the moon rises just at the moment that the sun sets. Yang sinking to the west and Yin rising in the east is one of the most powerful moments in which to make inner elixir. At that time you can face the north, the direction of deep tranquility, and reach out to the right to grasp the moon at the east horizon just rising and simultaneously reach out to the left to grasp the sun, just setting. It is a truly profound time for cultivation.

"But mostly the ancients came here to marvel at the Big Dipper and the North Star. It seemed to them that the earth, the sun, the moon, and all of the stars turned around the central North Star. More recent science has demonstrated that this perception is actually created by Earth's rotation. However, it remains true that Earth has a very special relationship with the North Star. Earth is constantly turning on an axis with the part of the heaven that lies in that direction. It is perceived as the most important place in the cosmos by many of the ancient cultures and early navigators. In the ancient Daoist view, the poles of Heaven and Earth are like the poles within the body. In the universe of yourself, the North Star is above you and the Big Dipper turns around your Heaven Elixir Field. In fact, many of the acupuncture points on the head are associated with stars. It is believed that the North Star is actually the doorway that leads beyond the local universe—the source of virtual beneficence and the purest of pure spiritual light and dark.

"When we meditate here in the presence of this immense universe it is very easy to absorb the Qi of the celestial realms into our earthen bodies—pure Yin, the body, infused with pure Yang, the universe. Our strength of spirit comes from the fact that the heavens are permeated with supreme wisdom and ultimate knowledge. When we open in the Qigong state, the virtue and beneficence of the heavens pour into our local embodied selves. We become more intelligent, more clear minded, more aligned with the innate tendencies of nature.

"When we practice, particularly at this time of day and especially in a place like this, the conditions are as good as they can get to optimize the most profound benefits of Qi cultivation. Benevolence and virtue pour through us like a cleansing celestial stream, bathing us in healing potential and the universal nourishment that fuels empowerment and fearlessness. So let's be quiet for a while. Here in the bright light of these stars, consider your universal nature."

We begin by initiating the Three Intentful Corrections, taking a few deep breaths, adjusting posture, and clearing the mind. We allow the immensity of the night sky to overwhelm us with wonder. The desire to think about the challenges of life back at home is just about gone. For a moment you think of what Yi Xin said about the stars and planets. You remember, prayerfully, your family and send off a declaration of well-being to all who suffer. Then your consciousness drifts. It is as if being in the light of these stars has blessed you. You are suspended between thoughts, concerns, and plans. In those moments it is almost as if your body has disappeared. Less aware of the body and its sensations, less aware of the nervous system's loyal and habitual readiness for something to happen, you begin to experience just the Qi. Dissolving in Qi you are out of time and place, dissociated from your personal history.

Your reasons for thinking and deliberation are pleasantly out of reach. In the silence—your vacation from complexity—you become a completely open channel for the flow of the universe. Instead of reaching out for peace you now find peace is present within you. The edge of yourself disappears, and you awaken to the experience of the boundless universe expanding into the fullness of your most whole being.

Next morning at the teaching session, our teacher Eternal Spring is standing in meditation as we enter silently. We all settle into a meditation state, some standing, some sitting. Every few minutes Eternal Spring changes the position of her hands as if she is sending messages to her inner self-healing nature or in a quiet conversation with higher forces. First she seems to be holding an invisible object, like a crystal ball, at about the level of the heart and she stares into it with great focus. Next she brings her hands together in the prayer position in front of the solar plexus where she remains in deep meditation for quite a while. She then forms the Daoist hand position for greeting and prayerfulness with the right hand in a soft fist and the left hand open covering or shielding the right—again in front of the heart. After a time it becomes obvious that she is pouring universal life force into the room and that we are bathing in it. Finally, she opens her arms, shoulders relaxed and palms facing upward. In this posture it looks as if she is holding a large invisible sphere of Qi that enfolds the upper part of her body—holding the universe in her arms.

Virtue

"You are aware of the states of water." Eternal Spring speaks slowly and poetically in her most soothing voice. "The solid state, ice, is the earth or body level of water. The liquid state, with its capacity to be either calm like a lake or tumultuous like a huge waterfall, is the same as the mind and emotions. As vapor, water rises to Heaven, and represents Spirit. There are many beautiful aspects of this image, and I invite you to explore these as a part of your practice.

"One of the guiding images for the ultimate phase of personal cultivation known as Dissolve in Qi is water. To Dissolve in Qi is to come home to your higher self. When you are in that great ocean of all being, you are unified with the body of all water.

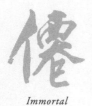

Immortal

Now, imagine that you are water that has evaporated and is drifting as a cloud. Imagine that you are aware of being separated from that unified ocean, feeling isolated. Then in a storm you fall to the ground and form a puddle. Then you evaporate again. You can barely remember being in the ocean, in that state of oneness. A wind carries you north and you fall as a snowflake.

"Children roll you into a ball of snow to make a snowman. Later you melt and penetrate the ground where you are absorbed by the roots of a tree. Within the tree you are transported as sap up the trunk into a branch and finally into sweet ripening fruit. You are picked and sent to market where someone buys you. When she bites into you she exclaims with enjoyment at the sweet, juicy taste. Suddenly, you are circulating within the body of a human being—first as blood and then as lymph. By now you have only the slightest recollection of being in your beloved ocean, but you experience a sense of longing to return to some vague yet alluring origin.

"Through perspiration you are evaporated into the atmosphere again. You feel yourself rising to gather with other bits of moisture from many sources into a beautiful billowing cloud. The cloud gets swept out over the ocean and you can sense that you are coming closer to some important moment, a reunion with the greater pool of all being. The ocean below is calm, the storm that you are a part of is not violent, more like a shower. Suddenly you are released from the cloud, free falling.

"It is a feeling of great exhilaration to be an individual drop of water, falling. But it seems like a long time since you were a part of something immense. Always, as a drop, you felt pulled to merge with other drops, longing for the sea. And now at last, as you enter the ocean, there is a slightly alarming sense of losing your identity as a single drop. Simultaneously there is the extraordinary sense of melting into this huge body of water and becoming one with it. Reunion with the One is indescribable.

"This is how dissolving in Qi works and feels. Throughout your life you have been in or moved through thousands of particular and even peculiar situations. You have longed to experience being one with the fundamental essence of all life. Through Qi cultivation you come closer to accessing your oneness with the boundless universal—the Supreme Ultimate, Tai Chi [Taiji]. Whether it is for healing or for greater intuition, you share this longing with many people. Through vigilance and constancy in your practice you may dissolve in Qi and when you do, you will feel the bliss of merging with all beings in the immense, unified ocean of the One."

Dissolve in Qi

Qi is pervasive. It is everywhere. Qi of stone, Qi of weather, Qi of wood, Qi of light, Qi of pure Spirit—all are Qi. Yet, the Qi of a sick and confused person is clearly different than that of an athlete or of a nationally revered heroic figure. When you were first discovering Qi, you were different than you are today. Through cultivation you have refined and clarified yourself to reveal your essence.

It is promised, when you remove all obstacles, open all channels completely to the flow of universal forces so that there is absolutely no resistance—then you become radiant. You generate the most profound and highly refined inner-healing resource, Golden Elixir. When you use this elixir effectively, you dissolve in Qi.

> *The Sage surrenders*
> > *to that which arises,*
> > *moment to moment.*
> *Knowing her ultimate nature*
> > *she clings to nothing,*
> > *no illusions of the mind,*
> > *no resistances in the body.*
> *She does not think about her actions,*
> > *they flow from the essence of her being,*
> > *she holds nothing back*
> > *living as if she has already embraced*
> > *her passage from this life.*

—LAO ZI, *DAO DE JING*, #50

This state is beyond stress free; it is a surrender to that which spontaneously arises by knowing that the entire force and wisdom of the universe is behind it. Imagine this for a moment and engage with it if you wish: acting from the position of oneness with all that is or could be—aligned and cooperating with the power of the whole universe.

Falling into the Embrace of Pure Light

It is not easy to discuss this phase of Qi cultivation. Many fear it because they feel that they might lose themselves and dissolve into the mystery. The Qi masters suggest that when we cultivate at the Ninth Phase of Qi Cultivation and Mastery we will merge with the One, the ultimate form of "Guarding the One." Lao Zi describes this phenomenon:

> *Looking into the dark Mystery brings clarity,*
> *Knowing how to surrender is the greatest strength.*
> *Cultivate your own light*
> > *and merge with the source of all light.*
> *This is the practice of eternity.*

—LAO ZI, *DAO DE JING*, #52

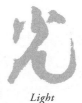

Light

To dissolve in Qi you will open to your ultimate nature. Your Spirit is already perfect, you can't change it. You can't *become* it because you already *are* it. You can only get out of the way and let it be. There is no way that someone outside of yourself can tell you or teach you how to do this. The great teachers do not tell you what to do, they show you how to be. When you meet such a teacher, he or she will see only your spirit. It is obvious that such a person has fallen into the embrace of pure light.

Qigong Method to Dissolve in Qi

Dissolve into Light

HISTORICAL REFLECTION Dissolving in Qi is less about doing any particular Qigong form or method than it is about being in and sustaining a state of direct association with Spirit—not only during your practice time but from moment to moment. However, there are specific methods you can use for focused practice. Dissolve into Light is a standing Qigong meditation that has had many names over many centuries. Like the method from the last chapter this standing form has been called Primordial (Wuji) Qigong. It too has the focus of supporting the practitioner in becoming One with the original nature of the universe. One of the more prevalent names for this type of deep HeartMind clearing practice is Yi Quan. In English, this translates as intention (Yi) practice or mind boxing. Guarding the One and Circulating the Light are the more advanced versions of this practice. Natural Flow Qigong is another more contemporary approach to Dissolve in Qi.

INSTRUCTION First do some body-oriented practices to warm up for this meditation. This could include the methods for the previous eight phases. Align the Central Tai Chi Channel and the three Elixir Fields. Stand with feet parallel about shoulder width apart. Sink just slightly. Allow the hands to form the ball of Qi at a comfortable place in front of either your Earth, HeartMind, or Heaven Elixir Field. Turn your attention to the concept of mind boxing, Guarding the One, Circulating the Light, or Natural Flow Qigong. Hold the focus. As often as you need to, check through the Three Intentful Corrections. After significant practice, if you hold this position for even a few minutes, you will feel the Qi. Pay attention to the Qi sensation. Slip into that state where you lose touch with the substance and personality of your local self and associate with your radiant self, your universal eternal being. Feel the drop of yourself as you unite with the ocean of all being.

You may choose among the hand positions shown—they are known as salutations or mudras—or make some up. The point is to find your most comfortable position to relate with an open system to the Qi, which infuses all beings and things. With practice, over time, you may gain the ability to focus so completely on the aspects of your own Qi, which is unified with the Qi of all beings and the whole universe, that you will dissolve into the One.

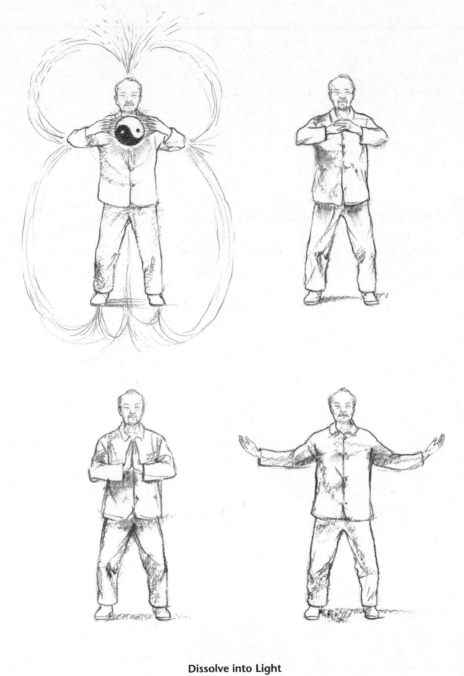

Dissolve into Light

One day one of my teachers, Chang Yi Hsiang, originally from Dragon-Tiger Mountain in eastern China, demonstrated some of the secret Daoist salutations and hand positions to help elicit higher states of consciousness. I had two very deep impressions. The first was that I could feel waves of energy or consciousness as if she was releasing messages from the thousands and even millions of serious Qigong practitioners who have participated in the field of all Qigong intention over all time. The second was remembering myself as a child in Cincinnati, Ohio. A group of friends and I used to make up hand signs just like these as we played together in our secret little camp under a group of lilac bushes in the backyard.

The Qi is everywhere.

Mind Focus Affirmation

Dissolving in Qi, I merge with the boundless universal field of being.

Phase 10: Transmit Qi

One with all beings and possibilities
I am moved to serve others
knowing that in the One
they are none other than myself.

—WU WEI, LEGENDARY QI MASTER THROUGHOUT
MANY MILLENNIA

Compassionate Service

After hearing of our encounter with Dr. Chen, a number of people ask to join us when we go to learn the Primordial (Wuji) Qigong (Chi Kung) practice that he promised to teach us. We retrace the path from our earlier visit. Just after we turn off the trail and begin the climb, one of the group suddenly begins experiencing a severe asthma episode. She coughs and gasps. Believing that Qigong has cured her asthma she has left her inhaler back at the training center. She is leaning against a large rock looking pale and panicked.

One of our group members immediately runs off to find Dr. Chen, who arrives very quickly. The woman's face has gone ashen, and it is obvious that her vitality is draining rapidly. Dr. Chen quickly takes hold of both her hands and begins rubbing the point between her thumb and first finger vigorously, on both sides. Then he turns her around, sits her down on a nearby rock, and works quickly on several

Transmit Qi

points on her upper back—striking the points vigorously with the tips of his fingers. His hand resembles the beak of a woodpecker, tapping in search of insects in a tree trunk.

Then Dr. Chen moves around beside the woman. In no more than a minute her condition seems to be easing a bit. Without touching her he uses the open palms of his hands, one in front over her chest area and one in the back at the same level. He begins to do what looks like Forming the Qi Ball. It is as if the Qi (Chi) that naturally passes between his hands is now passing through her body. We can see that Dr. Chen is deep in a state of personal practice as he works with her. A bit of color returns to the woman's face.

As he works, Dr. Chen carries on a simple, soothing conversational monologue. "Remember that the Qi of the entire universe is behind the flow of Qi through and within you. As we are here together, purposefully go toward the deepest, most relaxed state that you possibly can. Even if you were to lose your life, you know that you live forever, so fear is not a useful response right now. Visualize that your Qi channels are opening internally to the flow of healing resources. Allow my presence here with you to be of assistance. I am glad to offer my own practice for your benefit and for my energy field to mingle with yours to help reestablish inner harmony." Dr. Chen begins to do a movement with his hands that looks as if he is combing, smoothing, or massaging an invisible part of her body—about three to six inches away from the physical surface. He smoothes, in a downward direction, five or six times, and finishes by placing his hands carefully on her shoulders.

Within ten minutes of the beginning of the asthma attack the woman seems to have recovered. It was amazing to witness this very humble man help to turn the situation around so quickly. We finished the climb to Dr. Chen's hermitage; it is a beautiful, clear morning. On our last visit the cloud sea was billowing below. Today the mountains and valleys are open and clear. For about an hour we follow Dr. Chen in the Wuji form. Very quickly we are all humming with Qi and excited about the Inner Alchemy practice—reversing fire and water and reversing the flow of time. It seems as though it would not take long to learn this inspired Wuji form. We all have a sudden interest in Qi healing following the asthma experience.

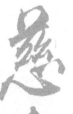
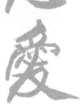

Compassion, Kindness

Back at the training center, when we begin class, the woman who had the asthma attack declares, "I just had the most amazing Qigong healing experience with Dr. Chen. It seemed like he was doing his Qigong practice with me present, his Qi was spilling over to help me. I could feel it. It was extraordinary. How can we learn that?"

Jade Unity nods slowly and responds:

"Qigong healing can happen in a number of ways. Here at the training center we have a tradition of focusing on an approach to healing that is a clear extension of personal cultivation practice. Some forms of Qi healing that are promoted draw upon internal energy with a loss or drain to the person or group who is providing the healing. Our way is to work with healing by either using intention to stir the Qi of the universe to affect the person who needs healing or by reaching a state where our own internal practice causes a natural overflowing of Qi that can have a positive effect on the person that needs help.

"Of all the teachers who have taught me about Qigong for healing I especially liked Old Master Wu who insisted that the most powerful healing comes from the universe. He taught that it is counterproductive to use your own life force for healing. He always spoke of healing as an effect of one's personal radiance and referred to the sun. The sun radiates without effort, according to its nature. When you have cultivated your Qi effectively over time, two things can occur. One is that your intention will become very focused and cause positive influences to affect those around you in a healing way. Or second, your Qi multiplies, accumulates, and overflows. In both cases you are radiating Qi. In neither case are you depreciating your own life force.

"Master Wu used to say, 'For healing just be like the sun, radiate healing resources by knowing that in the Qigong state you are removing constraints from the natural self-balancing nature of the universe. You do not have to do anything, just relax and be like the sun.' If you wish you can use your intention to direct the Qi to specific areas as we did in Direct Qi. Or you can place your hands on or near the person whom you are assisting."

Transmitting the Qi

As you now know, the greatest focus in Qigong for more than fifty centuries has been personal practice for self-improvement—from healing, health maintenance, and longevity to alchemy, transcendence, and spirituality. When your Qi has been purified, accumulated, stored, and transformed through your cultivation practice, you dissolve in Qi. When you dissolve in Qi, you become one with all beings and all possibilities. A natural effect of your immersion in and awareness of unity is compassion and service. In this you will achieve a unique and extraordinary relationship with life itself. Those who have achieved this level of cultivation express a natural wisdom and kindness.

Imagine being filled with pure Qi until a bountiful excess spills out to others as radiance and healing energy. As we noted earlier, one of the promises of the Qi is that your practice of cultivation automatically multiplies your access to celestial resources and heavenly influences including virtue, beneficence, wisdom, and compassion. As your Qi overflows, your radiance of these qualities pours out and triggers beneficial effects for others. We are all merged, it is now apparent from the findings of both physicists and systems biologists, in a single interconnected and universal field of being, energy, and consciousness.

A human being is part of a whole,
the "Universe."
Our task must be to free ourselves
from the delusion of separateness,
to embrace all living creatures
and the whole of nature.

—ALBERT EINSTEIN, PHILOSOPHER AND PHYSICIST, TWENTIETH CENTURY

Knowing that you are irrevocably interconnected in the fabric of the universe with all beings, compassionate service to others becomes spontaneous. In Qigong this phase is known as Qi transmission. It is an outflowing, emission, or projection of Qi, which expresses in many forms with a wide range of beneficial effects. You may find yourself feeling these effects just by standing near someone who has attained Qi mastery or by hearing that person speak. Various forms of Qigong healing and medical Qigong are aspects of the Transmit Qi phase as well.

Qi transmission, in the context of Qi cultivation and mastery, is not focused so much on becoming a Qi healer as it is on simply radiating the beneficial influences that arise from your own cultivation. Your own capacity to cultivate Qi can bring about positive benefits for others. This mysterious and pervasive universal resource is not limited within you. Qi is not just energy, it is also consciousness and the communication of subtle information, sometimes called signals or messages. Your own sincere practice has power and influence beyond the boundary of your body. At some point in your life you have likely met someone who radiated such a powerful sense of peace or vitality that he or she inspired you to think about your life in a different way. That is Qi transmission. This effect of Qi can have influence both near and far.

Transmission of Qi has little to do with exertion or effort. Simply hold the intention for healing during your Qigong practice; focus it on one or several others who are either nearby or far away. Relax. There is nothing to *do*. Instead, allow your cultivation practice to maximize the natural activity and flow of Qi within you, near you, and at a distance. This occurs automatically because of the natural potential within dynamic fields of energy and consciousness.

When your cultivation is genuine and sincere, when you can enter into and sustain the state of inner resistlessness, the Qi field is enhanced. Inner hindrance and constraint are neutralized by your practice, which allows for the optimal expression of the Qi. In the presence of another or when focused on another at a distance, especially with the conscious intention to generate a beneficial influence, the methods of the Transmit Qi phase can have profound effects.

The Masters render effortless service.
They do the work and then relax,
Neither expecting nor forcing any result.
Therefore, their influence is eternal.

—LAO ZI, *DAO DE JING*, #2

The transmission of Qi need not be overt. The most empowering healing occurs when there is no apparent healer. In Transmit Qi—whether it is focused locally or across a distance, one-on-one or in groups—the healing methods are based in personal cultivation with the intention to benefit others. Because we live in a culture in which healing is commonly perceived to come from doctors and hospitals, it is hard for some people to believe that healing comes from within.

You don't have to try to send the healing effect; just do your cultivation practice. If the conditions are correct, the benefit will arise. Trying, or even hoping for a greater effect, doesn't improve the situation. Instead, engage sincerely in your practice. The promise is that, without spending your own energy, you are triggering beneficial effects in the Qi field.

Qi transmission effects that assist others but do not deplete you operate along one or more of the following pathways:

1. Universal Qi passes through you as a channel to another person or persons.
2. The Qi of others is balanced and organized due to your harmonizing influence.
3. Healing Qi from the universe pours directly into the field of one or several other persons due to your intentful practice.

While more advanced medical Qigong, based in Chinese medicine, must be reserved for practitioners with a strong background in clinical practice of diagnosis and treatment, the Transmit Qi methods here are accessible to anyone who is cultivating Qi. These cultivation methods require no diagnosis, no treatment, no expectations, and no fees. In the Transmit Qi phase Qi is not manipulated with a clinical focus. Rather Qi is cultivated with a harmonizing focus. If the person transmitting is engaged in authentic cultivation and if the person receiving is eligible, healing will occur.

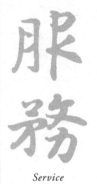

Service

Often, in classes, training sessions, or lectures people will experience pain relief, healing, or some personal revelation. Was this due to the energy of the group, the cultivation level of the instructor, or the eligibility of the person who received the benefit? The answer to all these questions is yes. As you will learn in Chapter 16, there are many levels of Qi, and it is nearly impossible to quantify how specifically the healing will occur in the transmission context. You will find in your own practice that the benefits of cultivation sometimes spill over with benefits to others. You don't need to analyze this or try to repeat it. It will arise spontaneously at the appropriate time. Similar to the findings in research on prayer and nonlocal intention, wanting or trying to create an outcome is likely to be less useful than simply holding the healing intention and allowing the larger universal plan to determine the outcome.

Ancient Roots

The roots of Qi transmission healing are planted in every tradition of Qigong. Origins from the shamanic era evolved into the Daoist and Buddhist traditions as compassionate service, and into the medical field as healing modalities to complement acupuncture, herbal therapies, and massage. Research on the shamanic traditions suggests that Qi transmission was common long before written history.

In the ancient text *Formula for Absorption of Primordial Energy,*[1] Master Youzhen writes, "To spread one's Qi in order to heal a sick person one must first examine where in the organs (*Zang Fu*) the problem is rooted. Then take in Qi through the mouth and place it into the patient's body. The patient faces the Qi master, but before he receives the infusion, he must calm his mind and cleanse his thoughts. After the infusion the patient should swallow the Qi. Thereby demons and evil forces will be expelled and bad Qi will be eradicated forever."

Swallowing Qi is a common phrase from ancient times meaning to practice Qigong and circulate Qi throughout the body. *Evil forces, demons,* and *bad Qi* can mean a range of things—a simple cold or flu can represent bad Qi. Evil forces are often merely disease-causing factors with physical manifestations such as excessive heat or dampness. Demons can be chronic emotional imbalances or, just as easily, they can be real demons and evil forces—for example, the negative influences of trauma imposed by violent, angry, or vengeful people. It is very important to understand that there is a strong directive for what the person who is receiving the healing must do to receive benefit: "before he receives the infusion, he must calm his mind and cleanse his thoughts." It is very rare in authentic Qigong for transmission to occur without some indication of how the person receiving the benefit can enhance his or her own health through self-practice methods.

It is difficult to determine the mechanisms for these effects. They remain a mystery. We know that distant healing effects do occur, but we do not know how they are mediated. Scientific debate in this area is intense. Some favor energy fields; others, fields of information or consciousness (see Chapter 16). In China, of course, distant healing (both near and far) is attributed to Qi, which is a mystery in itself.

In Daoism, the practitioner who has merged with nature, revealing his or her essential being and becoming one with the undifferentiated field of all possibilities—the Immortal—transmits Qi. This frequently is accomplished through compassionate service, healing, and blessings. In Buddhism, the bodhisattva who is devoted to the salvation and enlightenment of all beings also renders service through healing or generous acts that carry Qi as intention, teaching, transcendental messages, or prayers. In the practice of medicine, both hands-on methods and distant healing methods, individuals with the gift of healing or those who through their practice have cultivated a high level of skill, also have the capacity to express outflowing Qi.

Benevolence

Ethics of Qi Transmission

Qi transmission raises a profoundly moral issue. Medical philosophy as well as the spiritual philosophies of Daoism and Buddhism invite the practitioner to very high ground regarding values and respect for the evolutionary process of all persons. Not every person who has the skill to use Qi emission also has the spiritual maturity and judgment to use it for highest good. The ego, for better and for worse, can become involved.

A person who is doing healing without teaching others to access the Qi that is always present around them is cause for caution. Healing that is done without a strong teaching component to help others access self-healing is radically disempowering for the recipient. In many cases it is also dishonest.

Qigong is designed to give each person an open channel to a universal resource that is free and pervasive. Healing work, even by trained professionals, falls short of its highest calling when the healer neglects to encourage the health seeker to learn and practice self-healing methods and develop a personal universal connection.

Often the person who seeks healing deludes himself or herself with the belief that the essence of healing lies *outside* of oneself. This invalidates the profound possibility for self-healing and self-reliance that is promised in Qigong. I will always remember a particular woman who accompanied our group on a trip to China. As soon as we left China she said, "I really must start saving my money to go back and get healings from the Qi master." The physician at the regional hospital who had given her a Qigong healing treatment had stated very clearly, "When we do this work I am not actually healing you; I am assisting you to heal yourself. My work is to support you in maximizing your Qi." She experienced significant relief and was very impressed.

The doctor explained that she should use a few simple self-healing methods that he described. "With my assistance you have opened up to what is already there. As my hands are moving before you and around you, I am assisting you in coordinating your Qi field—finding the areas of discord and helping to bring them into harmony. I am reaching into your channels and organs with Qi guided by mind intention to remind you of what you can do for yourself. I am particularly interested in helping you to find the underlying emotions that deplete or stagnate your self-healing capacity. When you sigh or weep it is an important release of withheld or toxic Qi. The most profound medicine does not come from the doctor. It comes from the universe and you have direct access to it—personally."

Is it appropriate and responsible to put forth a worldview that suggests that the healing comes from the practitioner? Some people who use Qigong healing methods leave their clients with the impression that the healing comes from the healer—often for a significant fee. When we disempower an individual through a healing process that is not complementary to self-practice, it is not so much better than those in conventional medical fields who put forth the idea that patients must simply take medications or receive treatments and wait or hope for results if they want to be healthy.

Traditional Values of Medicine and Healing from Ancient China

Qigong healing comes in diverse forms. Before we explore the methods for transmitting Qi, review for a moment the deepest ideals of all the traditional Asian medical systems.

- Honor the Spirit, destiny, potential, and rights of the health seeker.
- Teach people to sustain their health and heal themselves through personal practices and lifestyle adjustments.
- When using any of the transmission methods, provide a context in which it is understood that healing treatment activates inner resources—the healer within.
- Support your community in creating health-improvement activities for citizens of all ages, from children to elders.

When these ideals are included in the context of Qi transmission, the person who receives the benefit of the transmission will always be empowered to engage in his or her own practice as the basis of the healing process. The healer in this context is a kind of hero in his or her community.

Personal Qi or Universal Qi

Some traditions hold forth the idea that healing energy comes from the reserves of the healer or physician. A second perspective suggests that healing energy comes from the universe and is triggered or directed by the intention of the healer. Both are true.

One of the most fascinating and disappointing experiences of my many trips to China was when a Qigong healer was to demonstrate his skill by making a fluorescent lightbulb light up without connecting it to an electrical source—just by holding it. A whole group of American physicians and scientists had come a long way to see the demonstration. To our amazed disappointment, it was announced that the healer had treated too many patients, had depleted his Qi, and would not do the demonstration.

This healer apparently depleted his personal Qi in his work. Healing that is mediated through personal Qi can be injurious to the practitioner and is not recommended without very specialized training. This is a very different sort of mastery than we are exploring. When you mediate the healing effect by cultivating your connection to the shared field of universal Qi—called Shen Qi, Heavenly Qi, or Cosmic Qi—there is no risk of depletion because the Qi that is transmitted is not personal—it is universal and boundless.

Qigong Tricks

One more note of caution. For some reason that frankly I do not understand, some people become involved in a very questionable approach to Qigong. In this approach seemingly impossible feats are demonstrated—and attributed to Qi mastery. I am a believer in the phenomenal possibilities associated with Qi cultivation. I have witnessed some awe-inspiring Qigong effects in the area of healing. I have had personal experiences confirming that Qi and Qigong have the potential to alter people's lives radically. This caution is not based on any doubt of the forces in nature that we refer to as Qi or the natural power of Qi.

However, there can be a fine line between what could actually be possible with Qi and what many have called Qigong tricks, a form sometimes referred to as Hard Qigong and associated with Kung Fu and the martial arts. There is a historic tradition in Chinese culture where demonstration of Hard Qigong mastery is encouraged. These demonstrations are usually done at weddings and holiday celebrations. In such demonstrations Qi masters break things, drill holes in bricks with their fingers, walk on sharp blades, lie on nails, or have large stones placed on their chests that are then broken with sledgehammers. This is all great fun and clearly a demonstration of highly skilled human beings with extraordinary personal capacities. Such skills clearly require a high level of inner coordination of function.

Empowerment

The problem arises when such demonstrations are proposed as evidence of healing skill. Certainly, there are Qigong practitioners with these Hard Qigong skills that also have authentic healing skill. However, some practitioners use these tricks as evidence of their ability to heal and teach others to do Qigong healing. There is no guaranteed relationship between Hard Qigong skills and healing. Unfortunately, I have known very knowledgeable Qigong teachers to use these tricks to lure students or patients. Some practitioners consider this a perfectly acceptable way to inspire students to practice with greater devotion.

The best source of information about Qigong is your own intuition and the knowledge you gain through your practice. When you practice Qigong yourself and access certain Qi skills, you become less of a target for inauthentic Qi entrepreneurs. The positive Qi healing effects of a group of sincere Qigong practitioners working together are certainly as powerful as those of a Qi healer with questionable skills. Authentic Qi healers do exist; I have studied with several. However, people with questionable motives take advantage of the naivete of eager and enthusiastic learners. The best strategy is to focus on your personal cultivation.

The Qi Transmission Spectrum

Your transmission of energy and life force to assist others will always be most effective when your own Qi is in harmony. At this, the tenth phase of cultivation and mastery, it is useful to have mastered the Earth phases. Likewise your sincere exploration of the HeartMind phases—Purify Qi, Direct Qi, and Conserve Qi—ensures that your ability to hold a focus and neutralize inner resistance will contribute to your transmission potential.

Within this context we will explore further Qi cultivation methods through which you can share the healing benefits of your Qi cultivation with others. In these healing methods the Qi is transmitted through your intentful cultivation of the universal field and all of its manifestations in nature. The beneficial influence flows from your access to the abundance of nature; Qi overflows from your cultivation practice.

Compassion and intention are the keys. Young children with little or no Qigong training can, because of their natural compassion, transmit Qi easily. If you simply bring your attention to Qi cultivation while you apply these methods, it can generate positive benefits. If you *try* to make something happen, results may be less accessible. Because you enter a state of deep relaxation and cultivation, and because you are not focusing on particular outcomes, the natural tendency of the universe to seek balance can be triggered to benefit others.

We will start with the hands-on and hands-near methods. Medical Qigong and Qi transmission healing both use Qi transmission massage and near-distant Qigong transmission. These focus on influencing the most local fields (within and very near the body) of energy, information, and consciousness. In addition to transmission methods that occur when we are with the person who receives the benefit, there are also fascinating transmission methods that project the Qi over a distance. Such methods allow us to do what the Chinese call *Qi Chang Gong*, "create a field of healing Qi." Essentially Qi Chang Gong occurs when people can trust that their own cultivation has an outflowing effect. This effect can be local or nonlocal.

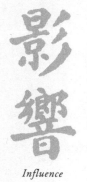

Influence

Every person who practices Qigong is contributing to a worldwide pool of purified Qi. As a part of our cultivation practice, we pour our intentions, healing declarations, prayers, and visualizations into this vast pool of all Qi. The rest is given. It is a promise that this pool can be tapped for healing.

One of the greatest promises of Qi and Qigong is that souls like yourself, with sincere and virtuous intention, can make a difference in the destiny of loved ones and strangers alike—even a difference in world events. Intentful transmission is profound.

There are at least five kinds of Qi transmission:

1. Hands-on
2. Hands-near
3. Near-distant with intention
4. Near-distant with instruction
5. Far nonlocal

In each of the Qi transmission methods we will discuss in this chapter, the general intention is to cause a beneficial effect in another or others in a context where your own Qi is conserved and protected. Your mind intention will induce the beneficial influence to flow from the natural universal Qi field. Visualize intentfully that your Qi cultivation triggers transmission of benefit. Declare silently and confidently, calling upon the promise of the Qi, that any disharmony of Qi—deficiency or imbalance—in the person or persons that you are serving may be resolved. Anticipate that your target person or group is open to an influx of healing Qi and universal wisdom. Declare that it is so, relax, and trust that you have done all that is necessary and that the universal Qi field will do the rest.

Beneficial effects arise directly from the universe's natural potential. This, plus the strength of your intention, creates the beneficial effect as Qi transmission. If you practice Qigong and have progressed in the cultivation phases, this multiplies the effect. The potential in the universe is limitless and ever present. Your potential, however, while limitless, is modified by the extent to which you have progressed in your practice and by your sincerity. Sincerity multiplies intent; intent enriches Qi cultivation; cultivation enhances transmission.

Qigong Methods to Transmit Qi

1. Hands-On

Hands-on transmission is accomplished with massage, pressure to points, or the holding of contact areas or centers. There are numerous methods, including Reiki, acupressure, Qi massage, and Polarity therapy, that are akin to hands-on Qi transmission. Hands-on transmission can be done one-on-one or in a group. Typically, there are two approaches. In the first the hands are usually stationary, holding particular points or centers so that the Qi is balanced or replenished. In the second, Qi massage, the transmission is accomplished in conjunction with a number of massage techniques. With shiatsu, acupressure, or Tuina, three forms of body therapy from Asian traditions, the Qi is transmitted as the pressure points are stimulated. With more Western forms of massage the practitioner holds a Qi cultivation intention during the massage session.

ONE-ON-ONE With the possible exception of herbal medicine, massage and body therapy are the oldest healing arts. People who do Qigong and Tai Chi (Taiji) in groups often offer massage to one another before or after the practice session. The Qi-based healing arts—also called energy medicine—are experiencing extraordinary growth in the West today. Professional physical therapists are becoming more aware of the potential of Qi cultivation. With a simple shift of intention and minor modifications in technique, these practitioners can enhance the physiological effects of their work by triggering a Qi healing effect. There are not only dozens of traditional forms of Qi or energy healing, but there are now versions that combine new findings in brain chemistry and neuroanatomy with the ancient Qi-based framework.

There is a simple rule in Chinese medicine that anyone can apply: find areas of soreness and focus your healing work there. These are called the ashi points, which means "ouch points." Find areas of soreness and give some gentle massage or pressure to the points. Add Qi transmission by initiating the Three Intentful Corrections and using the Ten Phases of Cultivation and Mastery while you perform the massage.

Running Energy Method. To transmit Qi by running the energy, you simply offer the service of placing your hands and then turn your attention to your own cultivation practice. Place your hands with great care on the recipient. If there is not a specific location of discomfort or dysfunction, simply make a comfortable connection and relax. Qi will automatically flow through you or from the universe to the receiver and begin to harmonize and balance healing resources within him or her. You don't

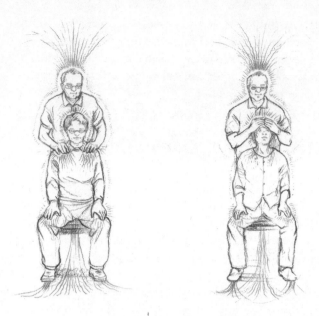

Running Energy—Give and Receive

need to know anything except that the natural tendency of Qi is to go toward a greater state of harmony when given an opportunity to do so. Also remember that the Qi that is channeling through you to the person arrives directly from the universe. It does not draw upon or deplete your own resources in any way. Just be present and focus on cultivation within yourself. Visualize the person you are working with in a renewed and perfect state of health.

One variation of the Running Energy method is the Two Qi method. In this, both parties are intentfully transmitting to one another. There are several approaches to this. One of the most common is sending Qi and compassion to the heart center or HeartMind. In this version your right hand is on your partner's heart and your left hand is covering your partner's right hand, which is placed over your heart. Once you are in the correct position turn your attention to your Qi cultivation practice. Adjust your posture, breath, and mind. Your partner should do the same. Rest for a while connected in this way. Alternatives are hands on each other's shoulders or simply holding hands.

Massage with Qi. When you apply massage, reflexology, or any form of bodywork in a state of Qi cultivation, the Qigong healing process occurs because your intention is to infuse Qi into the exchange. It happens automatically when you are in the focused Qigong state. By getting out of the way of the universe's natural tendency, you allow yourself and the person to whom you are giving bodywork to seek balance and harmony. Bringing Qigong to the exchange requires a shift from applying mas-

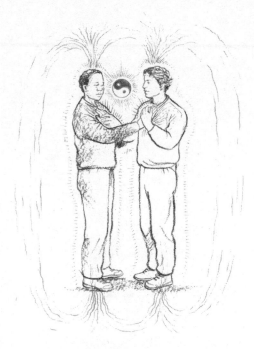

Running Energy—Two Qi

sage to applying massage in a state of elevated focus on Qi and cultivation. Use deep, slow, relaxed breathing, encourage the receiving person to use their breath. Enter the deep Qigong state. Visualize energy or positive effects from the universal field being infused into the exchange and benefiting the recipient.

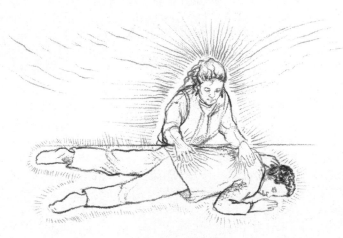

Massage with Qi

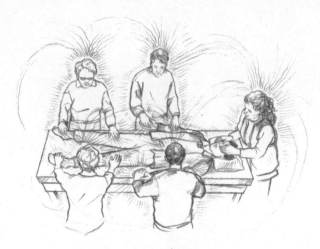

Five on One

GROUP-ON-ONE There are many ways of accomplishing Qi healing. In a group-on-one exchange, several people lay their hands on one person who is usually lying on the floor, a bed, or a massage table. There are numerous variations, depending on the number of people, but one method is where one of a group holds the head of the receiving person and another holds the feet. Place one hand on the sole of the foot or the palm of the hand and the other on the leg or arm. Simply make contact with the receiving person and focus on your cultivation practice.

GROUP-ON-GROUP This may be the most empowering form of Qi transmission. Why? Because, in group-based Qigong with a healing intention, both with and without touch (including prayer or distant healing), there is no single person set up as "the healer" who has greater access to the Qi than anyone else. Each person gives and receives of the Qi at the same time. The benefit that anyone in the group receives is contributed by all in the group. The benefit that anyone contributes into the process is potentially transmitted to everyone. As we have been learning, contributing to a group healing effect does not require much knowledge; however, it does require a strong degree of hearty intention.

Shoulder Circle. With the other members of the group make a circle. Then face right (or left) and place your hands on the shoulders of the person in front of you. The area under your palm is like a super energy crossroads. Important points on the Yang channels (which carry the Qi of Heaven through the gallbladder, small intestine, and triple heater channels) are like energy intake and output ducts right there under your hands. On your inhalation gather resources with the breath and visualize (or feel if you can) Qi collecting through the top of your head, and through all of your energy points. Collect that potential in your belly and torso by concentrating on the Earth. Visualize Yin and Yang merging in the HeartMind Elixir Field as a balanced Tai Chi.

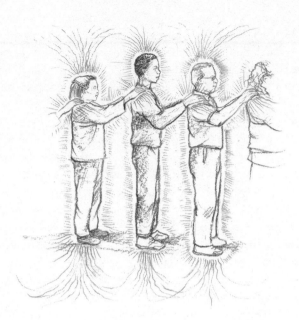

Shoulder Circle

On the exhalation express the potential of the gathered harmonious Tai Chi energy out through the heart, through the arms, and into your hands. Then transmit the Qi out through your Palace of Merit (*Lao Gong*), important Qi points at the center of each palm, into the energy channels of the person in front of you. Simultaneously, you are absorbing Qi from the person behind you. Everyone is drawing in Qi from Heaven and Earth. To multiply the effect coordinate the group's breathing. Express a deep sigh, "Ahh," on the exhalations. Notice that the sound multiplies the effect. You can further enhance the effect by sinking slightly with bent knees on the exhalation and rising on the inhalation—like a Qi pump.

Then do some vigorous rubbing of the shoulders, neck, and upper back. Use your thumbs and do some massage. Follow with some gentle pounding, with loose fists or cupped palms, particularly out along the shoulders. Finish by returning your palms to the holding points and doing three more sighs. Turn and repeat, facing the other way. Smaller groups can do a shoulder line instead of a circle. The shoulder circle works best, but it is hard to do with less than fifteen people.

The focus is to do this in the deep Qigong state. In our Qi cultivation practice, we make the medicine within. Through Qi transmission, we make a medicine among us. The group automatically draws upon the universal Qi field and multiplies the effect through shared intention.

Gate of Life and the Great Pillar. Create a circle. Stand close to the persons next to you. Try to avoid having very tall people standing next to short people. Place your

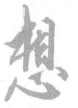

Visualize, Imagine

right hand (Lao Gong point) on the lower back of the person to your right, on the Gate of Life, which is located on the spine between the pelvis and the lower ribs. The person to your left will do the same to you. Place your left hand (Lao Gong point) at the place where the spine and shoulders intersect on the person to your left. This is named Great Pillar and is located just below the large seventh cervical vertebrae. It is the gathering point of all the Yang Qi channels.

Drift into a deep Qigong state. Feel Qi or visualize it entering the circle from Heaven and Earth and pouring into your heart (HeartMind). Feel or visualize Earth energy rising through the Gushing Spring point, in the ball of the foot, and Heaven energy descending through the Celestial Convergence point, at the top of the head. Knowing that all of these resources are gathering in the heart area, feel the current of energy and consciousness moving outward from your heart as you exhale, through your right Lao Gong point and into the Gate of Life in the lower back of the person to your right. On the inhalation draw Qi into your left hand from the Great Pillar on the upper spine of the person to your left.

On the inhalation lift your body upward just slightly by unbending your knees. On the exhalation make a strong "Ahh" sound, further expressing the energy from the heart and sink down slightly, bending the knees. Go deeper and deeper into relaxation. Remove your personality from the process, become a wide open channel for the circulation of Qi in the group. Feel this profound Qi engine, or visualize it, with its

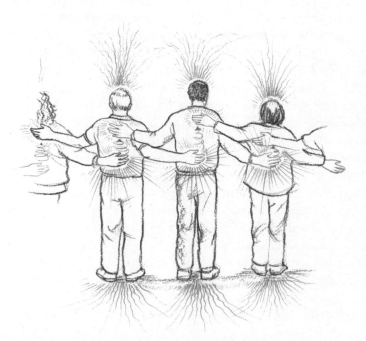

Ming Men (Gate of Life) Circle

energies circulating throughout the circle, into and up the spinal column, cleansing and energizing you and everyone in the circle.

Continue to acknowledge the influx of energies from the center of the circle into your hearts, and from Heaven and Earth through your head and feet. The rising and sinking, and the soothing chant of "Ahh" all contribute to the gathering and circulating of the Qi. After a while stop the sinking, rising, and chanting. Just feel the Qi engine running all by itself.

Lao Gong Circle 1. Step back so that it is comfortable to place your hands palm to palm with both of your neighbors. To do this symmetrically each person holds the left palm facing up and the right palm facing down. Connect hands and allow your arms to relax. The group is now holding hands with arms relaxed and dangling. This practice works on the same principle as the Gate of Life and Great Pillar practice. The current usually circulates to the right, although experience has demonstrated that some people feel the flow going to the left. Simply do your own practice and notice what you feel. Build up the group energy force by rising and sinking from the knees and chanting "Ahh" on the exhalation as the group sinks down. Give just a slight pressure to the palm and Lao Gong of both your neighbors as you exhale.

This method passes a powerful Qi current through the hearts of the circle participants. Feel energy pouring through your heart from the others in the circle, from the Earth and the Heaven. Each breath sends a surge of Qi that multiplies and refines the group Qi field to a pure and profound healing state. Enter effortless cultivation. In

Community

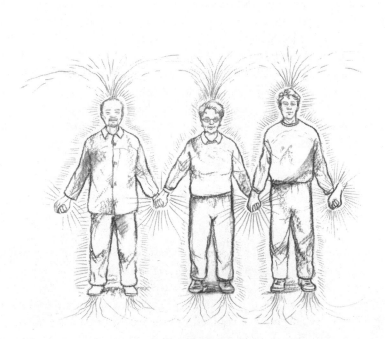

Lao Gong Circle 1

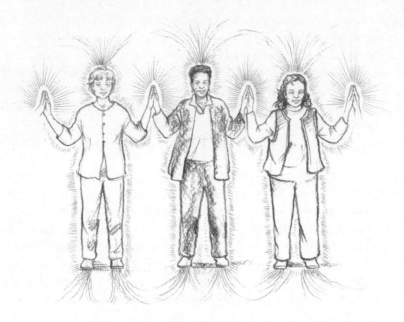

Lao Gong Circle 2

this state you transmit Qi without trying. Place your mind on the marvel of the Qi doing its natural work of healing and cleansing to sustain balance of the universe.

Deficient, hurt, or negative energy or emotion from any of the participants spills out of the circle and is pulled into the Earth or the Heaven as discussed in Purify Qi. A powerful field of healing influence (*Qi Chang*) radiates among you and then out from the circle to provide a beneficial and empowering influence on friends, loved ones, and anyone in need. Visualize and therefore activate the radiating field to avert accidents or catastrophes, soothe suffering, and interrupt or neutralize violent acts.

Lao Gong Circle 2. Now step back to create a wider circle. Raise your hands up so that they face the palms of your partner on each side, Lao Gong to Lao Gong. Continue to raise up on the inhalation and sink on the exhalation with the sound of "Ahh." Enter into and sustain the state from the last method. After a while stop the movement and the sound and carefully notice the sensations within you.

2. Hands-Near

Qi transmission using the hands near, not on, the body has stumped conventional science and yet people of many cultures and spiritual communities have been doing such practices for thousands of years. Many contemporary nurses and other health practitioners learn and practice therapeutic touch and healing touch methods, which provide healing without actually making contact with the receiver's body. One hospital I have worked with in Ohio has made it possible for all nurses to study these hands-near methods and use them freely with both in-patient and out-patient populations.

Quite a bit of positive research demonstrates that these methods are helpful in healing, reducing stress and anxiety, and improving patient satisfaction. However, as with all Qi-based modalities, Western science is not clear on how this works.

Hands-near Qi transmission, or emitted Qi, is a key feature of Chinese medical Qigong, along with Qigong Tuina, which is a hands-on massage method. Prana healing from the traditions of India and transmission techniques from shamanic traditions of American Indians also fit into this category. These cultures call the healing resource by different names—*Prana, Ki, Mana*—but the transmission methods are very similar. A highly refined contemporary approach to hands-near healing, with far-distant healing components as well, was developed by one of my favorite colleagues, Barbara Brennan, after many years exploring physics and doing NASA research. Her method is beautifully described in her landmark book, *Hands of Light*.

While many professionals study these methods for years, healing associated with the natural qualities of Qi is available to everyone. Rendering compassionate assistance is an extra benefit of your personal Qi cultivation practice. Because of the nature of Qi and intention, Qigong causes shifts in the healing field within and around you, which triggers positive influences for friends and loved ones near and far.

ONE-ON-ONE Enter the highest state of Qi cultivation that you have the ability to access. Your key focus is not diagnosing or treating the person that you are working with. You are simply being with him or her in your optimal state of cultivation and intention. This Qigong state removes obstruction to the natural tendency of the universe to come into balance within and around you. These hands-near transmission gestures are much like engaging in your own practice with another person present. In fact you should encourage the person you're working with to enter the Qigong state as well.

There are three basic stages of hands-near transmission—clearance, restoration, and coherence.

- Clearance—sweeping gestures—clears, purifies, breaks up, dispels, purges, pulls out, or removes accumulations of disturbed, spent, or extra Qi either generally or in particular areas.
- Restoration—sending and concentrating gestures—restores, tones, enhances, nourishes, or stimulates Qi in particular areas or throughout the Qi Matrix.
- Coherence—smoothing gestures that conclude the process—balances, harmonizes, coordinates, and integrates the field by aligning the whole system.

In each stage, you allow universal resources to be activated through your intention to help your friend, to either increase Qi or circulate stagnant Qi to rebalance Qi disharmony. Approach this with an open mind and heart. Just as in your own cultivation for personal improvement, Transmit Qi is very personal. Interestingly, in my own case, there have been many times when I was personally questioning whether anything was happening while the receiver of the transmission was actually experiencing a very positive effect. It may take some time to trust this process. However, you can rest in comfort that it has been used with positive benefits for thousands of years.

The Clearing Gesture: Sweeping. In most cases, particularly when there is pain and swelling or stuck, stagnant, and accumulated Qi, this vigorous sweeping gesture breaks up stuck Qi and whisks it away. At the end of the sweep, flick your wrist downward. You will find that some people are very sensitive to this and feel immediate relief. Encourage the person that you are working with to use the Three Intentful Corrections while you are doing the practice to enter into a deep Qigong state.

Hold in your HeartMind the promise that the natural urge of the universe is to find balance. When you cultivate Qi while performing Transmit Qi gestures, it helps to open the channels allowing trapped Qi to be released. Do this as much or for as long as it feels appropriate and then proceed to the restoring gestures.

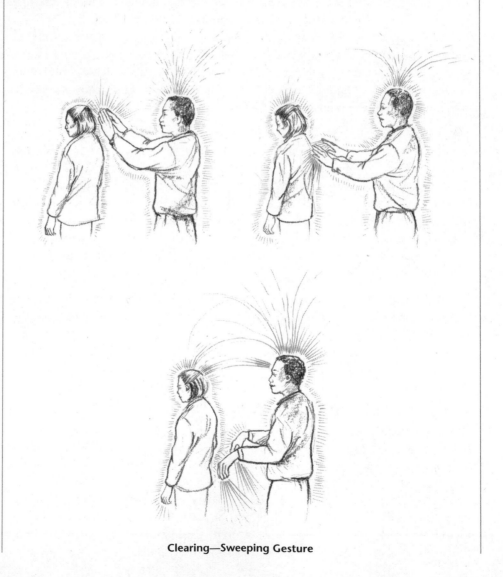

Clearing—Sweeping Gesture

The Restoring Gestures: Sending and Concentrating. When stagnant energy has been dispelled and cleansed it is appropriate to introduce fresh Qi into the system. If that is appropriate it will occur automatically with these gestures.

Sending is a gesture that you can do with one or both hands. Turn your hands toward the person you are serving and visualize that they are being filled with fresh, healing Qi. You can bathe the person in Qi; alternatively you can push Qi toward him

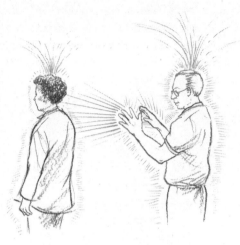

Restoring—Sending Gesture

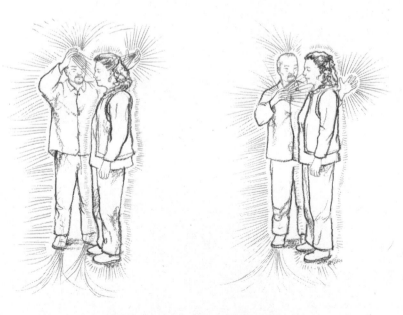

Restoring—Concentrating Gesture

倫次

Coherence

or her and then fluff the Qi. The idea is that healing resources will naturally fill the empty places where they are needed.

In concentrating, use the Forming the Ball of Qi position from the Discover Qi and the Transform Qi phases. Place one hand on each side of the part of your friend's body you feel could benefit from having its Qi restored. Move your hands apart and together and build up a field of healing energy between them—passing it through your friend's head, neck, torso, organs, elbow, hand, ankle, etc. Use a fluffing gesture as if you are gently squeezing and releasing a balloon or a pillow. You can also place your hands directly onto the body and run energy and heat into different parts. Your personal cultivation practice helps open the channels so that the restoring energy is enabled to flow.

The Coherence Gesture: Smoothing. This looks a little like the clearing gesture except that it is much smoother and slower. Instead of vigorous sweeping you are smoothing the whole field gently as if you were carefully combing and smoothing an invisible energy body or combing beautiful long hair. After having removed accumulated disharmony and restored fresh healing energy into the Qi Matrix, this gesture brings the whole Qi body into a state of coherence and integrity.

Simply do your own internal cultivation practice knowing that your sincerity and willingness to disassociate from complexity will naturally trigger your most refined level of Qi harmony and flow—in the presence of that person that you are assisting. The greatest benefit comes from the fact that you are going more and more toward the recognition, acknowledgment, and actuality of Oneness. The promise is that engaging in your practice as an actualization of your eternal nature causes the Qi to spontaneously maximize in and around you. The effect on the person that you are practicing with is spontaneous and frequently quite profound.

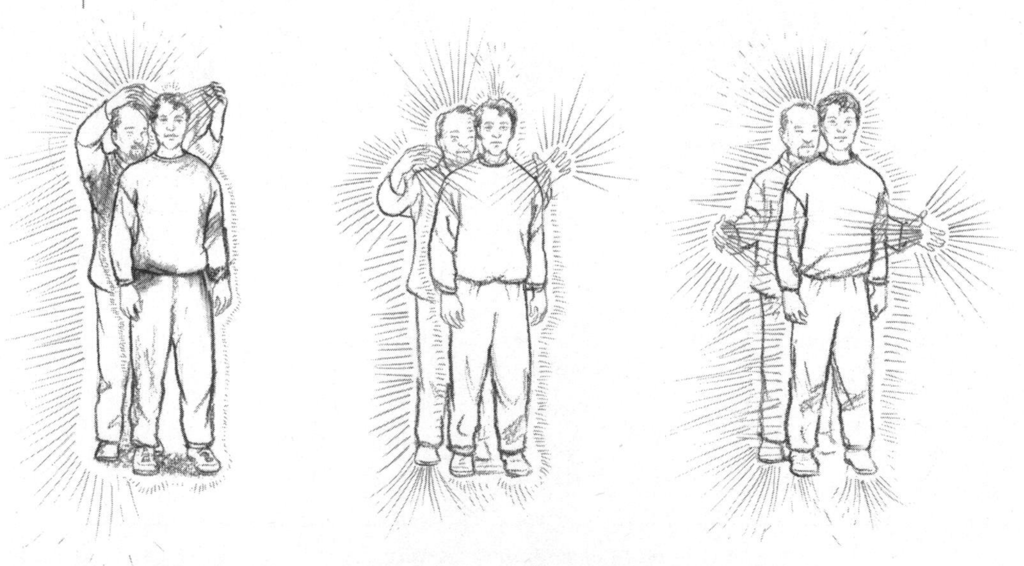

Coherence—Smoothing Gesture

ONE-TO-SEVERAL This technique also can be for group transmissions. It is quite common in China where charismatic masters do transmission with groups both small and large. In recent years there is quite a bit of debate as to whether the dramatic effects that occur within these groups are actually caused by the Qigong master or by the immense amount of emotional agreement among the members of the audience. In either case very positive healing can occur.

GROUP-ON-ONE Two or more practitioners can use the Clear Qi, Restore Qi, and Qi Coherence gestures with one receiving person. I witnessed this method at the Zhi Neng Hospital in Qing Huang Dao, where all participants—recipients and the transmitters—enter the deep and intentful cultivation state either doing hands-on or hands-near transmission. To enhance and coordinate the effect, they chant simultaneously, "Illness dispelled. Yes it is so." This practice reminded me of the healing services that take place in charismatic churches here in the West.

GROUP-ON-GROUP This is one of the classic methods for teaching people to feel Qi. Because there is such a dynamic energy when people learn and practice in a group, the Qi sensation from person to person can be more palpable than usual.

Lao Gong Circle 3. Proceed from Lao Gong Circle 1 or Lao Gong Circle 2 at the end of the section entitled "Hands-On," earlier in this chapter. Everyone holds the left palm turned up and the right palm turned down. Arms are in the bent-elbow position that is common for shaking hands. Place your right hand over the left hand of the person to your right. Allow the circle to adjust so that everyone is in a comfortable position. Feel the energy that arrives from the left and allow it to flow or pulse

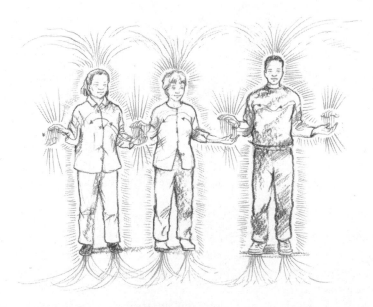

Lao Gong Circle 3

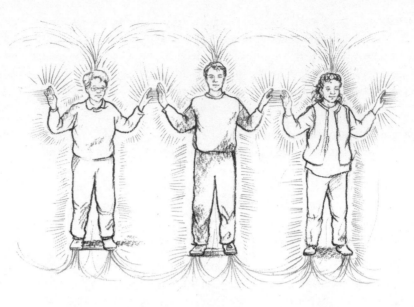

Lao Gong Circle 4

through your Qi Matrix to the right. If it feels to you like the current is going the other way, or if you find that the feeling is too subtle, do not worry. Worry is the enemy of Qi cultivation. It is absolutely impossible for this energy not to exist. The entire universe, including your own body, is made up of circulating and interacting fields of subtle energies and information. Relax and realize that this is so. Over time you will get a feel for the energy. When the group breathes together it enhances the effect; add the sound "Ahh" on the exhalation. On the inhalation raise up a bit. On the exhalation sink down. After repeating these steps a few times, stop and just feel the flow of healing resources.

    Lao Gong Circle 4. Raise your hands with palms facing right and left at head level. Step back a bit to create space for the circle to expand and to allow room to explore and experiment with feeling the Qi from the people next to you. Place your palms several inches from your neighbors' and proceed with your internal cultivation. Feel the sensation of the Qi as it circulates within you and throughout the circle. This force, traveling from, to, and through everyone has the potential to maximize healing and assist in clearing the Qi Matrix in all of the participants.

3. Near-Distant with Intention

You can transmit Qi without using your hands through a high level of focus and intention. This form of transmission usually takes place with the receivers fairly nearby. One of my favorite colleagues, Chiyan Wang, is originally from Xian, China, and currently lives in Santa Barbara, California. She is an excellent Qigong teacher and transmission healer. Among her skills is the method of sitting in a chair just a few feet from her clients and transmitting Qi to effect healing through focused intention.

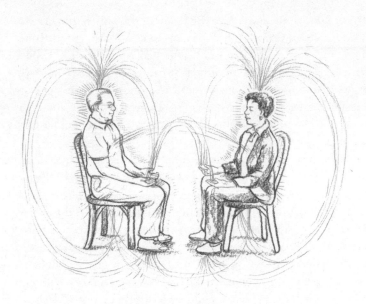

Near-Distant Two Qi

Near-distant can be interpreted as "in the same room." Beyond that space the transmission becomes far-distant. Any effect of intention that crosses a space—whether it be several inches, several feet, or many miles—is referred to as nonlocal intentionality in most of the research literature. The effect that is generated among people who pray together or practice Qigong together is a near-distant Qi transmission effect. However, such practices can have a far-distant effect as well.

ONE-ON-ONE TRANSMISSION While a professional healer would have the necessary training for both diagnosis and treatment, your most powerful healing tool is to relax and do nothing more than open to the natural flow of universal resources. The promise of the Qi is that the deepening of your cultivation practice has benefits that are not limited to yourself. Your practice, whether it is to address the separate phases of cultivation or simply to shift into the deep Qigong state, triggers effects in the field.

This transmission method is very much like prayer. In fact if you wish and if it helps you to sustain the Qigong state, use prayer or gratitude as a focus for your attention while you hold the intention that your practice will benefit those that you hope to support. If the universal arrangement of all key factors is such that your friend or loved one can benefit, he or she will. You can let the person know that it is your intention that he or she might benefit from your practice. If the person asks what to do, have him or her meditate or pray or visualize a state of vitality and comfort.

Rather than saying, "Now I will help you," say, "Let's cooperate to access benefit from the Qi field." You can do this at meals with loved ones, in intense family or group meetings, or at meetings with your colleagues at work. Simply transmit the intention that a person or the group will experience an influx of benefit.

LECTURE WITH QI One of the most powerful forms of transmission is known as Lecture with Qi. A lecture about Qigong (or self-healing or empowerment) delivered by someone in the Qigong state (or any state of heightened consciousness), whose intention is highly focused on a transmission of benefit causes an effect in our shared field of subtle energy or consciousness. The secret of Lecture with Qi is to be able to enter and sustain the Qigong state while speaking with great sincerity about the possibilities of Qigong and the promise of the Qi. It is typical for the speaker to suggest that the audience enter the Qigong state.

Everyone who has listened to an inspiring speaker is familiar with some level of this idea. In *The Healer Within* I reported on a lecture that I gave to fifteen hundred hospital executives. As I lectured, a group of people did a Qigong demonstration on the stage. The combination of listening to the soothing sound of the words about how to relax and experience inner healing along with seeing people practicing Qigong created several effects. One was that a number of people from the audience reported experiencing sudden relief from tension or fatigue. During the talk, the audience practiced together for a few moments to enhance the Qi Chang. Several executives from major hospitals who experienced the lecture and demonstration reported feeling that something unusually special must have happened in the room. They commented that they could "feel it."

I have frequent opportunities to lecture to large audiences. The subject is often Qigong or Qi and we usually practice some Qigong methods as a part of the experience. Almost always several people will approach me after a lecture and share that they had some sort of healing, from an ache or pain that was troubling them. Often some-

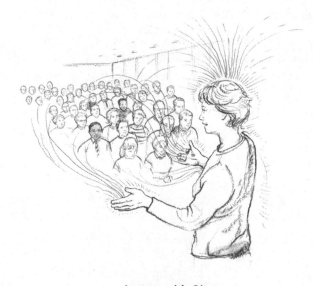

Lecture with Qi

one in the audience experiences a sudden overwhelming spell of weeping, an unexpected change of heart, or an unforeseen intuition about something that needed to be solved.

The natural tendency of Qi is to flow. When we do our practice, particularly with a group with sincere intention and in the company of an inspiring speaker, the Qi field can become very rich. The openness of the participants creates a potent dynamic in the field; healing, inspiration, and even miracles can result.

GROUP-ON-ONE AND GROUP-ON-GROUP Group Qi transmission is very much like prayer or directed meditation where the effect is focused in the same room or same area. A Qigong group focusing Qi transmission on one person is a common occurrence in contemporary China. Typically the participants practice sitting or standing Qigong. These transmitters focus on their own practice of Qi cultivation and the effects create a healing field of Qi—Qi Chang—which transmits a positive influence to the receivers.

This phenomenon can happen whether the practice is Qigong, prayer, contemplation, meditation, or even inspiring discussion of topics that all participants find interesting or meaningful. Any group support type of gathering maximizes Qi as well. Meetings where a group of people have all agreed to seek personal improvement, healing, or optimal future outcomes create a strong Qi field.

When I visited the Zhi Neng Hospital, I saw that among a practice group of three hundred people a number of individuals were lying on portable beds. This remains one of the most fascinating, practical, cost-effective, compassionate, and profound Qigong transmission practices I have ever witnessed. The very unwell person, with cancer or paralysis, who cannot participate actively within the group, joins the practice session and absorbs the transmission of Qi from the active practitioners. In conversations, I learned that these unwell persons relax completely and open up to the benefit of the Qi of the group—this is a *not doing* (*Wu Wei*). However, they also intentfully *do* something no matter how small—deepen their breath, wiggle their fingers and toes, or hold their hands together over their abdomen. Everyone creates the healing field and everyone benefits from it, especially those whose need is greatest. Due to the boundless nature of the Qi it is likely that Qi Chang Gong has marvelous benefits that we have not yet begun to explore.

4. Near-Distant with Instruction

It is very common for people to say that they feel the Qi is stronger when they practice with a group. Qigong tradition explains that this is due to Qi transmission from the instructor and the fellow students. The student or practitioner is in a more open state due to the effect of the group on his or her level of focus and intention. The presence of other students in a similar state creates a very rich pool of Qi resource. In addition, the instructor's Qi, transmitted from his or her own practice to help and inspire others, creates a powerful dynamic of energy and consciousness.

Sharing

ONE-ON-ONE AND ONE-ON-SEVERAL If you are instructing others, even in very simple Qigong practices, you can maximize the transmission if you can sustain your own practice as you teach. If you really pay attention to the instruction you receive from others, you will find that many instructors teach in part with transmission, whereas others are merely giving instructions. Both are authentic teachings, but when the instruction is infused with Qi it takes everyone to a higher level. As you give instruction, continually return to your own practice. As you answer questions allow the answers to arise from the field of ancient wisdom. As you correct the students also correct yourself—cycle yourself through the Three Intentful Corrections, consciously and constantly, from moment to moment.

If you are the student, understand that the benefits of Qigong are not generated solely within yourself. When you allow yourself to practice deeply and open your Qi Matrix to Qi transmitted from the teacher and from the field created by the group, you open yourself even more completely to the potential created by the relationship between Heaven, Earth, and all of nature. Because time flows in many directions, the rich Qi potential from past and future masters, practitioners, teachers, and luminaries is accessible to you at any time and in any location.

GROUP-ON-GROUP Many of the larger Qigong hospitals and institutes in China use a transmission method in which several or many instructors enter the Qigong state with the goal to maximize the field and enhance the learning and healing of the students and patients. At the Zhi Neng Hospital, the patients (called students) practice in a group with from ten to twenty instructors present. The main instructor stands on a platform with a microphone and speaks the instructions in a very soothing voice. Along the front of the practice area are a number of advanced instructors.

Their presence provides a visible model for the practice of course, but they are also transmitting Qi. Given their advanced practice, they are able to enter a highly focused Qigong state at a high level of cultivation. This creates an effect that is not limited within their own body or even within their local area. Because of the nature of Qi and the nature of a group practice of many sincere participants, the instructors are able to load the field with beneficial influence.

5. Far Nonlocal

The ancient Qi masters determined long ago that beneficial influences can be transmitted over great distances; more recently this phenomenon has been confirmed through science and research. As we will discuss, such influences must be mediated by fields of energy, information, or consciousness. Recently, physicists have uncovered the fact that such influences may actually be transmitted back in time to effect changes in the cause of events that can alter the future. In my practice of Chinese medicine I have had numerous patients who needed to have some additional treatment by transmission when they were out of town or having an emergency. In some cases I have worked with people who have called from far away and asked for help because it was impossible for them to travel to Santa Barbara.

In the last decade there has been a wave of scientific verification of the benefits of prayer—also known as nonlocal intention. My wife, Rebecca, is a prayer transmitter as well as a Qigong practitioner and instructor. People frequently comment that her prayers have helped them and as this phenomenon has become more known she has received more and more prayer requests. They like her Qigong instruction because it is prayerful. Prayer and Qigong may be seen as variations on the single idea of purposeful transmission of beneficial effect. There is no distance limit on the effect of either form of transmission.

A client of mine who was experiencing extreme health problems and having very little success from conventional medical treatment asked if I would send Qi to her. I agreed. As I did my own practice every morning, I would hold an image of Kathy in perfect health for a few moments along with a number of others that I was working with through intentful transmission. The most important benefit that she received was at night when she experienced relief from anxiety, panic, and sleeplessness. Several times she thanked me for sending Qi and asked if I had been transmitting healing energy to her at a certain time—usually in the evening or at night.

My early morning transmissions were apparently stored in the field until the evening when she needed the Qi most. When the recipients of Qi transmission are in a positive and open state and the practitioners who transmit Qi are able to reach an authentic state of Qi cultivation, the beneficial effect is not bounded by time or distance. There is a growing body of research that suggests that such effects can also reach into the past, so it is even possible that my transmission in the case above was actually having its effect back in time to the previous night.

In *The Healer Within* I reported on a case where the transmission effect was generated over thousands of miles with the mother of a physician in New York. I added her to my transmission list and mentioned at our weekly community Qigong practice group that those who wished to could use their intention during practice to transmit benefit to her. Confirmation came the next day when the physician called and encouraged us to continue, stating that his mother had suddenly improved. These effects have recently been granted a good deal of scientific study, as we will discuss in Chapter 16, and the findings have been very positive.

NONLOCAL TRANSMISSION BY AN INDIVIDUAL There are many ways to describe far-distant healing as a transmission method. In keeping with the theme of this book the primary guideline is to just do your practice and to create a beneficial influence through directed, effortless intention. Enter into the deepest possible Qigong state. Work through your practice of the Ten Phases of Cultivation and Mastery. As you do so, engage one of the following methods.

Bathe in Qi. This is really the same method as we discussed in the "Hands-Near" section—Forming the Ball of Qi. Instead of placing your hands around an area of the body of a friend who is present, visualize that you are holding a friend or loved one who is not present suspended between your hands. Turn to your cultivation practice, draw Qi into yourself using the breath and open the Qi Matrix. Collect Earth energy

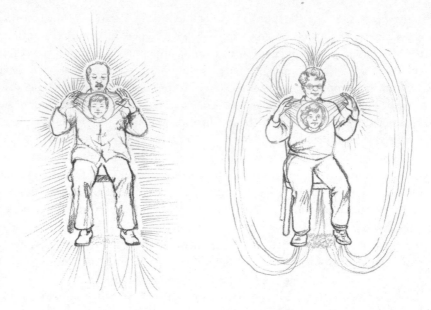

Bathe in Qi—Distant Healing

through feet and Heaven energy through the top of your head. Feel these resources converging in the middle Dan Tian where Yin and Yang merge—the HeartMind. Particularly on the exhalations, feel the Qi pouring out of the HeartMind into your hands and expressing from the Lao Gong points.

Feel the Qi field between your hands or visualize the Qi of Heaven and Earth filling the area between your hands where the image of your friend or loved one is caressed in healing Qi. Know that due to the nature of the universe and the promise of Qi, he or she is being bathed in healing resources. No matter how far away the person you are transmitting to may be, if you sincerely enter a deep Qigong state, that person can receive beneficial effect, especially if he or she is open to it.

Light Transmission Method. Prepare for this practice by absorbing, circulating, and cultivating Qi internally. As you go deeper into your practice bring the image of your friend or loved one into your mind's inner visual field. Knowing that the natural tendency of the universe is to seek balance and harmony, be aware that the balancing influence can manifest as radiant light and visualize that light shining upon the person you are focusing on. There are any number of ways to do this. Visualize the person glowing as if filled with light. Or imagine that the person suddenly receives an invigorating charge from Heaven, like a lightning bolt. You can also see the person bathing in the gentle glowing rays of sunrise or sunset. Acknowledge to yourself that seeing them infused with light equates with healing. Complete the practice by confirming internally, "So be it" or "It is so."

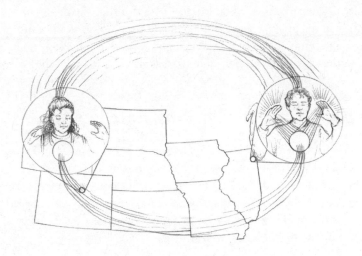

Light Transmission Method

When I do this with my students, patients, or family members it takes just a few minutes. It is a part of my meditation to sustain that state of inner quiet and go through an array of people—usually family members. I visualize each person in a natural setting unless he or she is always at home. I visualize purposefully and sincerely that the forces of Heaven and Earth are gathering potential. Then, with a gentle suddenness, I visualize that person, say one of my children, filled with a powerful light that is released from Heaven—like lightning—passing through him or her and into the Earth. For a moment I visualize that he or she is glowing.

You can also transmit Qi light in this way to groups. You may be moved to use Qi transmission for groups of people who are struggling in life or people who are experiencing sudden hardship or disaster. As you do your regular Qigong practice, think of the group that you are transmitting Qi to and know that there is more than enough power in the universe to provide for their highest good. It is not useful to expect any particular outcome. If a change for the better is appropriate, it will naturally arise.

NONLOCAL TRANSMISSION BY A GROUP In China, Qi transmission by groups is very common. The Qi Chang Gong, or "group-generated field with healing effect," is discussed frequently by the great contemporary Qi masters. In the West, some of the best research on nonlocal healing effects investigates this aspect of far-distant transmission. There are many documented cases involving groups of people with healing skill who have transmitted prayer and energy to people with health challenges. The findings show that those people who have been the targets of the transmission experience significant beneficial effects. In Qigong this kind of effect is transmitted when the group engages sincerely and with great intent on the practice of Qi cultivation. Every week at our

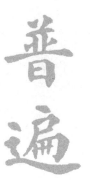

Universal

community Qigong practice session we close with this transmission method. We have, at that point in the practice, been doing cultivation methods for about one hour. To conclude, we transmit as a group to assist people in need, to intervene against violence, to reduce suffering, and to support national leaders in humanitarian decisions.

The Possibilities for Qi Transmission

It is obvious that there is a tremendous resource for our culture in taking a serious look at the Chinese tradition of Qi transmission to serve others. As science continues to confirm that these kinds of effects are possible, Qigong will play a strong role in actualizing the possibilities on a grand scale. The depth and richness of the Qigong tradition provides carefully crafted tools, as you can see, for a wide variety of contexts. These tools and methods are easy to learn.

The possibilities are limitless.

Mind Focus Affirmation

Transmitting Qi, I tap the potential of the universe to serve the healing and empowerment of others.

PART III

The Deeper Promise

Confucius instructed:
First, set your HeartMind on the One.
   Then listen,
      not with your ear,
      nor even with your HeartMind.
Listen with your Qi,
   the very essence of your ultimate self.
The ear can only hear.
The HeartMind is typically
   entangled in evaluation.
The Qi is completely open and receptive
   to every subtle level of being.

—Zhuang Zi, *Inner Chapters*, fourth century B.C.E.

The Practice:
Your Qigong and Tai Chi Owner's Manual

> He or she who seeks The Way
> and the Fullness of Life
> must practice the methods.
> Train sincerely
> with perseverance,
> and you will enter by the large gate
> to acquire the secret of Heaven.
>
> —AUTHOR UNKNOWN, *TOWER OF FRAGRANCE*
> *TRAINING SECRET*

Harvesting the Fruits of Qigong and Tai Chi

You have now seen how the three levels of Qigong (Chi Kung)—Earth, HeartMind, and Heaven—can be expressed in the phases of Qi (Chi) cultivation and mastery and compassionate service. Even the beginning levels of this system, the Earth phases of Qigong, promise to bring about tremendous changes in your life. Research in China and elsewhere has confirmed that the major clinical benefits of Qigong can result from methods that are relatively simple to learn and pass on to others. An enormous benefit in healing, personal productivity, learning capacity, work effectiveness, and general health is available to us with minimal effort. The more advanced methods of the HeartMind and Heaven levels are certainly worth pursuing yet a major revolution in health care and personal empowerment requires only the simplest practices.

Perhaps you have noticed that the practice methods we have learned, even in the later phases of cultivation, are neither complex nor time consuming. They do not require any special equipment or attire. Remind yourself of the Three Intentful Corrections. No matter where you are sitting, standing, or even lying down, you can implement these with almost no effort. And yet, by simply remembering and then using the Three Intentful Corrections, you begin making the most profound internal medicine—for no cost. Even as you deepen your practice, you will see that you can pursue advanced levels of Qigong in a context that is stress-free, easy, and fun.

Sometimes I am asked, "Are the complex and esoteric practices more effective or more profound than the simple practices?" Many people think that my answer will be yes. But, as Lao Zi said, "The greater outcomes are achieved with little effort." Nature achieves immense results without effort, and so can you. This is the third promise of Qi.

The Third Promise of Qi

The ultimate aim in Qigong is to attain the Qigong state, but it is not via the crowded, busy mind or the tense, confused body that we get there. The simpler the practice, the better. Plus, there is a greater benefit to our culture when practices are simpler, because more people can use them. The more people who benefit from Qigong, the greater our general health, inner peace, and overall productivity. The widespread use of the simple methods will generate far-reaching benefits across the domains of health care, business, and social services, as well as in our churches, schools, community agencies, and prisons.

THE THIRD PROMISE

Qi Cultivation—Qigong—is easy if you let it be.

Regarding the value of reduced complexity Lao Zi writes, "In pursuit of average goals, every day something must be gained. In the practice of the Way of Harmony, every day something is given up. When you align with natural forces, nothing essential is left undone." Here is your permission to pursue Qigong in a lighthearted manner with no self-judgment. Despite all the beautiful forms of Qigong that have accumulated over the centuries, your most direct path to the Qigong state remains simply focused intention and a relaxed body.

But what about mastery and the capacity to render the practices perfectly? These are, of course, noble pursuits. If you have ever witnessed a highly skilled master of Tai Chi (Taiji), you know it can be a breathtaking display. But the benefits of Qigong are not just available to those who seek mastery or perfection. In fact the greatest masters will tell you to relax your need for perfection, to simply seek your natural level of cultivation. The main goals are health, healing, enhanced personal productivity and creativity, longevity, and peace of mind. Qigong is intended as a tool for eliminating stress, not creating it.

This chapter will make your Qigong practice easier and more effective by addressing some creative ways to approach the phases of cultivation and the practice methods. In addition, we will explore some insights about teachers, teaching, and learning. Finally, because the Qi has the capacity to communicate and we have the capacity to listen, we will explore the voice of the Qi. Your practice deepens when you attend to what the Qi is communicating to you.

Approaching the Phases

Though many very traditional schools from China insist that their tradition is superior, there is no single, most authentic and inspiring way to learn and benefit from Qigong or Tai Chi. How can one out of ten thousand truths be *more* true? All the schools and traditions are profound, all of the authentically wise masters are, in fact, wise. What do the ten thousand forms of Qigong and Tai Chi have in common? Through synthesis, it is possible to embrace all of these separate bodies of great wisdom and then refine them, alchemically, to a concentrated set of basic principles— the Ten Phases of Cultivation and Mastery of Qi.

This approach is not intended as a rigid system for learning. It offers a way to organize and approach the knowledge, but you should feel free to modify and enhance the methods as well as the phases of cultivation. Everyone learns differently. Allow your fascination with Qi cultivation to pull you forward. If you find yourself operating outside of the model as it is laid out here, it is very likely an indication that you are developing an intimate and personal relationship with Qi as well as an enhanced capacity for intuition. Remember, the ten thousand forms of Qigong reflect ten thousand inspired revelations. Follow the path most likely to inspire your own revelation and personal breakthrough.

Using the Phases Sequentially

Approaching Qigong using the Ten Phases of Cultivation and Mastery creates a comfortable framework for learning and experience. The later phases are made possible by the skills and insights you learn in the early phases.

However, there is no reason why you should force yourself to master one phase before proceeding to explore later phases. The deepening of your skill in the areas of focus and intention, from the HeartMind phases onward, are the real keys to advancing even in the Earth level practices. Use the sequence of the phases within the context of free exploration.

Practice

Using the Phases Simultaneously or in Random Order

There is value in familiarizing yourself with the methods from the later phases—even if you are just beginning. The more you sincerely practice any of the phases, the more skilled you will become. Inevitably, the deepening of your practice comes through upgrading Qigong from an exercise or self-care technique to a more conscious way of being. This occurs much more in the HeartMind phases than in the Earth phases because the role of intention and will are ever expanding. In fact, exploring the later phases—particularly Direct Qi, Conserve Qi, Store Qi, and Transform Qi—provides a lesson in the necessity for holding the focus of attention and intention. Exploring the HeartMind phases before you have gained HeartMind skill will remind you of the value of the earlier phases. Jumping ahead in the phases can prove to be a terrific strategy for learning and progressing, allowing you to appreciate your growing mastery while reminding you of how much is left to access and explore.

Harvest

The Phases Transcended: Natural Flow Qigong

The most direct path into the heart of Qigong transcends the phases of cultivation. Natural Flow Qigong, which I have referred to frequently in this book, creates a direct connection with the ultimate Qigong state. Natural Flow Qigong is similar to the classic methods of practice Guarding the One and Circulating the Light. It includes all of the phases with no specific practice methods and no effort. By adjusting your relationship with the universal Qi field, by radically opening to natural flow—all of the gifts and benefits of Qigong are accessed instantaneously.

This is the simple, most difficult path—simple because it is easy to do for a moment; most difficult because it is very challenging to sustain when your life's conditioning is constantly distracting you. If you work with Qigong over time, eventually you can become adept at Natural Flow Qigong. Then like the ancient Qi masters you may begin to gain the capacity to remain aware of your ultimate, universal self in the midst of complexity. According to the ancients your universal self is always present. Giving expression to that presence of inner splendor transcends all levels, phases, and methods.

The Qigong Practice Methods

Like the phases of cultivation, the Qigong practice methods may be approached creatively and intuitively. There are a few key points that will make your use of the practices in this book more fun and accelerate your capacity to cultivate Qi effectively.

The practice methods for each of the phases have been carefully chosen. Each is a worthy representative of the many other methods that could help you to gain the benefits of that particular phase of cultivation. Each has been selected from among the beautiful historic forms developed over millennia, including Tai Chi, standing meditation, Tendon Changing Method, Bathing the Marrow, vitality medical Qigong, Primordial Qigong, and others. These forms, so carefully refined by generations of Qi masters, are programmed to take you right into the heart of Qigong. Using your intention and focus, you can use these methods to make contact with the heritage of the Qi masters who developed them.

The Multiple Applications of the Qigong Methods

The preliminary and warm-up practice methods that were introduced in Part I are not simply beginner techniques. All are methods that become more advanced as you deepen your practice. And the very advanced methods in phases seven through nine are not off limits to beginning Qi cultivators either. While some more martial methods require rigorous training, the primary guideline in Qi cultivation for personal improvement is to keep it simple and fun. The methods chosen to represent the phases are all very gentle and effective. At the same time they are easy to grasp and applicable as both beginning and advanced practices.

For example Gather Qi from Heaven and Earth (from phase two), the exemplary method for gathering Qi, is an excellent practice for circulating and purifying Qi as well. Bathing the Marrow, a method we explored in phase seven, Store Qi, is also a gathering and directing method. So don't get caught up placing these multifaceted practices into limited categories. The practice methods exemplify the particular phases of cultivation, but their benefits are not limited to the phase that they have been chosen to represent.

Guidelines for Your Practice

Historically, there have been many practice guidelines, and there are many excellent historical and contemporary books containing detailed instructions for practice as well. Some are focused on avoiding injury in very vigorous methods. Others prescribe elaborate lists of important precepts based on ritual or tradition to ensure success. The intention here is to support you in a practice that is easy, safe, and enjoyable. A very practical list of guidelines includes:

Keep your practice simple and fun.
Focus on relaxation.
Practice daily.
Use the Three Intentful Corrections throughout the day.
Find several practice spots—one inside and one in nature.
Experiment with doing your practice at different times of the day or night.
Feel free to modify and combine practices and make up your own routines.

Modify the practices to build strength.
Look for opportunities to practice with others.
Look for opportunities to work with advanced practitioners and instructors.
Stay within your comfort zone.

The Primary Caution for Qigong Practice

In keeping with our guiding principle of simplicity there is one point of caution: Always stay in the zone of comfort. If a practice causes discomfort, you have two options. First, modify the practice—either by proceeding more gently or by doing it sitting or even lying down. Second, avoid the practices that cause discomfort; just continue with other methods that have worked for you.

In appropriate cases there is a third option. With the support of a trusted instructor, and with great care, Qigong methods that cause discomfort can be practiced intentfully to expand your endurance, heal injuries, and promote flexibility. In this context it is still wise to go slowly. Rarely is it advised to push through a physical or emotional limitation. However, it is consistent with the philosophy of Qigong to approach and tease the limit. Playing gently at the edge of your limits, over an ongoing period of Qigong practice, can translate into a radical—but safe and comfortable—life transformation.

Typically, if a particular practice is challenging, you can simply modify it. Proceed at a 50 percent reduction or cut to 10 percent, and build slowly to 100 percent. Modification is a major key in successful Qigong and Tai Chi.

Seated and Lying Down Practices

All of the practice methods in this book can be done sitting. For some of the practices, it is more convenient to sit on a stool rather than a chair, for ease of turning and arm swinging. Or you may move to the edge of a chair.

There are no barriers to the use of Qigong. For people who are very ill, Qigong is an important healing tool. Sitting practice is very powerful and effective for rehabilitation, to treat injury, or after surgery. Seated Qigong is particularly applicable for elders, people who use wheelchairs, and even those in need of a break from their office or computer.

In severe cases the practices may be modified significantly for the reclining position. For the most severe cases where the patient is very weak or paralyzed, Qigong can be modified to use internal imaging of the methods through visualization. Research has demonstrated that simply visualizing yourself doing body movement causes an increase of metabolism and triggers healing effects.

Lying down Qigong practice is also a perfect way to begin and end the day. Many of us spend the last minutes of our day in an exhausted haze. Many of us begin the day with stressful thoughts about our to-do list. Consider ending the day and beginning the following morning by running through the Three Intentful Corrections and placing your hands to send Qi to your organs as in Direct Qi (see page 138). Or turn your attention to Natural Flow Qigong or Circulating the Light (see page 41).

How to Do the Practices

The location, state of mind and body, timing, and number of repetitions for your practice are all immensely personal. Some approaches insist that you face in a certain direction, be in a certain location, do a certain number of repetitions, do the practices in a certain order, and so on. In *The Healing Promise of Qi* we are using a more liberal approach. You are the best person to decide most of these practice issues. If you honor the inner teacher, your own connection with the wisdom of the universe, you will discover the perfect way to approach each practice for highest possible personal benefit.

Location and Timing

As you get deeper into Qigong you will find yourself looking for a special spot to practice. Always attempt to practice in a location that has the best exposure to natural resources—the best Qi. Whenever possible this should be a natural setting, which gives you an advantage because the Qi is automatically richer and fresher. The parks in China are crowded with Qigong and Tai Chi practitioners in the early mornings, before the rush of noise and pollution from traffic intrude on the natural environment. For me, there is a spot about a mile from my house where I can look one way and see the Pacific Ocean, and the other way to see the nearby mountains. Between November and March the distance from home to this spot is crowded with the monarch butterflies who spend the winter in the eucalyptus grove.

The Qi field that is created by a group (Qi Chang) can boost the benefits of your practice, so look for opportunities to practice with others. Many communities have Qigong and Tai Chi classes at the local hospital, in the parks and churches, schools, and community centers.

Tradition

You can even practice in airports. I do a lot of Qigong on airplanes. From San Francisco to China I generally walk to the back of the plane four to five times throughout the flight. Often there are others doing some form of Qigong or stretching there as well.

If you think you don't have a perfect place to practice, consider the accounts of master teachers in China who have been persecuted and jailed in challenging political times over many dynasties. They often share stories of practicing in confined spaces and testify that Qigong saved their lives in terrible times. This speaks to the remarkable self-sustaining power of Qi cultivation and its healing and life-saving capacity. It also speaks to the fact that the location for your practice can be just about anywhere.

Those who have discovered the power of Qi in their lives usually practice between forty and sixty minutes at a time, but it is important to understand that even ten or fifteen minutes is useful. It is best to practice for an amount of time that is agreeable to you. In China forty-five minutes to an hour and a half is typical. It is also typical for people to practice early in the morning. However, it is best to practice when you can; it is useless to try to practice when you can't. Many esoteric traditions suggest that you should practice in the middle of the night. While there are excellent reasons for doing so, it is better to plan to practice when you actually will; otherwise, the practice doesn't happen and the promise is lost.

State of Mind and Body

You will use the Three Intentful Corrections to begin your practice whether you intend to use particular prescribed methods or some sort of spontaneous Qigong, including Natural Flow Qigong. This means that it is best, as much as possible, to be in the Qigong state—with the body, breath, and the mind intentfully adjusted.

Intention, what the Chinese refer to as mind intent (Yi), initiates your practice. Mind intent is how you make the transition from what you were doing—resting, working, planning, worrying—to the practice of Qigong or Tai Chi. Once you are in the practice it is the mind (HeartMind) that will elect or choose which methods to use. As you are using the chosen methods it is your mind (HeartMind) that decides to deepen the focus; it is the intentful mind that elects to sustain the focus rather than drifting into preoccupation, worry, and regret.

Far more important for effective Qigong practice than particular forms are a relaxed body, comfortable breathing, and a sense of stress-free fun. The state of the body that is preferred in your practice is best characterized as easeful flow linked to awakened intention.

Number of Repetitions

Some people do vigorous practice first and move toward quiescent or meditative methods. Some do the opposite. For those who feel most comfortable with a systematic approach, the Ten Phases of Cultivation and Mastery are based on classic principles and the practice methods are easy to use in sequential order. Many people prefer to rearrange the order of these methods or to combine the practices with their favorites from other sources.

The number of repetitions always engenders an interesting discussion in Qigong circles. Many will tell you that their instructors have claimed that you must do a cer-

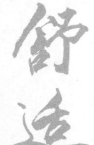

Comfort

tain number of repetitions to get the benefit. But everyone is at a different level of familiarity with Qigong and at a different level of personal endurance. The best approach is a personalized one. It just doesn't make sense for an exhausted person with a severe health condition to try to match the duration of practice of someone who is reaching toward peak performance. If you are getting started or if you are experiencing a severe health challenge, do only a little Qigong. If you have been working with the methods for a while and want to accelerate your progress, go ahead and do more.

There is one traditional method for the number of repetitions that is worth noting. There are Three Treasures associated with the three levels—Earth, HeartMind, and Heaven. Each of the levels has three phases. If you like the idea of being consistent with the traditions of China where Qigong originates, then use these numbers. To begin the Earth level of Qigong, use three repetitions, one for each level, Earth, HeartMind, and Heaven (body, mind, and spirit). As you do each one focus on and direct the benefit to that level of yourself: Gather Qi for the body, Gather Qi for the mind, and Gather Qi for the spirit.

As you deepen the practice, increase to six repetitions. This is representative of the HeartMind level. It definitely requires a certain focus to do six each of nine different practice methods. Then, as you advance to the Heaven level of your practice do nine repetitions. Intentful practice, using the nine methods of the nine phases for nine repetitions—particularly if you sustain a focused state of mind—will definitely take you into a very special experience and likely trigger a life-transforming encounter with the Qi.

How Important Is It to Do the Practices Perfectly?

It is possible to do the methods to a high level of perfection. This can be very beautiful and inspiring, but it is not necessary. I have found that people are more energized to reach for improvement if they are having fun than if they are being criticized, or are criticizing themselves, for failing to perform the practice perfectly. In Spontaneous Qigong, you get the benefits of Qigong without any form at all.

Frequently, people I have never met come to a lecture, workshop, or training session and tell me that reading *The Healer Within* helped them to regain their health. When they show me the methods that they have been doing, only a few out of hundreds are actually doing what I described in the book. Most have just understood the value of Qigong and have put together a set of practices that suits their needs—a set of practices that they enjoy doing. It is not so much special or particular methods that create healing but rather methods that feel right and are combined with an enthusiastic mind-set. The most beneficial methods are the ones that you actually use. As you use the practices suggested here and then go on to learn others, focus on deepening your attention and intent.

The Benefits of the Methods

As a doctor, scientist, and explorer, I have put a lot of personal energy into investigating the benefits of Qigong and Tai Chi. It is amazing how much is going on in the human system during these purposeful practices developed by the Chinese so long ago. Physiologically, the blood circulation is increased by Qigong, the delivery of oxygen and nutrition is accelerated, lymph moves more vigorously, immune cells are mobilized, and neurotransmitters associated with the self-repair capacity of the human system are produced and circulated. If there is a particular body part or function that needs healing, the use of movement, breath, massage, and mind focus can help direct Qigong benefits to it. An in-depth review of the benefits as well as the possible mechanisms through which Qigong and Tai Chi generate benefit are presented in the next chapter.

Within Qigong circles there has been a recent trend to claim that a particular method is for the benefit of the kidneys or that another method is good for the liver. I believe that this trend, based on the diagnosis or assessment of disease and dysfunction, tends to limit Qigong in an unfortunate way. In most cases Qigong methods have a broad range of benefits. An approach that confines and limits Qigong is contrary to the natural capacity of Qigong to open, release, and expand the capacity of the human system generally.

Medical Qigong has become very popular because we live in a time when people are deeply habituated to thinking of health care in terms of disease with medical solutions. Medical Qigong is often associated with doctors of Chinese medicine who determine a specific diagnosis in the terms of Chinese medicine and prescribe specific Qigong practices. It is typical of medical Qigong practitioners to work with Qi healing as well, as we discussed in phase ten, Transmit Qi.

In fact, many of the greatest forms of medical Qigong were not developed by physicians, but rather by sincere Qi lovers who followed the very basic principles of Qi cultivation. Guo Lin Qigong, probably the most famous method of medical Qigong, was developed by an artist. Another effective form of medical Qigong for back pain, used at the University of Maryland Medical School, was developed by a former violinist from China, Chan Zhang. And Jian-ye Jiang, the calligrapher and Tai Chi master who produced the beautiful calligraphy for this book, also teaches an excellent form of medical Qigong, Yin-Yang Medical Qigong.

Medical Qigong is worth your attention as an aspect of Qi cultivation, but even in China it is a very recent development. Keep in mind that most Qigong methods have multiple applications and a wide range of benefits. For example, the method in the Purify Qi phase benefits both the liver and the heart, according to Qigong tradition. It removes strain from the heart and dredges (cleanses) the liver. In addition, it opens or expands the center of the body, allowing for the influx of Qi. But, it also affects all of the organs, particularly the lungs, and circulates the Qi vigorously. In other words, this method purifies the Qi but it triggers many other benefits as well.

Choosing Methods to Enhance Benefits

With the idea in mind that a particular practice has specific benefits or limited benefits, people often ask me, "Which Qigong methods should I learn and use for my condition?" Typically, they believe that one particular method is more powerful than all others for their condition. If that were true there would not be thousands and thousands of methods.

I usually answer, "The best form of Qigong is the one that you enjoy. The Qigong methods that you like and the ones that you are likely to practice are the most powerful for you. It is fruitless to be encouraged to practice a method that you will not use because it is too long, too odd, or too confusing. Choose methods that you find inviting and that trigger a positive sense or sensation within you. Those will be the ones that you will tend to use and practice. It is through the practice that the benefits are gained." In general, most Qigong methods have a broad range of positive effects or influences.

More important than defining unique benefits for individual Qigong practices is learning how to modify the practices that you choose to accelerate their effectiveness to help heal a certain disorder, inner function, or part of your body. This is accomplished by using all of the powerful Qigong tools within your reach: your movement and posture, your breath, your hands (massage), and your intention (mind/-consciousness).

Select practices that you feel the most effectively activate and enhance the Qi. Then, using body movements and breath practices, circulate and direct the Qi to the area in need. Use mind focus to direct the Qi as well. Finally, use self-administered massage—both gentle and vigorous—to open the area for more robust Qi circulation.

What to Expect

Everyone will experience different signs of the activation of Qi. In years of teaching one of the things I have learned is not to tell people what they should feel. Spontaneous Qigong offers the fastest way for people in the early phases of exposure to Qigong to get a Qi sensation. This practice plus deep breathing with vigorous expressive sounds or sighs of relief ("Ahh!") rapidly and significantly activates the Qi. After we practice Spontaneous Qigong for a while, we stop, turn our attention inward, and explore the sensation of inner aliveness.

The question is, what do *you* feel and where do *you* feel it? The most important lesson in this experiment is that everyone reports a different experience. Some people say they experience tingling—in the hands or face, in the chest or abdomen, sometimes all over. Some people report that they feel spreading warmth, the release of tension in areas with tight muscles (particularly the neck and shoulders), or a lessening of headache or other pain. Some even report metaphysical experiences such as a sense

Benefit

of mild ecstasy, feeling high, or seeing lights or colors. Rather than tell you what you *should* feel, I invite you to explore what you *do* feel. If the teaching is based on what the teacher predicts you should feel, the magic of Qigong is already diminished. It is pretty amazing how many different experiences a few minutes of Spontaneous Qigong can bring on in a group of practitioners.

You may find it is easy to feel the Qi in your hands but difficult to get it into your feet. Eventually you will learn ways to move the Qi in all directions, to every area of your body and being. If there is a lot of energy in your head, but none in your abdomen, you will sense that to create balance you should explore Qigong for methods that help you move Qi down to the abdomen. These confirmatory signs of the awakening of the Qi are an important part of your evolution in Qigong.

Some people do not feel Qi as much as others. These people sometimes perceive this as a shortcoming. This type of self-judgment is one of the greatest enemies of Qi cultivation. On a trip to China, an Australian man in our group criticized himself for not feeling the Qi; he panicked that he had spent all this money to travel to China but was failing to learn Qigong. "You are healthy," I told him. "You get up early and are an energetic practitioner. You've got a great sense of humor that gets people laughing—this is very healing. Clearly you have great, ample, balanced Qi. Why don't you just relax and enjoy yourself?" Two days later, when we were waiting for the ferry to cross a river on the way to the scenic Yellow Mountains, he wandered off down the path. Later he came back all smiles and reported, "Just when I gave up on trying I had all of these sensations of the Qi in my fingers and in my cheeks."

The best answer for what to expect in Qigong is to have no expectations. If your mind is crowded with expectations, it cannot be free to perceive what else is really there.

Masters, Teachers, and Mentors

In the world of Tai Chi and Qigong, people typically rattle off a long list of their renowned master teachers. During my years of practice as a doctor of Chinese medicine, with numerous visits to China and thirty years of exposure to Qigong, I have met many teachers. With that said, I believe that the honor of having studied with a famous person is not an indicator of anyone's level of personal mastery. Certainly, the famous teacher can help to inform and empower, but this does not mean that his or her students will prove to be great or illuminated instructors themselves.

Some teachers pass on what they have been taught as if it is guaranteed truth. These teachers insist that you study and practice their methods exactly as they learned them. Tai Chi and Qigong traditions in this context, unfortunately, often discourage your own unique intuition and creativity in learning and practice. Even worse, many times a teaching that is passed down as truth is in actuality merely an opinion that is not true at all. Some such inaccuracies have been passed down for centuries.

Mentor

There are also teachers who pass on what they have experienced to be true, and suggest that each student also seek his or her own personal truth. This kind of teacher liberates students into their own direct experience, which serves as the source of the greatest learning. This kind of teacher acts as a gateway to the profound and views Qigong as a tool for accessing the raw essence of the universe.

A close colleague of mine had been studying Tai Chi with an esteemed master who after many years scolded her in front of a large group of other students for an oversight in technique. After much personal anguish she decided to stop working with this master. She then began to experiment with her practice. For the first time she practiced in her own way, not the teacher's. Within a few days she had a powerful revelation. "After eight years of vigilant study with little evidence of the personal experience of Qi," she recalls, "I had this profound and very personal experience of the Qi by following my intuition and by developing a more direct connection with the Qi."

Master Weng, my own favorite Tai Chi teacher, said about his own teacher, "The old man kept changing the form over the years and I realized he was adding in innovations from his own experience." The old man, known as the Leaping Butterfly Master, was renowned in the world of the martial arts. He served as the chief instructor for the police in Taiwan for many years. "We students were constantly getting the message that the basic principles of Tai Chi are like timeless immutable truths, but that the applications (the form, the technique) were dynamic and various."

In your own practice, you will most likely encounter numerous masters, teachers, and mentors, who will influence your experience of Qigong in different ways.

Masters

The master, in the most positive traditional sense, can lead you into a deep and profound relationship with your essential nature. The master is an open channel as long as the student performs, produces, and learns enthusiastically or sincerely. Chang Yi Hsiang and Zhu Hui, two of my most esteemed teachers, have both served as physicians in charge of major clinical facilities overseeing thousands of patients. Both command vast knowledge. And yet that knowledge always came toward me in the most caring way.

A master can save you an immense amount of time by passing along tried and true information. Such a person can give you access to a "transmission channel"—a direct connection to an ancient and authentic lineage of tradition, tools, and wisdom. The master can tell you what to do and what not to do, but he or she will also show you that Qigong is the method for awakening your own personal access to the universal resource. If you find yourself in a relationship with someone who promises to do the work for you, shake yourself awake.

A master who creates a transmission channel helps provide you with the means, but you must supply the effort in accessing this universal resource. The transmission

Master

channel is like walking into an ancient cathedral where the compassion, devotion, and community service of many generations is palpable. When working with some masters, your practice will tap into the lineage of teachers—a chain of departed spiritual luminaries that connects you back into ancient time.

There is, however, another side to the story. Because of the nature of the history of China many masters were forced by circumstances to become leaders of secret societies that focused on the martial applications of the Qi arts. As you can imagine, there are many masters who by necessity have worked in a training context of extreme rigor that the average student of Qigong and Tai Chi for healing may find overwhelming. You have to be the judge. Masters often reflect the styles of their own masters. Many have studied with harsh teachers and because of that influence also have a harsh teaching style. Be cautious; if you seek a gentle master teacher, feel free to pass if you find yourself learning from a more militant person.

Consider this: The greatest masters in any culture say one thing—that their knowledge comes directly from nature. Even Einstein, the master physicist steeped in the Western scientific worldview, claimed that his greatest insights came from drifting into intuitive states where he was directly exposed to the essence of nature. The most renowned spiritual leaders always point to Heaven, Earth, and nature as their source and suggest that their students seek direct experience of nature as well.

In Chinese medicine, we say that the doctor gives the treatment, but nature heals the disease. Nature is the ultimate master and teacher. The best earthly masters translate nature for us in a compassionate and loving context—even martial arts masters impart their message through encouragement and illumination rather than fear and guilt.

Ultimately the best master is one who inspires you to deepen your practice. In fact, it is the Qi itself that will become your most profound teacher.

Teachers

While every master is a teacher, not every teacher is a master. But it would be a terrible loss to the possibilities of Qigong and Tai Chi if we were to insist that every teacher be a master before we recognized the enormous benefits of his or her service.

Many teachers have been authorized through elaborate hierarchies of power in traditional Chinese lineages; others are empowered by their academic or political connections; still others are simply inspired individuals with little training. My favorite teachers are the people that I meet who are helping to fill the immense need for teaching Qi cultivation in everyday situations—people who have been energized to step up and satisfy the need for Qigong and Tai Chi in after-school programs; programs for children with learning or behavioral challenges; addiction prevention and recovery programs; facilities for those with cancer, MS, and other diseases; community programs for seniors; health clinics; and healing ministries at churches.

In the parks in China, the people who lead the practice groups are often uncredentialed citizens rendering service to their community. In China's nationwide Cancer Recovery Society and in Qigong programs at the Zhi Neng Hospital many of the teachers are recovering patients. These people have had powerful Qigong experiences and wish to give back through service.

If you do your practice on a regular basis and are inspired to share Qigong with others, I encourage you to consider acting as a guide, facilitator, or teacher. One of the most important kinds of instructors is a family member, a parent or grandparent who teaches Qigong or Tai Chi to a child. I will always be grateful for the influence my grandmother had on my experience of Qi.

For those who want to gain credentials, or to study with those who have them, there are many training programs available. At the International Integral Qigong and Tai Chi Training Program at the Santa Barbara College of Oriental Medicine we work with a number of training levels, including those appropriate for students of Chinese medicine and those for health-care professionals who need certification.

Widespread use of Qigong and Tai Chi will require many volunteers. One excellent definition of *teacher* is "someone who knows at least a little more than the student." This means that we are all qualified to teach something to someone. Ultimately, the greatest teacher is one who inspires you to deepen your practice.

The Importance of the First Teacher

When your first teacher is loving, compassionate, radiant, and inspired, you are blessed. It matters less whether this person is really an expert at Qigong or Tai Chi. The most important thing is that he or she supports you in your connection to the universal field of Qi.

When someone asks me, "How can I find a teacher and get started with Tai Chi or Qigong?" or "Do you know if Master So-and-So is a good teacher?" I recommend, that before that person begins with a teacher, he or she become informed through reading. A person can begin their learning through a book, video, or audio program.

The most important thing about the first teacher is that he or she not be someone who will exploit your urgent desire to learn Qigong (because of sickness or misfortune) or your exuberant innocence. Many people are infatuated with the notion that the power for healing lies outside of ourselves. Try to find someone who will encourage and inspire you to do your own practice to explore a creative relationship with the Qi.

Frankly, an enthusiastic amateur who is willing to be a mentor for you is a great first guide. This person will direct you to local practice sessions and workshops, books, and videos that will build up your knowledge base. This base of knowledge and experience will help you begin your exploration of Qigong and Tai Chi. It will enable you to feel comfortable and knowledgeable when you decide to seek more advanced teachers as you deepen your practice.

Finding Your Teacher

The important question is not who is your master or teacher, but rather are you inspired to engage in your practice. There are many books and Internet sites that can help you find a teacher. (See Resources for more information.)

When you meet with a prospective teacher, look for someone who radiates enthusiasm, positive spirit, and well-being. This is best noted in the brightness of the eyes, a healthy skin, sense of humor, and an energetic and buoyant walk.

The most disappointing stories are those involving people who were swept into a permanent relationship with a teacher who convinced them that they must learn a certain kind of Qigong or Tai Chi to have really authentic access to the Qi. The Qi is free! You are swimming in it. It circulates within you. It is not true that a certain form is better than all others. The reason there are thousands of forms is that many genuine Qi lovers have developed powerful new forms. Why not you?

Find a teacher that will support you in a personal quest to gain direct access to the universal field of Qi. This person will enhance, not suppress, your creativity and intuition.

Mentors

A mentor is someone who agrees to foster your growth and learning. A mentor does not have a particular agenda or teaching framework. In a mentored Qigong learning experience you will likely be encouraged to follow your own inner guidance by someone, often a friend, who has had success in following his or her own path. In China, grandparents, retired schoolteachers, and community-minded citizens often act as mentors.

I believe mentoring is the most far-reaching and empowering framework for Tai Chi and Qigong in the modern world. While students of mentors may not have access to master teachers, they do have access to powerful personal improvement tools. In this way, millions can be supported in accessing the Qi. And this will actually create a huge new pool of students for authentic masters in the future who could assist those who wish to go deeper or access the ancient lineages. I encourage you to seek a mentor and then become a mentor yourself. Ultimately the greatest mentor is one who inspires you to deepen your practice.

Learning from Books, Videos, and Audio Programs

It seems to be a common sentiment that a person can't learn Qigong or Tai Chi from a book, video, or audio program. My own experience belies this notion. Many people have walked up to me in practice sessions or at lectures with a copy of *The Healer Within*, with significant passages underlined, and have claimed to be inspired to use the practices just by reading the book. Some of these people have never had a lesson from anyone and yet have experienced significant positive healing effects. A few have started practice groups in their homes or their local community centers or churches. Some have given the book to their doctors; others *received* the book from their doctors.

Numerous excellent videos are available. Just recently a student at a training session demonstrated a very impressive form that she had learned from a video. Tai Chi is typically lengthy and complex, so briefer forms of self-healing Qigong are the easiest to learn from a video. While people who use videos would obviously benefit from personal instruction, there is a kind of miracle in the fact that they have been able to gain positive results of Qigong and Tai Chi without having to wait for a certified teacher or master to get started.

Personal Focus

The most direct path to fulfilling your preferred objectives in Tai Chi and Qigong is through focus, intention, and purpose. When you discover the direction that truly suits you in your cultivation practice, natural focus can arise. It is common for people to explore different approaches to Qi cultivation, to shop around before they find the right combination of methods, teaching, practice, and timing that naturally supports intentful focus.

As you mature in your practice, you will tend toward deeper focus. You will likely choose a teacher and develop a set of practices to explore to deepen your cultivation. You will likely select a usual time and place for practice that support you in deepening your cultivation. With all of these elements, mind intent, or focus, is the master key.

The Voice of the Qi

According to some contemporary thinking, Qi is information, the basis of all communication. The Qi is communicating with you. When nature is in balance, birds sing, and the breeze gently rustles the grasses or the leaves of the trees. When nature is out of balance—possibly seeking to reestablish harmony—the birds hide, the wind howls, and leaves are torn from the trees. Your own Qi is communicating with you as well. When you are well and functioning creatively, the voice of the Qi is singing, laughing, or comfortably quiet. When the Qi is singing you are joyful; you are able to concentrate and be in touch with your creativity. When Qi is in harmony, it whispers to you in affirmation and acknowledgment.

When the Qi is out of harmony, it speaks as well. If you are listening you can hear the voice of Qi as it whispers to you. It is easy at that point to make proactive or preventive adjustments. If you are not listening and the Qi must shout, it is too late for prevention. At the level of the body in disharmony—the Earth level—the Qi speaks as pain and illness. At the level of disharmony of the mind and emotions—the

HeartMind—Qi speaks as anger, compulsion, worry, doubt, fear, judgment, etc. What is the meaning of bodily pain or emotional distress? What is the voice of the Qi expressing or asking for? When the Qi is communicating about what you need, it will speak very clearly. However, most people are not very good at listening. Qigong can help.

At the Spirit level Qi is never in disharmony. Your Spirit is always waiting, residing in your heart, to speak as intuition and creativity. The voice of Spirit expresses in both the body and the emotions. It is Spirit that pushes for the resolution of pain and anguish. When we do Qigong it is, according to the ancients, a way to invite the Spirit to express. When we remove inner resistance the Spirit is uncovered, released, activated, and refined—it radiates.

According to traditional Asian cultures, physical or emotional disharmony is the voice of the Qi asking for help. Through Qigong we can become aware of this. Qigong can be enormously useful in restoring balance, both physically and emotionally. As the Qi is cultivated it allows for the in-pouring of universal and natural resources into the Qi Matrix.

One of the names for Tai Chi is shadow boxing, meaning that the inner focus and awareness of the practice create an opportunity for confronting the dark, shadowy side of your personality. This idea of facing up to your inner doubts and phantoms is a key to balance and peace of mind. When you deepen your practice with the intention of accessing inner peace, the shadow is what keeps the HeartMind in distress or compulsive thinking. Shadow boxing with a focus on purifying the HeartMind is an important pathway to resolution.

It is not unusual for Qigong to circulate Qi into blocked or stagnant areas, which can cause the release of pain or emotions. This process can be quiet and peaceful or it can be accompanied by emotional outbursts. If, for example, you have chronic anger or chronic sorrow, Qigong can create resolution by opening you up to shouting, forgiveness, or weeping.

It is possible for Qi cultivation to be the solution, over time, for all of one's life challenges. But this is rare. Qigong more often provides partial or temporary relief rather than complete resolution. It is important to know when Qi cultivation is not fulfilling your need or desire to resolve a problem. Qigong and Tai Chi can open the door of awareness for additional assistance. At some point you may benefit from participation in a support group, possibly a Qigong support group, or a visit to a practitioner of conventional medicine or natural healing. You may wish to call upon the skills of a psychotherapist, coach, or counselor as a complement to your Qigong practice. Your practice will help you to understand when you might be most effectively served by one of these services or a healer, shaman, rabbi, or priest.

Some of the significant developments in my personal practice occurred in this way. My first opportunity to give a lecture actually occurred through the caring insights of a preacher when I was twelve. When my dad passed away I was in a very impressionable state. The church leader asked me to deliver a brief presentation in front of the whole church. It scared me for a few minutes. Then I experienced the interest, love, and support of many people. They told me that I helped them and that my voice was clear in the back of the room. That support made a lifelong difference for me. One of my most important turning points was when an American Indian shaman by the name of Rolling Thunder interpreted a dream for me with great care. In the dream I chased a snake all night. Finally it climbed a tree and turned into a medicine bag. He said that meant I would be a doctor and healer. My life changed immediately and I have practiced Chinese medicine for twenty-five years. Over several decades a number of caring counselors have helped me to come to terms with the early death of my father and to reorient my life in the wake of certain personal traumas. Several men's groups have been a very powerful support and provided rich insight, especially into HeartMind Qigong.

The voice of the Qi helps us see the potential to complement and enhance the benefits of Qigong and Tai Chi with input, insights, and support from facilitators who can help us to evolve, learn, and grow. Over time, the practice of Qigong may eliminate our need for such professionals. After all, as we purify and empower ourselves, we become more capable of accessing resolution through our own practice.

When to Reach Out for Support

In the physical—the Earth domain—the best sign to watch for, as a trigger for reaching out for support, is that a health condition persists. For example if you have headaches and you practice Qigong for some time with no improvement, you might consider complementing your practice with input from an acupuncturist, physician, massage therapist, herbalist, homeopath, or biofeedback counselor.

Support

If the health challenge you are dealing with is not particularly serious, you can start with some form of natural healing. If the challenge is severe or if you suspect it could be serious, as in a rapidly changing skin lesion or sudden and enduring severe pain, then it is recommended that you see a medical doctor. A diagnosis from Western medicine can give you guidance, but this does not mean you should discontinue your Qigong practice. Qigong, Tai Chi, and medicine are complementary.

For the HeartMind—the emotional as well as the attitudinal—you can tell your Qigong is not fully supporting you when you spend your practice time making lists, analyzing opportunities, reviewing the transgressions of others, or planning strategies for "making things work." In ancient times the solution for mental overload was to retreat to the mountains and completely separate from involvement with family, society, and commerce. Such an opportunity can still help to quiet the busy mind. Most of us, however, are committed to worldly involvements and so we must be creative in developing strategies for facing and resolving discord and disharmony.

Psychotherapy, counseling, support groups, coaching, and numerous other strategies for personal growth and the resolution of inner distress are completely complementary to Qigong. The voice of the Qi may, if you listen, ask you to enhance your practice with some complementary strategies.

Ancient Systems of Natural Self-Healing of the HeartMind Psyche

In many ancient systems a promise exists that for every ailment of the body there is a remedy nearby. Nature, the voice of the Qi, fulfills this promise freely for those who listen and pay attention.

Right next to poison ivy in the Appalachian Mountains, there is almost always jewel weed (wild impatiens), which counteracts the poison ivy reaction. In the hottest climates, where sunburn is a fact of life, the aloe plant grows naturally with its soothing salve. Legendary Daoist Master Lu Dong Bin says, "Make the illness itself into your medicine." This not only indicates that the cure is present near the cause of the problem, it also suggests that, in fact, the disease *is* the cure.

There is a parallel promise for challenges of the HeartMind in Buddhism. According to the *Medicine Buddha*, there are 84,000 emotional challenges and 84,000 powerful antidotes to the inner poison of those emotions. For anger there is the antidote of forgiveness and loving kindness; for worry there is the practice of eliciting trust; for hate there is love.

In the Daoist thinking, there are five key emotions that form the root of thousands of mental, emotional, and attitudinal entanglements, which reside in the organs. Right alongside of these five key negative emotions, and residing in the organs as well, are the five resolving emotional qualities. First described in *The Yellow Emperor's Classic Book of Medicine (Huang Di Nei Jing)*, written during the Han dynasty around 200 B.C.E., this system of five—called the Five Phases or Five Elements—is the basis for many practices of Chinese medicine and Qigong.

These traditions reveal that the Qi is calling us to a deeper sense of how and why things happen in our lives. The invitation from the Qi is to use stress as a reminder of the value of practice. Illness and pain are also calls to practice. Even the positives, our victories, can be the voice of the Qi whispering messages to us to notice natural cycles, align with the natural forces that support well-being, and cultivate and refine a conscious relationship with the essential power of the universe.

信

Trust

HeartMind Medicine		
Organ	**Positive and Negative Emotion**	**Resolving Quality**
Heart	Joy and hate	Acceptance
Lungs	Caring and sadness (grief)	Inner strength
Spleen	Concentration and worry	Trust
Liver	Clarity and anger	Forgiveness
Kidneys	Courage and fear	Will

The Light of Science on Qi

That which is looked upon by one generation
as the apex of human knowledge
is often considered an absurdity by the next,
and that which is regarded as a superstition in one century,
may form the basis of science for the following one!

—PARACELSUS, SIXTEENTH-CENTURY EUROPEAN ALCHEMIST

In the thirty years of my involvement with Qigong (Chi Kung) and Tai Chi (Taiji), I have remained absolutely astounded that the ancient Chinese, with little modern scientific knowledge, discovered an essential universal resource that infuses everything, everywhere. This essential resource, Qi (Chi), became the foundation of Chinese science thousands of years ago and holds a strong place there today.

Qi has also attracted the attention of Western science. In 1997 the National Institutes of Health (NIH) declared acupuncture safe and effective for numerous diagnoses.[1] While the Chinese attribute acupuncture's healing effect to Qi, the NIH noted that Western science could not be certain just how acupuncture works.

One of the results that the challenge of Qi has had on Western science is that it has stimulated speculation and dialogue across a number of fields. These dialogues have triggered two monumental shifts in Western thinking. One is the realization that the model of isolated disciplines—such as psychology, biology, and physics—has been a problem and that cross-disciplinary conversation and research yields exciting results.

Interdisciplinary interaction is typically facilitated by a common denominator. The Chinese Qi or subtle energy has become a scientific common denominator. Second, scientists are beginning to realize that we live in the post-Einstein era of quantum physics but have continued to fall back on pre-Einstein science in the areas of physiology and medicine. As a culture we use the energy- and information-based sciences to make phone calls and transport data, but we practice medical science as if the natural laws of energy that allow for cell phones, the Internet, and television do not apply to human systems.

Long before Einstein, the ancient Chinese were doing medical research that was completely consistent with modern physics. This fact is having a major impact on contemporary science and causing radical new trends. We are finally beginning to use the framework of quantum era physics to investigate medicine, healing, and human potential. From its earliest history, Qigong has been associated with a mysterious and wonderful inner medicine, the Golden Elixir, which is based in Qi and the universal field of potential. The ancient theory that Qi is everywhere has both frustrated and stimulated the Western science community, which has a strong aversion to unsolved mysteries. To solve the mystery of Qi, Western science must experience a radical transformation. Research in Asia and Western countries has led to speculation that Qi could be a multidimensional factor that may link specific components of the local world with unspecific and immeasurable fields of cosmic proportion into a dynamic, unbounded, and unified web of life.

The Chinese, determined to tap this immeasurable field for its power and benefits, created the practices of Qigong and Tai Chi. From this process of exploration and refinement, ancient scientists in their secluded mountain observatories developed formulas (see page 11) to work purposefully with Qigong to maximize function. As you will see by the end of this chapter, these formulas are confirmed in the findings that are emerging from recent explorations in contemporary Western science.

Here is the ancient formula for health and longevity that has been based on the Qi:

Inner Harmony = Qi Flow = Health and Longevity

This first principle of Chinese medicine is the foundation of the Qigong paradigm. Although it sometimes appears that the ancient and the contemporary views of optimal function are nearly identical, there is in fact a major difference between the two. In the Western model there has been little awareness that an individual can actually affect whether his or her inner function is harmonious or not. However, in the ancient model there has been, for at least three thousand years, an awareness that an individual can affect the level of coherence of inner function with an elaborate yet simple set of practices that require little effort.

The ancient formula that acknowledges our capacity to cultivate coherence and optimal function through purposeful practice is:

Practice + Intention = Inner Harmony = Qi Flow = Health and Longevity

This flow, which the ancients determined creates and sustains health, has, it appears, numerous equivalents in the Western worldview. Western science has begun to investigate what the Qi actually is and what some of the more subtle dimensions of flow might be. New Western research is helping to engage the same sort of cross-disciplinary dialogue that has been so robust in China, which means that Western science is poised on the brink of a radical transformation, and Qi is a powerful common denominator. China's ancient formulas for flow and function may be restated in the light of contemporary science (see page 266).

Qi in Western Science

The West was not always so resistant to the concept of an invisible force that was believed to create and sustain life. In the Western traditions there were many names for such a dynamic universal resource. But around 400 B.C.E., after many thousands of years of shamanism, there was a shift away from appreciating "the mystery." Aristotle began to institute what many call "rationalism," which deplores the unknown. By the era of Descartes, Bacon, Galileo, and Newton (fifteenth through the seventeenth centuries), the mystery had become an enemy, a problem to be solved. From the beginning of the common era through 2000 there were numerous versions of the unseen life force. People who held the view that an invisible force underlies biology were called vitalists.

EUROPEAN EQUIVALENTS FOR QI	
Hippocrates	physis, vis medicina naturae
Greek Tradition	pneuma
Paracelsus	munia
Van Helmut	magnale magnum
Robert Fludd	magnetic fluid
George Stahl	anima
Mesmer	animal magnetism
Reichenbach	odic force

The mechanics of physiology and biochemistry promised to solve the mystery of life and relieve suffering. A great part of this promise to relieve suffering has been fulfilled, at least in medicine, by a fountain of so-called medical miracles. The mystery, however, remains unresolved. And Qi has remained an unacknowledged and untapped resource until very recently.

Obviously, the biochemical revolution was a reasonable path with very positive results. Fortunately our science is now sophisticated enough to return its attention to the invisible essence that the Chinese call Qi. After all, electricity is an invisible force, as are Newton's findings in gravity and the laws of thermodynamics. We are deeply involved in a world of many well-understood energies. Understanding Qi has great promise.

Benefits of Qi for Western Science

The typical Western approach is to have one equivalent per phenomenon. An inch has just one equivalent in millimeters. It is very unsettling to the Western mind to have to think that Qi could have a multilayered or multidimensional set of equivalents. This explains why the Chinese word *Qi* cannot be translated into English. Not only is the concept of Qi enormously far-reaching, but it also tempts the Western worldview to evolve toward a multidimensional view of the human being and the world at large—not an easy evolution.

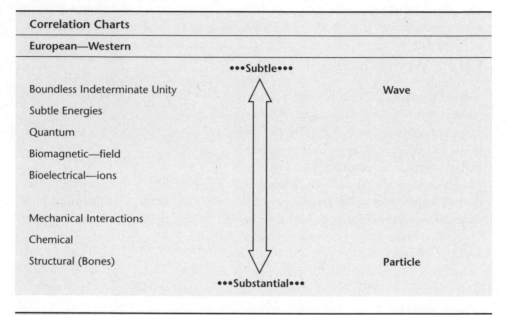

Correlation Charts

European—Western

•••Subtle•••

Boundless Indeterminate Unity   Wave

Subtle Energies

Quantum

Biomagnetic—field

Bioelectrical—ions

Mechanical Interactions

Chemical

Structural (Bones)   Particle

•••Substantial•••

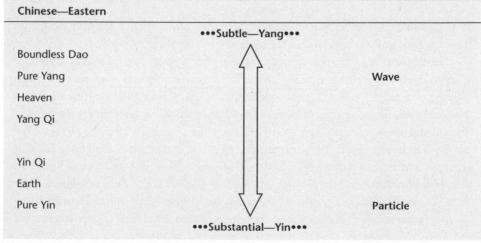

Chinese—Eastern

•••Subtle—Yang•••

Boundless Dao

Pure Yang   Wave

Heaven

Yang Qi

Yin Qi

Earth

Pure Yin   Particle

•••Substantial—Yin•••

What is typically called the body/mind split emerged in sixteenth-century Europe to help science eliminate ambiguity and create an even more rational framework for science. Recently, in spite of all the successes of this rational science, the body/mind split has been found to have created problems as it has become institutionalized in health care, education, and other fields. The unifying concept of Qi from the ancient Chinese challenges this split and recommends that it be healed.

The largely material and one-dimensional (physiological/biochemical) human being that science has been fixated upon for hundreds of years, and all of the progress of conventional science, will not suddenly be left behind. However, it is very likely that within a short time diverse fields of inquiry, from physiology to quantum physics and consciousness, will be linked by a single unifying fundamental theory. It is unlikely that Western science will call it Qi, but research is mounting in many fields that points to this multidisciplinary and unifying trend.

I wrote several articles in the late 1980s suggesting that exploring the Chinese concept of Qi might actually inform and enhance the scientific investigation of the West. As a result I received a number of invitations to present on Tai Chi and Qigong to groups of physicists and cell biologists. I wrote *The Healer Within* with the goal of framing Qigong for application in clinics, schools, community agencies, and churches. From that book, hundreds of local practice sessions were born, many of which continue today. Schools and colleges have created special courses. Even prisons have begun to use Qigong. And many physicians and doctors of chiropractic, osteopathic, and Oriental medicine have given the book to their patients. Clearly, understanding Qigong in Western terms assists in making it available to a wider group of students and practitioners.

The HeartMind in the Western World

In the mind/body context we in the West are confronted with a huge and seemingly unanswerable question: Where in the body is the mind located?

The Chinese are very clear on this: the aspect of universal mind that is associated with your self resides in your heart. That is why there is only one word for both heart and mind in the Chinese tradition—HeartMind (Xin). And that is why we learn in Chinese medicine and Qi cultivation that Spirit (Shen) resides in the heart. The ancient and revered *The Yellow Emperor's Classic Book of Medicine* (*Huang Di Nei Jing*)[2] states, "The heart is the imperial organ. The radiance of the Spirit stems from it." The cluttered and confused mind is in the heart. It compromises the radiance of Spirit. As the HeartMind is cleared of pain and confusion, the radiant Shen is expressed.

Scientists have begun to confirm the ancient insights of the original Daoist Qi cultivation masters. Rollin MacCraty from the Institute of HeartMath in the San Francisco Bay area, states, "The heart is to the spirit what the brain is to the mind."

The innovative research of MacCraty and his colleagues on the nature of the heart, discussed in *Science of the Heart*, is a significant force in bringing the light of Western science to bear on the concepts of the ancients.[3] In *Science and Human Transformation*[4] William Tiller, of Stanford University wrote, "Even more important than the Brain/Mind interface is the Heart/Mind interface. The Heart is the vehicle for Spirit entry into the body and is the key center on which to focus to initiate your inner coherence process."

The Western Equivalents of Qi

There are at least four equivalents in Western science for Qi. At the physical or Earth level, coherent and integrated function of numerous physiological mechanisms equals health and vitality. For many decades we have known that there is a dynamic relationship between, for example, the nervous system and the organs systems, but the level of complexity that science is now beginning to recognize is truly amazing. This knowledge is leading to more focus on the effects of intentionally enhancing coherence among the physiological functions that amplify the human capacity for self-repair. Coherence of function may be a physiological equivalent of Qi. This is not to say that blood, enzymes, and brain chemistry are Qi, but that their functionality may be one of the components of Qi.

The second equivalent is internal energy. Because the Chinese declare that Qi flows throughout the body in channels that are not distinct physiological structures, Western science speculates that Qi might be equivalent to bioelectricity or other internally circulating energy frequencies. This would make Qi equivalent to the accumulation, discharge, and flow of electrical impulses that operate the heart, the ionic charge that opens and closes the channels of entry and exit to the cell, or the ionic discharge that carries neurological impulses along the neurons.

Third, the Chinese also claim that Qi is not limited to or contained within the body and that the edge of the living human being is not delineated by the surface of the body. Research has shown that there are frequencies and fields of energy that surround as well as penetrate the human system, including magnetic fields and infrared radiation. This has led to new research in what is now being referred to as the biofield.

Spectrum of Equivalents for Qi in the Western View		
Scientific Domain	**Qi Equivalent**	**Three Treasures**
Physiology	Structure and chemistry	Jing
Bioenergy	Internal energies—ions	Qi
Biofield	Field of energy—magnetism and light	Qi
Quantum	Limitless information and consciousness	Shen

The Chinese have long believed that there is a kind of transcendental or spiritual light associated with life. Research has now shown that photons—particles or packets of light—produced by human cells are stored in the human body in the form of light.

This nonlocal aspect is the fourth equivalent of Qi. The Chinese historically have believed that mind and consciousness are unbounded in either space or time. Many Western physicists currently are exploring the nature of fields of information, consciousness, and the mind as well as what many call a *cosmological constant*—a form of subtle energy that is pervasive throughout the universe. It is likely that these quantum fields are equivalent to the universal Qi field acknowledged by the Chinese.

The multidimensional nature of the Qi; the multidimensional nature of our Western equivalents of Qi; the multidimensional Three Treasures that we have found so useful—all seem to be converging to deepen our understanding of the Qi. When the inquiring, the curious, and even the doubting mind is satisfied through this kind of scientific investigation, the door to Qigong can open even further.

Balance + Harmony = Coherence

The Chinese tell us that health is a result of balance and harmony in the Qi. In the West we have begun to say coherence equals optimal function. It is reasonable to say, then, that coherent function is equivalent to the Qigong state of balance and harmony. In the West, until very recently, this concept of inner cooperation or coherence was limited to structural and biochemical interactions, with just the slightest acknowledgment of internal energy currents. The Chinese, on the other hand, have always embraced the notion of energetic interaction among the components of the multidimensional being, including the interaction of the energies of the Earth self and the energies of the Heaven self, which merge in the HeartMind.

As we turn the light of science on the Western equivalents for Qi, we find that coherence, created through practice and intention, is required to reach that optimal or potentiated state. This is a direct equivalent to balance and harmony. In our exploration of the equivalents of Qi, coherence will be a primary point of focus.

Physiological Equivalent of Qi: Structure and Chemistry

Until very recently, in the Western world, the material/physiological aspects of our multidimensional being got all of the attention. As a result there has been fairly detailed documentation of ancient healing methodologies such as Qigong and Tai Chi, but only from the *physiological* perspective.

Excellent research in both China and the United States has demonstrated definite beneficial effects of Qigong on numerous specific diagnoses and on the human physiology generally. The Qigong Institute in Menlo Park, California, has collected more than sixteen hundred abstracts of research on Qigong. These abstracts, from numerous conferences in China and the rest of the world on cancer, diabetes, aging, and other areas, show a preponderance of positive findings.[5]

We know that deepening the breath accelerates circulation of the lymph and relaxes the nervous system. Relaxing downshifts the brain-wave frequency toward the alpha state, the level associated with natural self-repair. Relaxing also shifts the neurotransmitter mix out of the adrenaline mode, which actually diminishes healing potential, into the cholinergic, self-healing mode. Adjusting the posture fosters optimal circulation of fluids in all of the circulatory systems. Moving the body gently pumps the lymph and other fluids and mildly accelerates metabolic function and oxygen diffusion. These are all fully researched physiological mechanisms that are triggered by Qigong,[6] Tai Chi,[7] and Yoga as well as mindful walking and swimming.

Qi and the Mind/Body Connection

One of the most dramatic recent breakthroughs in the physiological domain is the effect of the mind, mediated through the nervous system, to influence function of the immune, endocrine, and other systems. This is representative of some of the earliest investigation into coherence and integration among body systems that were formerly considered to be isolated. Beginning in the 1940s, and especially through the 1970s to the 1990s, a landslide of research demonstrated the incredible power of stress and mood—states of the psyche—on health and disease. These findings pointed less to surgical and pharmaceutical strategies for healing and more to strategies for integrating mind/body. The mind's effect on immunity (psychoneuroimmunology) got the most attention; however, it was obvious that the effect of the mind on heart function, psychoneurocardiology, and other areas were just as important.

As the new research poured in, it became apparent that our contemporary culture had no practical tools to resolve mind/body challenges. Fortunately, the practices of the ancients—Qigong, Tai Chi, and Yoga—are applied mind/body practices that have been carefully refined for centuries. You can generate every one of the biological effects from the list in the next section if you consciously elect to attend to your breath, your posture and movement, and your mind. The elixir within includes not only energies, but also the coordinated and coherent function of the physiological system.

One noteworthy component of the physiological effect of Qigong is directly related to actual chemical energy. Glucose (sugars from food) and oxygen in the presence of a chemical called ATP (adenosine triphosphate) create metabolic energy—ergs. This energy does the work of the physical and biochemical body—muscle activity, organ function—from the perspective of Western science. Is this metabolic energy the Qi?

No, Qi is much more than physiological energy if it can hold the planets in place around the sun. Ergs are only one small aspect of the diverse and far-reaching Qi.

Mechanical and Biochemical Effects

- Qigong initiates the "relaxation response," which is fostered by any form of focus that frees the mind from its distractions. This decreases the sympathetic function of the autonomic nervous system, which reduces heart rate and blood pressure, dilates the blood capillaries, and optimizes the delivery of oxygen and nutrition to the tissues. This state is known as homeostasis, which is equivalent to the "balance and harmony of Yin and Yang," in the language of Western science.
- Qigong alters the neurochemistry profile toward accelerated inner healing function. Neurotransmitters, also called neurohormones and information molecules, bond with receptor sites in the immune, nervous, digestive, endocrine, and other systems to excite or inhibit function to moderate pain, enhance organ capacity, reduce anxiety or depression, and neutralize addictive cravings.
- Qigong enhances the efficiency of the immune system through increased rate and flow of the lymphatic fluid and neuroendocrine activation of immune cells.
- Qigong improves resistance to disease and infection by accelerating the elimination of toxic metabolites (metabolic by-products) from the interstitial spaces in the tissues, organs, and glands through the lymphatic system.
- Qigong increases the efficiency of cell metabolism and tissue regeneration through increased circulation of oxygen and nutrient-rich blood to the brain, organs, and tissues.
- Qigong coordinates and balances right and left brain hemisphere dominance promoting deeper sleep, reduced anxiety, and mental clarity.
- Qigong induces alpha and, in some cases, theta brain waves, which reduce heart rate and blood pressure, facilitating relaxation, mental focus, and even paranormal skills; this optimizes the body's self-regulative mechanisms by decreasing the sympathetic activity of the autonomic nervous system.
- Qigong moderates the function of the hypothalamus, pituitary, and pineal glands, as well as the cerebrospinal fluid system of the brain and the spinal cord, which manages pain and mood as well as optimizing immune function.

Science

Physiological Coherence Is Equivalent to Qi

All of these physiological mechanisms together are an expression of the potential for coordinated interaction or coherence of the human system—balance and harmony. Coherence within these systems obviously increases internal communication through information exchange and the improved function of biological and mechanical interactions. Science has recently accelerated its investigation into how coordinated interaction among these systems potentiates function and healing.

When you are in the Qigong state, or the state of inner coherence, the lymph vessels that end in the fluid-filled spaces between the cells actually begin doing their own Qigong and Tai Chi—just as we do in the methods we learned, particularly in Circulate Qi.

The ends of the lymph vessels reach out and surround some of the interstitial water (between cells) and pull it into the lymphatic system. Rhythmically, they reach out, embrace water, and pull it in. When you are stressed this mechanism is stalled, when you are relaxed and coherent this mechanism is active. This is a positive image for your practice—when you do Qigong or Tai Chi in a state of relaxed focus, millions of lymph vessels are practicing with you throughout your whole body. The sense of well-being that occurs when you do your practice and the benefits of improved organ function, improved sleep, or relief from pain are all signs of this and many other coherent functions throughout your system.

Physiology and the HeartMind

The focus and intention in Qigong practice are generated through the HeartMind. This causes coherence, first in the heart, which is then communicated through the brain and then the nervous system to create cooperative function—coherence—among other organs. In Chinese medicine the heart is like a beneficent ruler that coordinates the organs, which are like ministers or officials within the kingdom or community of your body.

Coherence is particularly enhanced by entering into a state of inner peace, trust, and calm that can be fostered through feelings of love, compassion, and acceptance and is evident in the extent to which the heart rhythm affects the balancing of the autonomic nervous system (sympathetic and parasympathetic). It is further reflected in a slowing of the brain-wave frequency toward the alpha rate and the shift of the neurotransmitter profile, which spontaneously activates and enables the immune system.

Investigation at the Institute of HeartMath and other research centers has uncovered the fact that the heart directs the brain rather than the brain directing the heart.[8] There are far more neurons that carry impulses from the heart to the brain than the brain to the heart. This upsets the former assumption that the brain was the center of "intelligence" and director of all body function. High coherence among the organs triggers healing, which is most often initiated when the pulsing rhythm of the heart reaches a state of calm and trust.

The Three Treasures and Three Brains

For decades foresightful scientists have suggested a three-part brain. One approach to this is the concept of the three-level brain—brain stem, midbrain, and cortex. Another suggests the importance of right brain–left brain harmony, similar to the Three

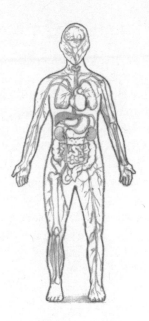

Physiological Equivalent

Treasures—Yin, Yang, and balance. Another view suggests that there are three brains throughout the body, in the three Elixir Fields (Dan Tian). Recent studies have shown that neurotransmitters are produced in the gut (belly) as well as the brain. It is rapidly becoming apparent that the "gut feeling" points to a brain in the lower Dan Tian. This was a major revelation to Western science toward the end of the twentieth century. Even more recently it has been found that the heart also produces neurotransmitters—atrial peptide, oxytosin, and others. You may recall the strong relationship between water and fire (kidney and heart, Yin and Yang) in Inner Alchemy Qigong. Science has now confirmed this relationship. The actual physiological relationship is not yet clear but researchers believe that atrial peptide creates a direct link between the kidneys and the heart. The number of neurological pathways between these three brains—gut, heart, and head—suggests an immense amount of communication among the three centers.

It is now apparent that each Dan Tian has an equivalent in these neurohormones. Not only does the Qi accumulate in the three Dan Tian, but these areas—belly/Earth, heart/HeartMind, brain/Heaven—are now seen as key centers of neurotransmitter productivity and interaction. Through Qigong and Tai Chi, the gut brain, heart brain, and head brain can be cultivated toward a state of coherence. The first of the Three Intentful Corrections adjusts the three Dan Tian, which contain the three brains, to access greater coherence and maximize function. This overlap of new physiology and ancient Chinese Qi science is likely to gain a lot more attention in the near future.

Bioenergetic Equivalent of Qi: Internal Energies

Around 1906, William Einthoven, a Dutch physician, discovered that an electrical charge builds up in the heart and discharges, which causes the heartbeat and the flow of the blood through the arteries and veins. This information was used to assess heart function through electrocardiography. We now know that the heart energy is just one small portion of a complex internal bioelectrical circuitry.

More recently, in research funded by the NIH, Dr. Robert Becker, author of *The Body Electric*, found a direct current (DC) perineural control system[9] in which high-conductance areas of the body correspond with the traditional acupuncture points of the Chinese ancients.

In addition, Dr. Bjorn Nordenstrom, from Norway, has proven that ion currents flow through preferential ion conductance pathways (PICPs) that are remarkably similar to the Chinese Qi channels.[10] These pathways make up what he calls the vascular-interstitial closed circuit (VICC) wherein energy flows in the mineral-infused fluids in the vessels (vascular), connective tissue, and extracellular (interstitial) spaces. This finding is consistent with the work of Albert Szent-Györgyi, who won a 1937 Nobel Prize for the discovery of vitamin C. He found that an interactive conductance system of internal water and protein crystal lattice form an "energy transmission continua."[11]

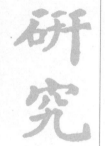

Research

In recent studies published by the National Academy of Science a stimulus from an acupuncture point on the small toe (bladder channel) created an effect in the area of the brain associated with sight.[12] This effect on the eyes and sight confirms ancient Chinese medical theory. There is an even more interesting finding of this same team from the University of California and several universities in Korea: the signal gets to the brain faster than would be possible through known neurological circuitry suggesting that a wave is propagated through the internal matrix (perhaps Nordenstrom's PICP) to deliver the stimulus to the brain.[13]

The Universal Elixir: Water

Your body's internal matrix, sometimes called the living matrix (a possible physical complement to the Chinese Qi Matrix), is approximately 70 percent water. That water is infused with electroconductive metals—iron, manganese, magnesium, sodium, potassium, even silver and gold. Body electricity is conducted in this medium. When you adjust the posture and move the body gently, you balance and harmonize the internal water throughout the matrix—the water-filled tissues and passageways of the body. This internal array of rivers and oceans is propelled and circulated when you deepen the breath, when you contract the muscles, and when you relax. Water is the bridge between the physical and the energetic domains in the human system—the interface between the living matrix and the Qi Matrix.

The connective tissue (CT), which is like a woven fabric throughout the body, is infused with water. Connective tissue surrounds the whole body like a jumpsuit, it surrounds all of the muscles and muscle fibers and holds the organs in place. This living matrix of water and tissue forms structures that transmit electricity, which generates magnetic fields.

At the same time, this water is cleansing you internally by carrying metabolic by-products out of the tissue spaces and delivering the immune cells to their destinations. Drinking significant amounts of pure water is equivalent to taking in a powerful medicine. In fact, in alchemy, both Asian and European, water is central; it is called the universal elixir. In addition, pure water is produced from every cell as it spends energy. This is a key formula for life; you learned it in school and no doubt forgot it right away. Oxygen plus glucose (sugar) with ATP (a catalyst) yields ergs (biological energy) and carbon dioxide and water ($O_2 + C_6H_{12}O_6 >$ ATP > Ergs = $CO_2 + H_2O$). This water is produced in the cell during the process of generating and utilizing energy.[14] Amazingly, the body produces metabolic energy (ergs) plus pure water. The water then becomes the conductor for internal bioelectrical energy. Clearly, water and energy are deeply engaged in the mystery of life.

Rearranging the hydrogen bonds to enable water to dissolve and carry higher concentrations of minerals, some scientists suggest, makes water more conductive of ions and other inner energies. One of the things that Qigong masters claim to do is using Qi to change water into medicine. I believe that in the near future we will discover that internal water can be purposefully structured and potentiated through intention and other aspects of Qigong.

A Pervasive Energy Generation and Conductance System

The fabric of the connective tissue (CT) web is pervasive. In addition to the outer sheath of the muscles known as the myo-fascia, this subtle yet extremely strong tissue, sometimes like silk and other times like thick sheets and cables, is everywhere. The nerves are sheathed in connective tissue (perinural CT) as are the vessels (perivascular CT), the lymphatic system (perilymphatic CT), and the bones (periosteum). The CT holds the bones together, attaches muscle to bone, and holds the organs in place. It is infused with highly conductive internal water and is arranged in a framework that is recognized by conventional science as a liquid crystal lattice.

Not only does the lattice of connective tissue conduct energy, but it also generates energy. In his excellent book, *Energy Medicine*,[15] James Oschman illustrates these points in a detailed list of the properties of the living matrix. Of the conductive nature of CT he notes, "The connective tissue fabric is a semi-conducting communication network that can carry signals between every part of the body and every other part." Of the energy-generating capacity of the CT he writes, "Each movement and each compression of the body causes the crystalline lattice of the connective tissue to generate bioelectronic signals." Literally every movement of the human body, particularly purposeful movements based on highly evolved traditions of healing and empowerment, creates and circulates energy and information in both the structural living matrix and the Qi Matrix.

This physiological processing and distribution of biochemical factors and interactions is activated and sustained through a complex interactivity of energy and information. This bioenergetic circuitry can be enhanced in its function through all of the components of Qigong and Tai Chi—breath, posture, movement, relaxation, and even self-applied massage.

Coherence and Bioenergy

Coherence in the bioenergetic component of oneself is evident in the practices from the phases of cultivation—particularly in Direct Qi. When you place your hands over the organs while you relax and breathe, you may feel a sense of warmth or flowing. The flow may be from your hands inward to the organs, or outward from the organs into your hands—either is the expression of the energy system seeking harmony or tending toward coherence.

In Transmit Qi, when you place your hands onto another person's body, you will learn to feel a pulsing within them, a regulating of temperature or an intuitive sense that a greater level of inner coordination has been reached. Coherence in the internal energetic system triggers a parallel shift toward coherence at the biochemical level and in organ function.

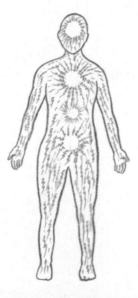

Inner Energy Equivalent

Bioenergy and the HeartMind

The Chinese Qi masters teach that purposefully cultivating the Qi to merge the influences of Heaven and Earth in the HeartMind center potentiates healing, health, longevity, and peak personal potential. While it is too early for Western science to confirm such a theory, we do know that the impulses of the heart rhythm transport information to the brain and other organs. At the Institute of HeartMath, Dr. MacCraty and his colleagues have determined that the effect of the heart on the brain and other organs is instantaneous. Using what is called the heartbeat evoked potential technique, they have found that the heart rhythm pulse wave is transported instantaneously through the body fluids long before the impulse arrives through the nerves or through the mechanical wave of the heartbeat.[16]

The heart's capacity to create coherence between itself and the brain demonstrates the very real and practical power of the heart. With the observation that the influence of the heart's rhythm transmits instantaneously as an energetic wave, Western science awakens to the Qi of the ancient Chinese and to their insights regarding the HeartMind.

Biofield Equivalent of Qi: Fields of Energy and Light

A basic law of nature and physics tells us that when an electric current flows through a conductor, a magnetic field is created in the surrounding space. The beating (charge and discharge) of the heart creates a magnetic field. The discharge of neurological impulses throughout the nervous system creates a magnetic field. The ion conductance in the vascular interstitial circuitry creates a magnetic field. The bioelectronic signals generated by body movement and then circulated within the web of the connective tissue and its water-infused lattice structure create a magnetic field.

These biofields are a key Western equivalent for Qi. Like bioenergy, the biofield is insubstantial; however, it is not contained within the body—it radiates. In the West we understand that this field exists, but we have never really explored ways to enhance, refine, or cultivate it. In contrast the Chinese ancients did so before written history.

In the contemporary era, excellent Western theories for internal energy conductance and the consequent associated fields began to emerge with the writings of Harold Saxton Burr in the mid-twentieth century.[17, 18, 19] Burr was a great pioneer in bioenergetics and introduced what he called "life fields." It is reported that the trees around his house were hooked up to life field detection devices. I'll never forget getting my copy of Burr's *Blueprint for Immortality: The Electric Patterns of Life* in 1972. I digested it with a great sense of relief. Satisfying my linear Western mind regarding body energy liberated my abstract and intuitive mind to embrace the Qi.

While training at the School of Chinese Medicine in Hawaii, I was assigned to feel the energy between the thumb and the first two fingers when we inserted the acupuncture needles as a way of transmitting Qi into the needle. I always questioned whether I was just imagining the sensation until I met Lu Yan Fang, chief scientist at the laboratory of the China National Institute of TV and Electro-Acoustical in Beijing. She demonstrated her research on the emission of infrasonic (acoustical) waves, emitted from the hand of a Qigong practitioner between 6 and 16 hertz (Hz). Her research was impeccably controlled for all possible interfering frequencies with an extremely efficient isolation chamber in which the research subject's emissions were measured.[20] Interestingly, the frequencies emitted during these studies fell in the alpha range of brain activity (8–14 Hz), which triggers spontaneous healing and self-repair within the human system.

Several researchers have detected magnetic fields around the human body. In the United States John Zimmerman (using the superconducting quantum interference device)[21] and A. Seto in Japan (using a special magnetometer)[22] have demonstrated that human bodies, particularly individuals who focus on healing through high-level intention, emit pulsing biomagnetic fields (7–8 Hz Zimmerman; 8–10 Hz Seto). These frequencies fall within the alpha level of brain-wave activity as well. The earth also vibrates at this frequency, 7.8 Hz. In Qigong, aligning with the energy of the earth brings the body frequency into coherence with the earth's natural vibrations.

About 20 percent of the studies in the Qigong Institute database are on external Qi emission, which is in most cases based on transmitting effects from one person (the transmitter) to another (the recipient).[23] These methods are similar to those discussed in the Tenth Phase of Cultivation and Mastery, Transmit Qi. It is apparent that the effects of such Qi transmission methods are mediated through a field of energy, information, or consciousness. We know that the human system does radiate frequencies. It is much speculated that such effects must be due to these fields, which fall in the 7–14 hertz range. It has also been discussed that the magnetic near field is only an aspect of our energetic being and that even farther-reaching fields of subtle energy, information, and consciousness are involved as well. Clearly the moon affects all oceans, all women, and most men, as does the sun, so we already know that the fields of nonlocal planetary bodies have a constant effect on us.

The Institute of Noetic Sciences has aimed the Western model of investigation at Qi fields with two rounds of rigorous research. Data is in on the first round in California and in process for the replication trial in Beijing. Qi emission practitioners, mostly traditional Chinese medical Qigong doctors, performed a protocol to enhance the growth rate of human cell cultures in a highly controlled environment and a highly controlled research model. In the first trial, chief investigator Dr. Garret Yount found more healthy colonies in the treated samples compared to control untreated samples, suggesting that some not yet understood Qigong transmission effect definitely does occur.[24, 25]

In similar research at the University of California at Irvine, human cells were used to quantify a distant healing effect, in this case with Prana (the sister of Qi from India). The cells were subjected to gamma radiation, which kills about 50 percent of them over a period of several days. The control samples are subjected to the gamma rays only. The cells that receive the distant healing treatment are in three groups—treated before and after gamma, treated only before gamma, and treated only after gamma. Compared to the 50 percent survival of the control samples, there is a 68–73 percent survival for cells treated after gamma, 78–83 percent survival for cells treated preventively, and 89–92 percent survival for cells treated both before and after the subjection to the gamma rays. It is interesting to note that prevention is more effective than treatment.[26]

Humans Are Light Beings

One of my favorite characters in the research for the Western scientific equivalents of Qi is William Tiller, Ph.D., of Stanford University. He got my attention at a conference in Arizona when he introduced several Qigong studies from Shanghai, China. Electromagnetic energy and infrared emissions had been measured in Qigong practitioners.[27] Dr. Tiller declared, "The human body is not just a chemical and electrical machine, the human body is a light machine."

The earliest biophoton (biological light) research was done by Dr. Fritz Popp, in 1984, who found that light is emitted from the cells of cucumbers.[28] Tiller noted that the photon emissions spread in the region of infrared to ultraviolet, with the mitochondria within the cells being the radiation source. Tiller later worked at Stanford University with Dr. R. R. Zhang to conduct experiments that confirmed photon emission from the hands of Qigong practitioners.

In the summer of 2000 I was invited to present at a special think tank on subtle energy and uncharted mind, which was cosponsored by the Esalen Institute and the Institute of Noetic Sciences. It was an honor to teach Qigong to the luminary physicists, biologists, and physicians present at that meeting. Among them was Dr. Roland Van Wijk, a colleague of Dr. Popp's, from Holland.[29, 30, 31] He reconfirmed that internal water is the bridge between the material self and the energetic self. He spoke of his research at the University of Utrecht. In that study, cells from a heart were thoroughly desiccated. The cells completely dissociated from one another and were spread on a medium in petri dishes. After a number of hours these dissociated heart cells began to reestablish communication and reach a kind of coherence. Finally they began to pulsate as if they were still assembled in a living, beating heart—apparently communicating through a field of energy, information, or consciousness.

But the most remarkable thing that Dr. Van Wijk revealed was new research on stored energy and light. "Living bodies store energy," he said. "We use a device that measures biophotons [light] to determine the viability of agricultural seeds, the health of cows' milk and many other practical applications. We also can use this device to

Equivalents

measure the stored vitality and energy quotient of humans. This can be done by assessing the biophoton emissions of the skin, but the easiest way is to measure the light in the breath. The capacity to store light is increased when the system is in a state of coherence." As a doctor of Chinese medicine on a quest to understand Qi and Qigong I began to get goose bumps.

In Chinese medicine we learn that the health of the Spirit (Shen) can be perceived by a brightness in the eyes and a radiance of the face. Do we have a way to increase our inner coherence to enhance our energy field or our luminescence on purpose? Apparently, Qigong offers us a way.

Our science is undergoing a radical rebirth with these findings about energy fields and radiant emissions. It is a very major step for science to conclude that the interactivity and coherence of our material internal parts can create electromagnetic, infrared, and ultraviolet fields of energy and light. The Chinese would argue an even more provocative point: instead of being a body that creates a field, we are actually originally a field that creates a body.

Coherence and the Biofield

John Zimmerman's work showed the electromagnetic field to be more extensive in people who had the capacity to affect the fields of others through healing. Chinese research found that people who had a certain amount of mastery in Qi cultivation had a greater capacity to express or emit Qi. The extent of the field is correlated with the extent of inner coherence. Those who have the skill to bring the various aspects of their multi-dimensional self into coherence create the more robust fields. Dr. Van Wijk and his associates have found that the capacity of living systems to store photons (energy in the form of light) increases when the system is in a higher state of coherence.

Clearly coherence can be generated from the physical level through to the energetic level and, conversely, from the energetic through the physical. Given that we associate mostly with our physical self, it is convenient that we have access to tools for cultivating coherence that have a basis in the physiological. Movement, breath, and relaxation very quickly shift the human system toward coherence in the presence of intention and focus. Physiological coherence creates an internal state that contributes to coherence in the bioenergetic system and the biofield as well.

The Biofield and the HeartMind

In the theory of Qigong, internal Qi can be accumulated and cultivated until it spills out of the body. The Chinese suggest that this can happen without spending or losing one's own Qi. Instead, as we discussed in Transmit Qi, the high quality of the personal field can cause beneficial effects in others. The hands are one of the most active places for this to occur because the Qi of Heaven and Earth meet in the HeartMind Dan Tian and pour out the arms and through the hands.

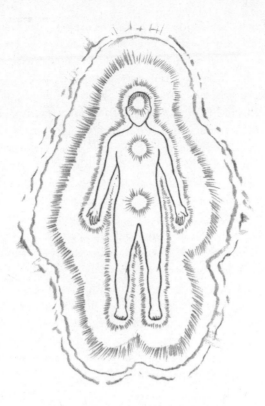

Near Energy Field Equivalent

It has been found that the field of the heart can reach to eight feet from the body. A 1994 *Scientific American* article on the use of the superconducting quantum interference device (SQUID) notes that the field of the heart is five thousand times stronger than the field of the brain, which calculates to approximately eight feet.[32] It is part of Qigong tradition to say that a person has "big Qi." Sometimes this refers to people who simply are well-trained martial artists. More often, however, it refers to people who consistently serve others and who are compassionate and wise expressions of the HeartMind.

The Quantum Equivalent of Qi: the Boundless Domain

The Chinese masters found, in the deeper levels of Qigong practice, that each individual is actually woven into a deep connectivity with the whole cosmos.

Pierre Teilhard de Chardin, a priest-scientist who lived in China for many years, had this to say: "No one can deny that a world network of practical and psychic connections envelops and penetrates deeply within each of us. With every day that passes it becomes a little more impossible for us to act or think otherwise than collectively."[33, 34] He named this interconnection phenomenon the Noosphere. In Qigong science this subtle interconnectivity is pervasive throughout the universe.

The Chinese suggest that, in addition to its local manifestations, Qi is boundless in space and time. This indicates that the ancient Qi masters figured out some of the limitations of Newton's mechanical model of the universe long before Albert Einstein. During the era of Einstein's revelations, space and time were displaced as the fundamentals of physics. This gave birth to quantum physics and there was vigorous debate about what would replace space and time as the foundation of science. Einstein predicted in his theory of relativity that matter, energy, and light were in a relative relationship.

It was not long before practical research determined that light could actually manifest as either particle or wave. Further, it was discovered that among the factors that determined whether light manifested as a particle or a wave was the effect of the observer or the experimenter. Many argued that the role of consciousness was fundamental in the realm of physics. With his uncertainty principle Werner Heisenberg determined that conscious observation of an event in research would so significantly alter the event that the research findings would automatically be rendered uncertain. This became known as the observer effect; clearly consciousness is a key component of scientific research and of personal experience.

Heisenberg and Niels Bohr were debating provocative issues in the new quantum theory when another of the great physicists of the era, Wolfgang Pauli, made the declaration, "The only acceptable point of view is to embrace both physics [natural world] and psyche [consciousness] as complementary aspects of the same reality."[35] While many people still find it hard to believe that consciousness would be a key to the physics of the universe, it is fascinating to note that the Chinese knew this at least a thousand years before Columbus sailed off to prove that the earth was not flat.

Since the original mind/body split, originating with Descartes, there has been a major taboo against scientific study of the mind and consciousness. Science got the body to explore—and until the advent of psychology and the neurosciences, the mysterious, invisible consciousness went to the church. In recent years, however, it has become obvious that the mind/consciousness is not in the brain. Neuromuscular memory has been demonstrated, a fact that locates aspects of mind in the tissues. The capacity of DNA to hold the code that remembers how to sustain an individual's unique qualities in the constant replacement of living tissue puts the capacity for memory in the genetic material, which is pervasive throughout the body. The intuitive relationship that people have with their animals or that is shared by twins suggests that certain aspects of mind or consciousness are not limited to the body.

Qi as Mind and Consciousness

William James wrote, "There is a continuum of consciousness into which our individual minds plunge as into a mother sea." Carl Jung and Joseph Campbell helped reveal that groups of people separated by entire continents can still be closely associated. Jung called this the collective unconscious, a kind of world mind. Campbell did extensive research that confirmed Jung's ideas.

Experts from neurobiology to psychology, from anthropology to physics have been asking, "Where in the world is the mind?" The original Chinese scientists, ancient Daoist investigators, were very clear: the mind is everywhere. Evidence of a boundless field of mind has been demonstrated in studies on prayer and nonlocal intention. Studies with random-numbers generators have demonstrated significant effects in small, large, and even global samplings that suggest a field of global transpersonal consciousness. Studies with groups of meditators have revealed a capacity through group intention to decrease deaths, injuries, and violence over great distances.

This research demonstrates that the effects do not fall off as distance increases, and there is no time lapse. The effects are instant over small and great distances. In fact, it has been determined in some research on remote viewing and random-numbers generation that consciousness or mind can actually "know" the outcome of an event before the event occurs, called time-reverse phenomena. Research in physics has shown that when photons are traveling at the speed of light in opposite directions, they are in communication. This reflects an instantaneous effect that is transmitted at twice the speed of light.[36, 37]

What is the mediating infrastructure for such phenomena? Perhaps it is some mysterious and as yet unexplained manifestation of a field of consciousness or universal mind.

Einstein predicted a phenomenon that might also be at play here—the cosmological constant. Contemporary cosmologists and field theorists have found that there is significant value in exploring the vacuum energy or dark energy that the cosmological constant predicts. It is a uniform super-low-density energy that permeates the entire universe and is everywhere. Sounds like Qi! It is many times weaker than the weakest known force. Recent research has suggested a refinement of this theory, which has been called quintessence,[38] based on the fifth element in the Greek system, an ephemeral force that holds the moon and planets in place. Sounds like Qi! Some researchers speculate that the cosmological constant or quintessence could be associated with the capacity for a signal or influence to communicate instantaneously, whether within the small universe of the human body or the large universe of the cosmos.

It may not be accurate to speculate on the application of the human or personal effects of concepts of cosmological proportion. However, just as the Chinese have carried on their dialogue about Qi for century after century, our physics is carrying on this dialogue as well. In China the inner experience has always been extrapolated to cosmological proportions. In the near future we may find ourselves becoming more comfortable speculating on how personal experience reflects the boundless cosmos as well.

Possibility, Probability, Actuality

The basics of quantum physics, stated simply, suggest that for every event that actually occurs there are nearly innumerable probable events (probability waves) that arise from an infinite pool of possibilities. This includes cosmological events, personal events, and the immeasurably small subatomic events that comprise larger events. Probabilities arise from an indescribable, boundless ocean of completely undifferentiated possibilities. Many people believe that, particularly in the context of our lives and in the domain of our experience, it is consciousness that determines which probabilities will become actualities. As one contemporary quantum physicist, Amit Goswami, puts it "quantum possibilities wait until consciousness is ready to collapse them into actuality."[39]

The ancients operated on the assumption that this model is workable; in fact the framework of Qigong was developed with this model in mind. Dao is that infinite, unified ocean of indeterminate possibility. This is where the mystery comes in. The Chinese understood the overall picture, but instead of trying to solve it or control it they accepted it as an unsolvable mystery. Intention and practice in Qigong foster a direct association with this natural process in a context where we gain an ever-deepening capacity to align with the natural course of events.

Holonomic Theory

Quantum mechanics states that we are not separate entities. Everything is woven into a single interconnected fabric. As a result, the language of science reflects on the whole. This dialogue originated with ancient Greek science and language. The word for *whole* is *holos*, which means "everything." Our words *holistic, holy, holiday, hologram,* and *holocaust* derive from this. In the most simplistic terms *holos* refers to this boundless interconnected pool of possibilities.

Holonomic theory acknowledges that any individual or portion of that individual is woven into the whole. The example often used to describe this is the holographic image, a special image or picture (graph) that has the very unique quality of displaying the whole image even if you cut it into small pieces. The idea is that no matter which part of the whole universe is being investigated, including you or a portion of you (even the atoms that make up your cells), the whole is present. In practical terms, holonomic theory is another way of stating an ancient Qigong proverb, "I am in the universe and the universe is in me." The Chinese knew holonomic theory intuitively. Qi pervades the One (the cosmos). Each individual's Qi is derived from the One. Each individual is a small universe.

Qi Chang Gong

In China, the concept that Qi is unlimited is not at all unusual. You can sense this in Qigong and Tai Chi. When you practice with a group there is a distinct awareness that it is easier to do your practice, and the internal effect of your practice tends to be more evident. Qi Chang Gong works with the idea that Qi and its field of influence is limitless. Qi Chang Gong is the practice of Qigong to produce, with others, a field of healing influence. In addition, however, Qi Chang Gong can be applied across great distances. I have written extensively about this in *The Healer Within* and several magazines.[40]

A Qi Chang, the group-generated healing field, is created when people practice together in groups. Patients (students) at the Zhi Neng Hospital work with this concept by bringing those who are severely ill, including those with advanced cancer and paralysis, into the practice group to absorb healing Qi. This effect, the Chinese know, is not limited to a local influence. The Qi is everywhere and the effect of Qi Chang Gong can reach over great distances. This means that people can practice together without being in the same place. In fact the Qi Chang—healing field—of all who practice Qigong is always present because there are always people doing Qigong in the world.

Your Qigong practice initiates a wave of intention that travels through the quantum field of information, consciousness, or the quintessential energy associated with the cosmological constant to trigger effects in friends, family, and even strangers at any distance. The research on prayer and an innovative program called the Global Consciousness Project are practical demonstrations of this in Western research.

Prayer: Nonlocal Intention

The most prolific writer on distant healing effects and the science that attempts to explain it is Dr. Larry Dossey, M.D.[41, 42] In one of my favorite debates about the multidimensional domains of Qi, Larry and I, along with a number of other serious students of "these things," concluded that it is counterproductive to translate Qi as energy because it is more than just energy. Research with prayer has demonstrated that a beneficial effect can be transmitted over great distances with neither the loss of strength nor the loss of time that would be typical of energy.

Several studies have demonstrated the healing effect of prayer over significant distances. Randolf Byrd, M.D., in the most often referenced research, studied 393 patients in the coronary unit at San Francisco General Hospital. The patients were divided into two groups—the "home prayer" group and the "not remembered in prayer" group. The group who received prayer had five times less need for antibiotics; they were three times less likely to develop pulmonary edema and twelve times less likely to need artificial assistance with breathing (endotrachial intubation). This is a very significant beneficial effect. This study was published in a respected peer-review medical journal.[43]

In more recent studies of distant healing and AIDS patients, Elizabeth Targ, M.D., at the California Pacific Medical Center, completed two very successful trials. The positive finding in the first with twenty participants was confirmed in a replication trial with forty participants. The distant effect of healing intention was significant in a number of areas. Compared to the double-blind controls, the distant-healing participants had three times fewer new AIDS-related disorders, lower AIDS severity scores, fewer hospital days, fewer doctor visits, and less general distress.[44, 45]

Clearly, major beneficial effects are propelled by intention and transmitted across distances. While we are not clear whether this effect is transmitted by fields of energy, consciousness, or information, it is clear that something wonderful occurs. The Chinese would remind us that this all occurs through a pervasive universal field of Qi.

Global Consciousness Project

In 1987, in the mail one day, I received a copy of *The Margins of Reality*[46] by Robert Jahn and Brenda Dunne. I devoured the book in just days. It was a book about Qi from the perspective of Western science. Jahn and Dunne did their amazing research through the PEAR project—Princeton [University] Engineering Anomalies Research.

The authors described a series of experiments using random-events generators that could measure the influence of waves of consciousness or very low-frequency energies, transmitted by human intention. The most interesting of these is typically accomplished with a mechanical device called a random mechanical cascade apparatus. The subject in the experiment uses focused intention to influence the landing pattern of nine thousand small balls that cascade downward over 330 pegs into nineteen collection bins. As the balls trickle downward they tend to collect in a curve with the highest number in the center. The general law of averages suggests that this would occur evenly over hundreds or thousands of trials. But what Jahn and Dunne found was that the subject or operator could, with focused intention, influence the direction to the right or left of center that the majority of the balls would fall.

The PEAR laboratory has continued with research on the influence of consciousness using much more sophisticated digital random-numbers generators. One interesting study is called the Global Consciousness Project (GCP). Roger Nelson, the chief researcher, has placed forty random-numbers generators at various points around the world. The study constantly reads what is considered to be the consciousness of the human race, or perhaps even of the entire living planet, by streaming data into the GCP data management center.[47]

Nelson reports that, after approximately three years, there are now more than fifty events that he and his team have investigated. The embassy bombings in Africa in 1998 just after the initiation of the project, the death of Princess Diana, the Y2K celebration, and major earthquakes in Turkey are among the events that derived significant shifts in the random-numbers generators from around the planet. The tragic events of September 11, 2001, registered a "strikingly significant" effect. Based on the data collected, Nelson notes that the overall effect that has been revealed could only occur by pure chance one time in ten thousand repetitions of the entire experiment. Either the global field of consciousness is very real and very significant or Nelson's experiment is actually the one in ten thousand that would occur purely randomly.

World Tai Chi and Qigong Day

The single most impressive Qi Chang Gong event takes place in April on World Tai Chi and Qigong Day, which was originated by an innovative Tai Chi teacher named Bill Douglas. It is associated with the weeklong celebration of World Health Week of the World Health Organization (WHO).

The effect of Qi Chang Gong is to increase and enhance the Qi field. In April of 1999 World Tai Chi and Qigong Day included ten thousand participants in eighteen countries. In April 2000 twenty-five thousand people in fifty countries took part. By April 2001 the numbers had increased to seventy-five thousand people in eighty countries. This Qi Chang, a worldwide field of healing and empowering influence, is growing by 100 percent per year. Given the remarkable healing effect of small groups, we can only guess at the benefit that this group field will generate in the future.

Time Reversal

One of the most fascinating things to me in Qigong has been the Chinese fascination with longevity and immortality. Immortality does not mean living forever in the body you have today; it means becoming aware of your eternal nature. Interestingly, Lao Zi addresses this in the context of light in *Dao De Jing*, #52: "using your own radiance, return to the source of all light; this is the practice of entering eternity." In Qi cultivation this process is initiated at the practical level of health and healing. However, in the more advanced methods of the Heaven phases, healing, longevity, and immortality come through returning to one's primordial or prebirth nature and by merging with the timeless field of universal Qi. Many Qigong practices are focused on reversing time and returning to the prebirth state when there was no stress, no complexity, nothing to know, nothing to plan, and nothing to remember.

Scientists recently have determined that our long-held perceptions of time are not entirely correct. The arrow of time does not just travel forward in accordance with the clock and the sun, it also travels in the opposite direction. I found this out while presenting at the Esalen-Noetic Sciences conference on energy and consciousness. My roommate was the distinguished physicist Helmut Schmidt, who developed the digital random-numbers generator (DRNG) at Boeing in 1969. This device produces sets of random numbers that allow scientists to investigate nonlocal and quantum effects. I was amazed to find that Schmidt's work reflected the concepts that were so prevalent in the worldview of the ancient Chinese Qi masters. Talking to Dr. Schmidt is a little like talking to Lao Zi. For example, we were discussing the nature of Qi when he said, "When exploring the science of Qi, emphasize the mystery—anything else that you name it is probably wrong." In his research Dr. Schmidt demonstrates that mind or consciousness influences the chance process in nature so that an outcome can reflect intention.[48, 49]

Schmidt's findings were further confirmed by Russell Targ,[50, 51] a physicist who conducted CIA research on remote viewing, and Dean Radin of the Boundry Institute.[52, 53] In discussions with these three luminaries of contemporary science it became obvious that a significant amount of research data suggests that an influence can travel from the present to influence the past or from the future to influence the present. It has been found that this influence is potentiated by coherent function, aligning inner resources through mind focus and intention.

The possibilities that arise from this research are mind-boggling. Healing may not actually be simply physiologic. In the light of time reversal, healing could just as easily be caused by an influence going into the past and altering the development of health status before a disease occurred. The set of probabilities that had been on track to cause the actual disease would be altered by a signal or message that travels into the past to trigger an alternative set of probabilities. This would prevent the disease before it began, establishing a new history, a new set of "actualities," for the person that begins to manifest in the past but is reflected in the present and the future.

In an applied sense this means that in our practice of Qigong and Tai Chi we may be influencing the past to affect the future or that our practice in the future has an effect on our present. Let this sink in. Your practice today may influence the past to alter your future. Deepen your intent to deepen this possibility. As your practice advances in the future, that more powerful influence may be having an effect on you now. This Qigong effect could translate into new choices or behaviors. Or it could simply inspire you to increase the quantity or quality of your Qigong practice.

As this picture formed in my discussions with Schmidt, Targ, and Radin it became apparent that as probabilities become actualities it creates what is called our world line—a sequential set of probabilities that are actualized. The time-reverse effect suggests that, through intention, an alternative set of probabilities actualize creating a new world line—a new you. This is exactly what the Chinese promise in Inner Alchemy and the cultivation of the Golden Elixir, the spiritual medicine that creates peace of mind and a direct association with the timeless nature of life and your ultimate self. The Primordial Qigong introduced in Chapters 12 and 13 is specifically programmed to trigger this time-reversing effect.

Love

In the highest levels of Qigong the practitioner uses intention to become one with all life. The Dissolve in Qi phase is essentially this—to melt into the universal field of Qi, to deeply associate with and accept oneness with everything. This is love.

Interestingly, the physics writers I have drawn upon most in my exploration of the Heaven level of equivalents of Qi all talk about love. One of the first and most interesting things William Tiller said about the practical application of his findings in

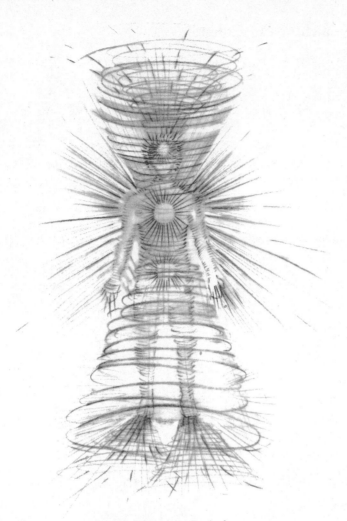

Nonlocal Quantum Equivalent

physics was, "We have an inherent capacity to resonate to the frequency of love, except for one thing—fear creates resistance in our circuitry."

Love in all its forms—compassion, devotion, appreciation, gratitude, caring—creates inner coherence. Love describes interacting with openness. The physicist Amit Goswami suggests that the reality of quantum mechanics at the human level is love—where the "boundaries of the self are transcended through the experience of unity in spite of apparent separateness." *Shen*, the Chinese word for "Spirit," is often translated as "unconditional love." In the ultimate sense personal Spirit is associated with the One. In the most advanced forms of Heaven Qigong, sometimes called Shen Qigong, one enters into a form of practice where the self merges with the One. This could easily be interpreted as merging with love.

The Quantum and Coherence

These universal interactions suggest that the Chinese idea of the One—and the relationship we can elect to have with the One—is accessible. We cannot decide to make the universe more coherent. The universal field is already coherent. However we can, through our practice, align with or enter into coherence with the inherent power of the universe. When your Qigong practice advances to a level of coherence with the One, all other levels—physiologic, bioenergetic, and biofield—come into coherence as well. It is at this level that one of the most provocative promises of the Qi is fulfilled. In the most profound sense, Qigong allows us to operate with the assistance of the power of the entire universe.

The Quantum HeartMind

Consciousness, it appears, may be the primary or fundamental factor in our experience of what we know as the cosmos or the world. It also appears that each person's consciousness may actually be derived from or infused with the universal field of consciousness. In the Chinese tradition this is all consistent with the idea of the pervasive Qi of Heaven, which enters the individual and resides in the HeartMind as Shen.

When we overcome the illusion of separateness that causes fear and worry, the heart opens or becomes clear and the influences of Heaven and Earth pour through into our lives, our work, our families, and our communities. Purposeful Qi cultivation can eliminate inner resistance; the forces of the universe are then free to flow. This is an expression of the One. Complete surrender to all that is—that is openness to the One.

The Multidimensional Human

Ancient Chinese science has contributed to our capacity to understand what looks like the limitless nature of our being. It appears that each of the levels of our self may be nested or embedded in the other levels. This can be viewed from the bottom up as is typical here in the contemporary science of the West, or from the top down as in the more intuitive sciences of the ancients.

The Multidimensional Human		
Physiology	Earth	Internal, material, local
Bioenergy	HeartMind	Internal, nonmaterial, local
Biofield	HeartMind	Internal/external, nonmaterial, local
Quantum	Heaven Qi	Internal/external, nonmaterial, nonlocal

Nesting: Embedding

Of the four Western equivalents of Qi, only one is material. Yet, for most practical applications, particularly in health and medicine, Western science has been fixated on the material aspects of our being. Considering that only the smallest material portion of the multidimensional world and only a minor aspect of the multidimensional human has been explored, the future of Western science is guaranteed to be awesome. Breakthroughs in energy and consciousness promise to transform the human experience.

Bottom Up: Western Science

The body—physiology and biochemistry—is the conductive ground for the inner bioenergetic circuitry, which generates the biofield. These together provide the local framework for the interface of quantum/consciousness, which is boundless and timeless.

Top Down: Ancient Science

The boundless and timeless ocean of Qi (quantum field) creates the personal Qi Matrix (biofield) which infuses the channels and centers (Dan Tian), which in turn builds and maintains the physical body (structural and biochemical interactions).

This nesting integrates the parts into a whole—woven together with Qi. In our practice of cultivation we can either work from the Heaven level down or from the Earth level up. Heaven down is not generally that easy to accomplish for people from our Western background in the material world. Natural Flow Qigong, Circulating the Light, and Guarding the One are examples of this. Fortunately, we can also cultivate from the bottom up. This approach to Qigong is easy and open to everyone. Creating inner physiological coherence among the heart, brain, nervous system, and other organ systems enhances the flow of ions that maximize the capacity and robustness of the biofield. In addition, our coherent biofield very likely creates a positive interaction with the universal field, the quantum domain, and our eternal nature.

The New Science Formula for Personal Cultivation

While the multidimensional human represents a big challenge for science, excellent practical tools for self-cultivation practice have been refined and improved over centuries. Without absolutely conclusive science, we can access the promise of Qi through the tried and true methods of the ancients.

Earlier we briefly explored the ancient formula for health and longevity. The emerging new formula that reflects the equivalents of Qi from the contemporary sciences of biology and physics is:

Inner Coherence = Information Exchange = Optimal Function

Western culture is beginning to recognize that it is possible to enhance inner coherence through methods developed by the ancients (as well as some more recently developed self-improvement methods). Here is the new formula for the use of personal practice to potentiate optimal function:

Practice + Intention = Coherence = Information Exchange = Optimal Function

The ancient Chinese would declare that we can manage our relationship to the universal Qi to improve our lives through the practice of Qigong and Tai Chi. Western science is beginning to confirm this. The ancient Chinese would declare that by doing the cultivation practices we engage our whole multidimensional self. By intentfully merging our Heaven self with our Earth self we create the illuminated life. With current trends in energy medicine and quantum science we are, it seems, close to this same discovery in the West. Will Western science solve the mystery through sophisticated scientific methods? The ancients would predict that it is unlikely that we will ever find the answer to the ultimate question known as *Tai Xuan* (*Tai Hsuan*)—the supreme mystery. Better to love the mystery through our cultivation of Qigong and Tai Chi.

The Supreme Ultimate

Tai Chi, the Supreme Ultimate,
  the immense absolute,
  is the expression of the Great Harmony
  —the balance and mutual support of Yin and Yang.
Whether boxing with your shadow
  or engaging in the complexity of life and things,
  the Supreme Ultimate
  within and around you
  secures the potential for harmony and ease
  in every moment of the eternal present.

—WU WEI, LEGENDARY QI MASTER THROUGHOUT
MANY MILLENNIA

We produce the most profound medicine within us. This fact alone is one of the most remarkable medical breakthroughs imaginable. In Western culture this radical discovery is very recent. In China, however, this same breakthrough happened thousands of years ago. A wide awareness of this healer within will change how we care for and maximize our health as much or more than the mapping of the human gene will advance medical technology. Add to this the fact that the newest research in heart disease, diabetes, cancer, and even addiction confirms that simply increasing personal health activities prevents and heals disease. The personal,

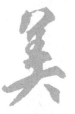

Beauty

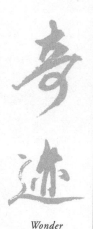

social, and economic promise of activating the medicine within is astounding. The best of modern medicine, plus the miracle of our ability to optimize our self-healing capacity, bring us closer than ever to the longevity and vitality that the Qi (Chi) masters promised in the writings of the ancient dynasties.

With the knowledge of the ancients that the basis of life and health is invisible energetic interactions and the transfer of subtle life information, it becomes obvious that the future of our personal lives, as well as the future of our culture, is being radically reshaped. All of science, including medicine, is in a phase of exuberant transformation as we embrace the implications of quantum physics. This exciting picture culminates with the fact that there are practical and accessible tools that we can utilize at almost no cost to help us take advantage of these incredible opportunities for health and personal empowerment. Clearly, the promise of the Qi, inherent to Qigong (Chi Kung) and Tai Chi (Taiji), is immense.

From individual to culture wide, from youth to old age, from economic to philosophical, the practical applications of Qigong and Tai Chi can come to bear on a multitude of human challenges. In this intriguing scenario, the absolute necessity of the expert—the doctor, the technician, the healer—is creatively diminished. Experts won't disappear, but each of us is empowered to access healing and personal optimization directly. This promises to be one of the most life-changing findings in our era. Instead of a breakthrough based on a new product that you must buy or a new technology that you must access through an expert, you can become the expert yourself in the purposeful management of your own Qi, in your own home, in your own time, for no cost.

The Tai Chi of Qigong and the Qigong of Tai Chi

As we have discussed, Qigong and Tai Chi have an intimate relationship. Tai Chi, while many insist it is a martial art, is clearly a kind of Qigong—move the body intentfully, manage the breath, and clear the mind. Tai Chi is not just a form of exercise or fitness enhancement, however; it is a rich philosophical concept—Supreme Ultimate —the harmony of Yin and Yang. In fact, Qigong has these aspects of Tai Chi as its goal. Tai Chi, the concept, has implied the promise of healing and personal power in the Chinese culture from eras previous to writing. The black and white Tai Chi symbol is so ancient that its origin is unclear. Tai Chi represents a whole range of things from the symbolic description of the birth of the universe and the harmony of cosmic forces to the foundation of Chinese medicine and philosophy and the popular, applied health-improvement exercise method used by millions in the parks early in the morning.

Tai Chi and Qigong as applied methods for healing and self-improvement have been used in times of peace and in martial conflict. They have been used in health care, in schools, and in the workplace. They have been used with children and elders.

And they have been used personally at home, in solitude, as well as in massive public practices. Pick from the wide array of challenges across numerous contexts in contempoary culture and it is likely that Tai Chi and Qigong can be applied as inspiring yet practical tools for resolution.

Tai Chi is a very special form of Qigong and Qigong is in most cases an exploration of the Supreme Ultimate—Tai Chi.

Cultivating the Supreme Ultimate in Contemporary Culture

Perhaps it is a coincidence. Just as our culture is becoming fascinated with longevity and peak performance, the Asian traditions for cultivating natural inner resources have become more accessible. Just as our health-care system is discovering the importance of self-care as a complement to medical treatment, the Qi cultivation arts are rapidly gaining popularity. Just as our need for low-cost stress management and injury prevention programming in business is peaking, the self-healing methods of China and India are becoming more accessible. And just as innovative programming has become critical for our schools, senior centers, and social service agencies, Qigong and Tai Chi are becoming prevalent and available.

Cultivating the Supreme Ultimate—the harmony of Yin and Yang—obviously has ancient roots. More important, cultivating the Supreme Ultimate has significant relevance in contemporary culture as well. To conclude our time together we will look at the Tai Chi of a few of the most prevalent areas of life—some personal, some culture wide. These concluding thoughts will speculate briefly on a future vision for the application of intentful Qi management and the implications for Qigong and Tai Chi in key areas of our lives: courage and honesty; relationship, conflict resolution, and sexuality; money; power and leadership; winning; belief; personal and world peace; and love.

The Tai Chi of Courage and Honesty

Through your practice, it is promised, you will have continued revelation and insight about the nature of the universe. Fearlessness, which leads to the ability to be honest with oneself and others, has at least two primary roots in nature. First, when you trust in the characteristic flow of nature's activity it becomes easier to surrender to that which spontaneously arises. In this state of openness and resistlessness the flow of natural, universal resources through you is maximized. In this maximized state every inner function is enhanced. The relationship between yourself and the world moves toward coherence—balance and harmony. While you may not be invincible, with the resources of nature so fully flowing within and through you, you are definitely more aligned with what is and therefore more powerful.

Even more compelling, your practice may take you into the awareness of boundless unity—the One—which is so frequently noted in the quantum discussion. When you tap this state, even for a moment, it begins to rewire you. If the experience of unity overtakes you, it changes everything. This is the state that is described by the great spiritual traditions as enlightenment, nirvana, bliss, ecstacy.

Those who have had near-death experiences also point to this state, recounting that they are transformed by their knowledge of the domain beyond this life. The deeper states of Qi cultivation actually refine your relationship with the aspect of yourself that survives death and is attuned to the link between your eternal nature and cosmic unity. Following enlightenment and for many who have returned from a brush with death, this sense of unity or oneness becomes the foundation for radical honesty and courage.

Qigong and Tai Chi are designed not just for healing the body, but also for merging with nature and channeling the raw force of the universe. As your practice advances through the Ten Phases of Cultivation, you may find yourself playing with the possibility of reacting less to old fear patterns and the habit of lying to yourself and others. Particularly as you transform your practice from a health exercise to an authentic and penetrating form of deep and provocative personal renewal, you will automatically transit to a more empowered state in which courage and honesty will express from you with greater and greater ease.

The Tai Chi of Relationship, Conflict Resolution, and Sexuality

In the Qi traditions of healing, the focus is on collecting, protecting, and transforming Qi. In the martial Qi traditions a primary focus is training to respond from balance to manage external forces. In both cases the goal is balance and harmony—the state of Tai Chi.

In every sort of relationship—social, professional, and intimate—the principles of Qi cultivation create the potential for greater success. Wise use of the concept of conserving Qi in relationships that are draining can lead to personal renewal. However, this is only possible when behaviors are changed. Qi cultivation can create the internal strength to be clear in relationships and even in the use of the powerful Qi conservation word—no. It is not unusual for people to realize that a challenging relationship is at the root of their ill health. The practice of Qi cultivation can help to reprioritize healing and energy management through honesty and clarity in relationships.

In conflict, at home or at the workplace, the Tai Chi principles of seeking balance and redirecting energy can help to create resolution. The practice of Tai Chi and Qigong helps to reaffirm these principles and build an inner awareness of how to bring them to life. Sometimes the concept of balance will lead conflicting parties to an awareness of a fair way to resolve conflict. Alternatively, knowledge of these values can help a cultivation practitioner to know when it is counterproductive to sustain a relationship. Given that our relationships are directly related to the HeartMind through emotions and feelings, it is unlikely that the true value of Qi cultivation will show up in our relationships until the practice has evolved to the HeartMind phases.

In sexuality the applications of the Qi cultivation arts can be utilized to have more sex and better sex as well as to deepen intimacy and improve relationships. As discussed in detail in the Conserve Qi phase, the Qi cultivation arts can support lovers in conserving Qi. Women who attend to the conservation of Qi, particularly during the menstrual period, sustain their health and increase their personal effectiveness as a positive side effect. For men who are able to gain the capacity to retain their sexual resources while participating in dynamic sexual relationships, the benefits are having more sustainable personal energy while actually creating greater satisfaction for their loved ones.

The Tai Chi of Money

The Supreme Ultimate approach to money is promising in both the personal and cultural domains. The primary ingredients in making money are health, energy, stamina, creativity, and insight. Is this an interesting coincidence, or was this planned by the architect of the universe? The ingredients necessary for making money are the very ingredients required for managing and enhancing Qi. Qigong and Tai Chi are power tools for enhancing health, energy, stamina, creativity, and insight.

First, your path to become a practitioner of Qigong and Tai Chi requires little expense. There are no necessary supplies or equipment to begin and sustain a practice in Tai Chi or Qigong, no special outfits, uniforms, or shoes. You can practice with a teacher or you can practice by yourself. You can congregate to learn and practice with others at community centers, YMCAs, spas, or retreat centers for some minimum cost, or you can congregate with friends to practice at home or in the park for free.

Abundant

Second, because Qi cultivation helps to sharpen and enhance any skill and assist in solving any challenge, your practice can become a part of how you improve your personal capacity to be more alert, learn faster, complete projects, suffer less from stress, have more energy, have new ideas, and put ideas into action. These can all translate into better jobs, more responsibility, more creativity, and more money coming in. What puts you ahead in any aspect of the workplace or the marketplace? Energy—Qi!

There is a more culture-wide relationship of Qi and money. The citizens of the United States have been spending more than $1 trillion a year on what we usually call health care—actually disease-based medical intervention. This number rises at an annual rate of 10 percent to 15 percent. Yet the Department of Health and Human Services (DHHS) and the National Institutes of Health (NIH) declare that 70 percent or more of disease is preventable. We produce the most profound medicine within us for no cost, and yet we have neglected to use it. Perhaps you have done the calculations using the 70 percent and the more than $1 trillion of expenses—more than $700 billion can be saved or reallocated for roads, schools, tax reductions, peacekeeping, humanitarian causes, or military preparedness. Why aren't we doing this?

The most amazing thing is that you don't have to do anything but your own Qigong or Tai Chi practice to leverage these benefits. In just ten years the number of people who are accessing natural healing in the United States has increased by more than 100 percent. Tai Chi, Qigong, and Yoga are a major portion of this growth. The most amazing figure is that the NIH has increased the budget of its National Center for Complementary and Alternative Medicine by an incredible 3000 percent in the last ten years. Much of this increased budget is directed at research on self-healing methodologies that are founded in managing and enhancing Qi.

Both money and Qi are resources. We can elect whether we spend, conserve, accumulate, invest, or waste them. They can either flow and enhance us or become stagnant and deficient. When we engage in Qigong we tend to conserve Qi, increase the flow of Qi, and store up and accumulate Qi. We will also have greater health that costs less medical dollars and we will be more energetic and creative, which contributes to greater earning and innovation capacity.

The Tai Chi of Power and Leadership

Power is what the entire framework of Qigong and Tai Chi is about. Qi cultivation is aimed at engaging the immensely powerful force of nature. In the Qi cultivation context, power is not typically used to overcome or dominate. In fact, even the most powerful martial artists live by a code that says "the greatest warrior is the one who can resolve the conflict without having to fight." When we align with the natural force of nature, the definition of power shifts from the idea of overwhelming or exploiting to cooperating and collaborating. Everyone—athletes, businesspeople, professionals in all fields, cultural icons, and government leaders—can align with and channel the flow of universal power into their work, their play, and their community service.

For a rare few, the ability to align with the power of the natural flow of events seems to come naturally. For the rest of us, aligning with the flow of nature requires that we develop the skill to *recognize* that universal power—Discover Qi—and then carefully *cultivate* the capacity to align with the natural flow. That is the essential purpose of the Ten Phases of Qi Cultivation and Mastery. Tai Chi was created and named with just this idea of aligning with the Supreme Ultimate nature of the universe in mind.

Those in the position of power and authority achieve the greatest outcomes by noticing what is imminent and aligned with the natural trends or forces. In his poem #17 Lao Zi wrote, "The great leaders and sages foster actions that achieve positive results but boast little. The people say, 'We have achieved this ourselves.'" When you, the great leader of your own life, cultivate a deep knowledge of the natural flow of energy and resources in your corner of the universe, you can then align with that natural power to achieve your greatest successes. This may or may not translate as opulence, wealth, or excess. But it always translates into inner harmony and optimal personal function.

The Tai Chi of Winning

Have you noticed that the great athletes and the major players in business have been using this Qi language of *flow* and the *zone*? When all of the training and practice have been accomplished and the moment of truth arrives, the greatest athletes will tell you that they let go of all thought, relax completely, trust that their capability has been fully exercised and polished, align with the flow of universal forces, and enter the high performance zone. Time seems to slow down, a sense of peace comes over them, and they achieve the impossible. Winners are naturals at cultivating the Qi.

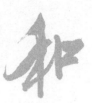

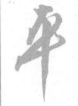

Peace

The greatest athletes of every era tell this same story. Even the ancient Greeks who developed the Olympics cultivated personal strength along with their alignment with the forces of nature—called the Gods. They even lived in special retreats where they not only used bodily exercise but also received massage and used inner awareness to tap into the natural forces of the universe. The great win was to be in the Olympics and participate in high-level engagement with others who had achieved advanced levels of skill. Most contemporary Olympians say that the big win is to get to the Games. Achieving the gold medal is an added benefit, a positive side effect of the process of learning to work toward coherence of body, mind, and spirit.

For centuries in China the most popular sport was Kung Fu, now known as *Wu Shu*. The basis was Qi cultivation. It is true that this sport was sometimes used in combat with the aim of winning by overcoming the opponent. However, for the bulk of the Kung Fu activity in China over many dynasties, the primary goal was to overcome the worst of oneself with the best of oneself—to align with universal forces to attain focus, clarity, immediate responsiveness, and inner power. This is the definition of the Supreme Ultimate—Tai Chi—to align with the essence of balance and harmony in the situation. That is the win. Taking first place is secondary to experiencing the Supreme Ultimate.

In fact Tai Chi is often called shadow boxing. When you practice Qigong and Tai Chi early in the morning, your body casts a long shadow. But that is only the most obvious aspect of boxing with one's shadow. In practice one overcomes one's separation from the Supreme Ultimate of balance and harmony by mastering laziness, self-judgment, inflexibility, fatigue, and physical limitation—one's own shadow self. In the conflict one overcomes separation from balance and harmony by mastering fear, self-doubt, and hesitation—the shadow self.

The principles are the same in sports and business. The ultimate athlete and the ultimate business innovator—the winners—are the ones who reach coherence between universal forces, personal focus, intention, and the dynamics of the moment-to-moment situation (the game, the marketplace). The stakes don't have to be huge. Everyone is in the game of life and everyone's life is a business. Tai Chi and Qigong prepare us to align with the Supreme Ultimate to help to assure the win.

The Tai Chi of Belief

Love

Beliefs are the foundation of almost all of our emotions and actions. It is at the very foundation of Qi cultivation to seek an understanding of the world and the flow of invisible resources that infuse all beings and things. In the history of Qigong, entire schools of thought have proposed philosophical and theoretical frameworks for getting at the true essence of life and experience. One of these was called the True One (*Zhen Yi*); another was known as the school of Complete Truth (*Quan Zhen*).

While both of these traditions went through periods of what we might call dogma, they also experienced periods in which they were operating from direct revelation of universal principles. Direct revelation nourishes belief. This was much like our contemporary physicists who discover new insights about the nature of the universe using mathematics. Ancient Qi masters used Qigong and deep states of inner observation. Interestingly, ancient and contemporary scientists came to similar findings: the universe and everything in it is composed of dynamic interactions of energy and consciousness. This provides a powerful foundation on which to build one's life and beliefs.

Your beliefs are usually taught to you through exposure to repeated ideas and behaviors or, unfortunately, through trauma. Through your Qigong practice over time you can—if you are practicing in an authentic state of awakened awareness—begin to notice what is actual about your world and compare it to what you were taught. It is not easy to find the faults and errors in your own patterns of being. This is one of the reasons people who seek healing and refined awareness practice together and look for opportunities to support one another. Cultivating the Supreme Ultimate allows you to arrive in a stronger relationship with beliefs that are accurate and to begin to cast out those beliefs that were caused by false teaching, traumatic experiences, rumors, or phantoms.

The Tai Chi of Personal and World Peace

One of the most obvious aspects of the Supreme Ultimate is internal and external peace. If just a little practice creates an experience of inner peace, what then might be the long-term effect of practice with sincerity and intention. Balance and harmony within and with the universe—coherence—create higher function, clearer thinking, and the ability to make better decisions. These all contribute to inner peace. Inner peace has the natural effect of pouring out—as transmission—for the benefit of others.

There is no guarantee that your inner peace is going to actualize peace in the world, but it is completely guaranteed that people who have attained inner peace are peaceful with one another. There is no more likely path to world peace than the fostering of inner peace for all of the people in the world. While you may not be able to cause peace in others, you can definitely work toward causing peace in yourself. This contributes to the critical mass of peacefulness in the world.

The Tai Chi of Love

As we have discussed, there is proof from science and from the great spiritual traditions that there is just the One, the Great One (Tai Yi). Even though we are exposed from moment to moment to overwhelming sensory evidence that there are many parts to this world, our quantum science is clear—there is just one boundless and unified field. Qi is diffuse and pervasive; it penetrates all beings and things. It permeates the boundless field of all possibilities, all probabilities, and all realities. To become aware of the One, cultivate your awareness of the essential aspect of the universe that is everywhere—Qi. As your Qigong practice advances from health-improvement methods to the practice of the Supreme Ultimate, a revelation of the unified nature of the universe will come to you. As you become aware through your practice that you are one with all that is, love and compassion for all that is will spontaneously arise within you.

The HeartMind is the meeting place of the forces of Heaven and Earth within you. Yin Earth and Yang Heaven are like lovers. They rush together and merge into one in your HeartMind. The love Yin and Yang have for each other creates your life. They seek harmony through you. Your being is an expression of the natural love that is innate in the Qi.

It is not so hard to imagine that love would spontaneously increase as you move toward balance and harmony through your practice. Given that the Spirit (Shen) resides in the HeartMind and is more fully revealed as you eliminate conditioning, habits, and beliefs to reveal courage and honesty, it is not so hard to imagine that love would increase as the layers that cover over the radiance of your eternal nature are peeled away. You are an expression of Supreme Ultimate, and therefore it is not so very hard to understand that love would increase as you release your latent splendor.

At the annual conference of the National Qigong Association in 1999, one of the great contemporary Qigong masters, Li Jun Fen, said, "True Qigong awakens understanding in the heart, so people can have a *natural* life rooted in unconditional love. Qi is never separated from love. Through the practice of Qigong, true love is always with you—the joy of the lightness of being is always with you. A healthy mind coming from the practice of Qigong cooperates with the flow of Qi in the body. In the end, one realizes that it is not that the heart and the mind are used to make the Qi flow effectively. It just happens naturally, of its own accord. Then life and love are never apart from the Qigong state."

The Tai Chi of Conscious Evolution and the New Human

At their very best, Qigong and Tai Chi are evolutionary tools. We may use them simply to accelerate healing, sustain vitality, and optimize function—these alone are profound. The deeper promise is that Qi cultivation is a transformative technology, a tool for personal evolution that can actually be used to mine for the gold of the deeper, more essential self. The deeper levels of Qigong are called *Nei Gong*, meaning inner cultivation. Nei Gong is essentially Inner Alchemy (Nei Dan), through which we can transform the raw ingredients of our conditioned and habituated self into the Golden Elixir—the most profound medicine—that can help to heal the body, mind, and emotions and ultimately reveal the radiance of the eternal nature, Spirit. The primary ingredient in the elixir is Qi; the primary process for making or firing the elixir is purposeful Qi cultivation—Qigong.

Evolution

These deeper levels of Qigong are not reserved for the privileged or the famous—everyone has access. The possibilities are nearly limitless for anyone willing to put forth the necessary intention and focus. Rather than being complex and impossible, personal evolution is accessible through Qigong. It is promised that the Qi can be purposefully cultivated to achieve harmony. The three primary promises of Qi follow:

1. Qi is free, it is everywhere, and everyone has direct access to it through simple methods that are easy to learn and practice. Qi can be cultivated purposefully to resolve any challenge or enhance any function.
2. Every person who uses Qigong to cultivate Qi consistently experiences some form of health improvement and personal access to greater energy and power.
3. Qi cultivation—Qigong—is easy if you let it be.

And as you have surely discovered by now there are innumerable additional promises of the Qi that are inherent to the intentful practice of Qigong and Tai Chi.

The HeartMind and Conscious Evolution

Conscious evolution cannot happen without consciousness. This suggests that the HeartMind levels of Qigong are central. Personal evolution is focused primarily on the area of changing conditioned patterns of behavior. How does Qigong change our way of being? First, spontaneous changes occur in health and vitality. But this is not particularly conscious, except for the fact that you must actually use the practices, which requires a conscious decision to do so.

In the HeartMind phases of cultivation, success in the practice is dependent on awakened self-observation and focus. Simply remembering to be grateful and manifesting compassionate actions constitute a powerful first level of this. A more challenging component of conscious evolution is making choices that shift behavior and alter beliefs. Being and acting differently is the essence of transformation. It is both internal, as in thinking and believing differently, and external, as in changing conduct and actions.

Qigong is a powerful tool for exploring and actualizing change. In the quiet of your practice you know what you are thinking and believing, but only if the HeartMind is focused and you are practicing in a deliberate state does this foster authentic transformation. It is easy enough to go through the motions. When you discern that your consciousness is drifting or jumping about, you can know that conscious evolution is out of reach. However, if you gain dominance over your consciousness through intention (Yi) and will (Zhi) and actually make those changes toward the expression of your most essential self, conscious evolution is occurring.

If you find in your practice that your life conditioning and habitual beliefs are distracting, you can still benefit from the Earth level of the practice—your health and vitality can still improve. Fulfilling the higher intention of conscious evolution, however, may remain out of reach until you can break through to clarity of heart and mind. To truly clear the HeartMind of its compulsion to evaluate and then react is the Supreme Ultimate aim of Qigong and Tai Chi.

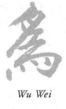

Wu Wei

The Call to Conscious Evolution

How many reasons do we have to make this evolutionary transformation? Living in a new millennium; the stress of high-paced lives; the presence in our environment of diverse forms of chemical, electrical, and social pollution; our desire to discontinue ingrained and self-sabotaging behaviors; our longing for a life of meaning; the mandate that peace can be achieved only by peaceful people—these are a few of the more motivating ones.

In the past humans evolved without thinking about it, as an automatic feature of biological life and historic events. Today, we have crossed into a new era. The human race has begun to have an effect on its own evolution—not always in positive ways. The more hopeful philosophers of our time predict that we will begin to consciously evolve—to make purposeful choices and decisions that have the potential to improve our future. How will we do this?

Futurists report that there are two potential futures. In one, predominating trends carry us along to predictable but undesirable future destinations. In the other, we purposefully plan for a preferred future that we will create through intention and action.

It is inevitable that a "new" human will arise. Will we elect to create preferred futures or just accept that which follows on current trajectories with the passage of time? Conscious evolution is certainly desirable; it may even be necessary for long-term survival of human life. If conscious evolution were impossible or extremely costly we would likely have to drift with the trends currently carrying us along. But purposeful evolution of individuals and groups is neither impossible nor costly, particularly with the widespread use of simple yet powerful personal improvement and health-enhancement technologies like Qigong and Tai Chi.

With more than 100 million people practicing Qigong and Tai Chi in China and the potential for millions more in the United States and around the world, it will be fascinating to see how well we will use these tools to consciously determine and pursue our preferred future.

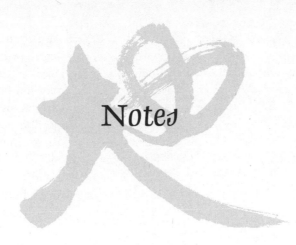

Notes

Chapter 1

1. Lao Zi. *Dao De Jing (Tao Te Ching)*. Numerous translators. Please refer to Recommended Reading under "Translations of Lao Zi and Zhuang Zi."
2. Ni, Maoshing. *The Yellow Emperor's Classic Book of Medicine (Huang Di Nei Jing)*. Boston and London: Shambhala, 1995.

Chapter 2

1. Jahnke, Roger. *The Healer Within: Using Traditional Chinese Techniques to Release Your Body's Own Medicine*. San Francisco: HarperSanFrancisco, 1997.
2. Please refer to the Recommended Reading section under "Classic Chinese Works on Cultivation" for a complete citation of *Compendium of Essentials on Nourishing Life, Prescriptions Worth a Thousand Ounces of Gold, The Great Clarity Discourse on Protecting Life, Record on Nourishing Inner Nature and Extending Life, Book of the Master Who Embraces Simplicity*, and *The Visualization of Spirit and Refinement of Qi*.
3. Ornish, Dean. *Dr. Dean Ornish's Program for Reversing Heart Disease*. New York: Random House, 1990.
4. Covey, Steven. *Seven Habits of Highly Effective People*. New York: Fireside, 1990.
5. Zhuang Zi. *Inner Chapters*. Translated by Gai-Fu Feng and Jane English as *Chuang Tsu: Inner Chapters*. New York: Vintage Books, 1974.
6. Cleary, Thomas. *The Secret of the Golden Flower* (*Tai Yi Jin Hua Zong Zhi* by multiple Chinese authors). San Francisco: HarperSanFrancisco, 1991; Wilhelm, Richard. *The Secret of the Golden Flower: A Chinese Book of Life* (*Tai Yi Jin Hua Zong Zhi* by multiple authors). New York and London: Harcourt Brace Jovanovich, 1962.
7. Ware, James. *Alchemy, Medicine and Religion in the China of A.D.* 320 (translation of the *Bao Pu Zi*, by Ge Hong. Usually translated as *The Book of the Master Who Embraces Simplicity*). New York: Dover Publications, 1966.
8. Lao Zi. *Dao De Jing (Tao Te Ching)*. Numerous translators. See Recommended Reading.

9. *Daoist Canon (Dao Zang)*, the collection of all the existing classics and scriptures of Daoist heritage, including cultivation, ritual, Qigong, and medicine. Several classics from the *canon* are listed in the Recommended Reading under "Classic Chinese Works on Cultivation."

Chapter 3

1. *Seven Slips of the Cloudy Satchel: Daoist Encyclopedia (Yunji Qiqian)*. Referenced from Livia Kohn, *Taoist Meditation and Longevity Techniques*. Ann Arbor, MI: Center for Chinese Studies, University of Michigan, 1989.
2. Ware, James. *Alchemy, Medicine and Religion in the China of A.D. 320* (translation of the *Bao Pu Zi*, by Ge Hong. Usually translated as *The Book of the Master Who Embraces Simplicity*). New York: Dover Publications, 1966.
3. *Book on Precepts (Zhonjie Wen)*. Referenced from Livia Kohn, *Taoist Meditation and Longevity Techniques*. Ann Arbor, MI: Center for Chinese Studies, University of Michigan, 1989.
4. *Scripture of Divine Nature (Suling Jing)*. Referenced from Livia Kohn, *Taoist Meditation and Longevity Techniques*. Ann Arbor, MI: Center for Chinese Studies, University of Michigan, 1989.
5. *The Method of Extending One's Years and Increasing Knowing (Yunnian Yisuan Fa)*. Referenced from Livia Kohn, *Taoist Meditation and Longevity Techniques*. Ann Arbor, MI: Center for Chinese Studies, University of Michigan, 1989.
6. Kohn, Livia. *Taoist Meditation and Longevity Techniques*. Ann Arbor, MI: Center for Chinese Studies, University of Michigan, 1989.
7. Cleary, Thomas. *Book of Balance and Harmony* translated from Master Li, *Dao Qun*. New York: North Star Press, 1989.
8. Cleary, Thomas. *The Secret of the Golden Flower* (*Tai Yi Jin Hua Zong Zhi* by multiple authors). San Francisco: HarperSanFrancisco, 1991; Wilhelm, Richard. *The Secret of the Golden Flower: A Chinese Book of Life* (*Tai Yi Jin Hua Zong Zhi* by multiple authors). New York and London: Harcourt Brace Jovanovich, 1962.

Chapter 4

1. Satchidananda, Sri Swami. *The Yoga Sutras of Patanjali*. Buckingham, VA: Integral Yoga Publications, 1997.
2. Please refer to the Recommended Reading section under "Classic Chinese Works on Cultivation," including Sima Chengzhen's *Discourses on the Essential Meaning of the Absorption of Qi* and *Discourse on Sitting in Oblivion*.
3. Please refer to the Recommended Reading section under "Classic Chinese Works on Cultivation," including Sun Simiao's *Prescriptions Worth a Thousand Ounces of Gold*, *Handbook of Methods for Nourishing Life Sun* and *Visualization of Spirit and Refinement of Qi*.
4. Kohn, Livia. *Early Chinese Mysticism*. Princeton, NJ: Princeton University Press, 1991.

Chapter 14

1. *Formula for Absorption of Primordial Energy*, referenced from Livia Kohn, *Taoist Meditation and Longevity Techniques*. Ann Arbor, MI: Center for Chinese Studies, University of Michigan, 1989.

Chapter 16

1. NIH Consensus Opinion on Acupuncture, National Institutes of Health (NIH), 1997.
2. Ni, Maoshing. *The Yellow Emperor's Classic of Medicine (Huang Di Nei Jing)*. Boston and London: Shambhala, 1995.
3. MacCraty, Rollin. *Science of the Heart: Exploring the Role of the Heart in Human Performance*. Boulder Creek, CA: HeartMath, 2001.
4. Tiller, William. *Science and Human Transformation: Subtle Energies, Intentionality and Consciousness*. Walnut Creek, CA: Pavior Publishing, 1997.
5. Qigong Database (Internet, CD-ROM). Kenneth Sancier, editor. Menlo Park, CA: Qigong Institute (http://www.QigongInstitute.org) 2000.
6. Qigong Research References (from most recent year):

   Cherkin, D. C.; D. Eisenberg; K. J. Sherman; W. Barlow; T. J. Kaptchuk; J. Street; and R. A. Deyo. "Randomized Trial Comparing Traditional Chinese Medical Acupuncture, Therapeutic Massage, and Self-Care Education for Chronic Low Back Pain." *Archives of Internal Medicine* 161(8):1081–8 (April 23, 2001).

   Sancier, K. M. "Search for Medical Applications of Qigong with the Qigong Database." *Journal of Alternative and Complementary Medicine* 7(1):93–5 (Feb. 2001).

   Mills, N., and J. Allen. "Mindfulness of Movement as a Coping Strategy in Multiple Sclerosis: A Pilot Study." *General Hospital Psychiatry* 22(6):425–31 (Nov.–Dec. 2000).

   Scherer, T. A.; C. M. Spengler; D. Owassapian; E. Imhof; and U. Boutellier. "Respiratory Muscle Endurance Training in Chronic Obstructive Pulmonary Disease: Impact on Exercise Capacity, Dyspnea, and Quality of life." *American Journal of Respiratory Therapy in Critical Care Medicine* 162(5):1709–14 (Nov. 2000).

   Lee, M. S.; B. G. Kim; H. J. Huh; H. Ryu; H. S. Lee; and H. T. Chung. "Effect of Qi-Training on Blood Pressure, Heart Rate and Respiration Rate." *Clinical Physiology* 20(3):173–6 (May 2000).

   Luskin, F. M.; K. A. Newell; M. Griffith; M. Holmes; S. Telles; E. DiNucci; F. F. Marvasti; M. Hill; K. R. Pelletier; and W. L. Haskell. "A Review of Mind/Body Therapies in the Treatment of Musculoskeletal Disorders with Implications for the Elderly." *Alternative Therapies in Health and Medicine* 6(2):46–56 (March 2000).

   Yocum, D. E.; W. L. Castro; and M. Cornett. "Exercise, Education, and Behavioral Modification as Alternative Therapy for Pain and Stress in Rheumatic Disease." *Rheumatological Discourse in Clinics of North America* 26(1):145–59, x–xi (Feb. 2000).

   Lehrer, P.; Y. Sasaki; and Y. Saito. "Zazen and Cardiac Variability." *Psychosomatic Medicine* 61(6):812–21 (Nov.–Dec. 1999).

   Farrell, S. J.; A. D. Ross; and K. V. Sehgal. "Eastern Movement Therapies." *Physical Medicine of Rehabilitation Clinics of North America* 10(3):617–29 (Aug. 1999).

Sancier, K. M. "Therapeutic Benefits of Qigong Exercises in Combination with Drugs." *Journal of Alternative and Complementary Medicine* 5(4):383–9 (Aug. 1999).

Mayer, M. "Qigong and Hypertension: A Critique of Research." *Journal of Alternative and Complementary Medicine* 5(4):371–82 (Aug. 1999).

Iwao, M.; S. Kajiyama; H. Mori; and K. Oogaki. "Effects of Qigong Walking on Diabetic Patients: A Pilot Study." *Journal of Alternative and Complementary Medicine* 5(4):353–8 (Aug. 1999).

Takeichi, M.; T. Sato; and M. Takefu. "Studies on the Psychosomatic Functioning of Ill-Health According to Eastern and Western Medicine: Anxiety-Affinitive Constitution Associated with Qi, Blood, and Body Fluid—Diagnostic and Therapeutic Methods." *American Journal of Chinese Medicine* 27(2):177–90 (1999).

Lee, M. S.; C. W. Kang; H. Ryu; J. D. Kim; and H. T. Chung. "Effects of ChunDoSunBup Qi-Training on Growth Hormone, Insulin-like Growth Factor-I, and Testosterone in Young and Elderly Subjects." *American Journal of Chinese Medicine* 27(2):167–75 (1999).

Loh, S. H. "Qigong Therapy in the Treatment of Metastatic Colon Cancer." *Alternative Therapies in Health and Medicine* 5(4):112 (July 1999).

Pandya, D. P.; V. H. Vyas; and S. H. Vyas. "Mind-Body Therapy in the Management and Prevention of Coronary Disease." *Comprehensive Therapies* 25(5):283–93 (May 1999).

Wu, W. H.; E. Bandilla; D. S. Ciccone; J. Yang; S. C. Cheng; N. Carner; Y. Wu; and R. Shen. "Effects of Qigong on Late-Stage Complex Regional Pain Syndrome." *Alternative Therapies in Health and Medicine* 5(1):45–54 (Jan. 1999).

Van Dixhoorn, J. "Cardiorespiratory Effects of Breathing and Relaxation Instruction in Myocardial Infarction Patients." *Biological Psychology* 49(1–2):123–35 (Sept. 1998).

Lee, M. S.; C. W. Kang; Y. S. Shin; H. J. Huh; H. Ryu; J. H. Park; and H. T. Chung. "Acute Effects of ChunDoSunBup Qi-Training on Blood Concentrations of TSH, Calcitonin, PTH, and Thyroid Hormones in Elderly Subjects." *American Journal of Chinese Medicine* 26(3–4):275–281 (1998).

Reuther, I., and D. Aldridge. "Qigong Yangsheng as a Complementary Therapy in the Management of Asthma: A Single-Case Appraisal." *Journal of Alternative and Complementary Medicine* 4(2):173–83 (Summer 1998).

Li, W.; Z. Xing; D. Pi; and X. Li. "Influence of Qigong on Plasma TXB2 and 6-keto-PGF1 alpha in Two TCM Types of Essential Hypertension." *Hunan Yi Ke Da Xue Xue Bao* 22(6):497–9 (1997).

Wirth, D. P.; J. R. Cram; R. J. Chang. "Multisite Electromyographic Analysis of Therapeutic Touch and Qigong Therapy." *Journal of Alternative and Complementary Medicine* 3(2):109–18 (Summer 1997).

Sancier, K. M. "Medical Applications of Qigong." *Alternative Therapies in Health and Medicine* 2(1):40–6 (Jan. 1996).

Wang, C. X.; D. H. Xu; and Y. C. Qian. "Effect of Qigong on Heart-Qi Deficiency and Blood Stasis Type of Hypertension and Its Mechanism." *Zhongguo Zhong Xi Yi Jie He Za Zhi* 15(8):454–8 (Aug. 1995).

Tsai, T. J.; J. S. Lai; S. H. Lee; Y. M. Chen; C. Lan; B. J. Yang; and H. S. Chiang. "Breathing-Coordinated Exercise Improves the Quality of Life in Hemodialysis Patients." *Journal of the American Society of Nephrology* 6(5):1392–400 (Nov. 1995).

Tang, K. C. "Qigong Therapy—Its Effectiveness and Regulation." *American Journal of Chinese Medicine* 22(3–4):235–42 (1994).

Zhang, W.; R. Zheng; B. Zhang; W. Yu; and X. Shen. "An Observation on Flash Evoked Cortical Potentials and Qigong Meditation." *American Journal of Chinese Medicine* 21(3–4):243–9 (1993).

Lim, Y. A.; T. Boone; J. R. Flarity; and W. R. Thompson. "Effects of Qigong on Cardiorespiratory Changes: A Preliminary Study." *American Journal of Chinese Medicine* 21(1):1–6 (1993).

7. Tai Chi Research References (from most recent year):

Li, J. X.; Y. Hong; and K. M. Chan. "Tai Chi: Physiological Characteristics and Beneficial Effects on Health." *British Journal of Sports Medicine* 35(3):148–156 (June 2001).

Wong, A. M.; Y. C. Lin; S. W. Chou; F. T. Tang; and P. Y. Wong. "Coordination Exercise and Postural Stability in Elderly People: Effect of Tai Chi Chuan." *Archives of Physical Medicine and Rehabilitation* 82(5):608–12 (May 2001).

Naruse, K., and T. Hirai. "Effects of Slow Tempo Exercise on Respiration, Heart Rate, and Mood State." *Perception and Motor Skills* 91(3 Pt 1):729–40 (Dec. 2000).

Lan, C.; J. S. Lai; S. Y. Chen; and M. K. Wong. "Tai Chi Chuan to Improve Muscular Strength and Endurance in Elderly Individuals: A Pilot Study." *Archives of Physical Medicine and Rehabilitation* 81(5):604–7 (May 2000).

Lin, Y. C.; A. M. Wong; S. W. Chou; F. T. Tang; and P. Y. Wong. "The Effects of Tai Chi Chuan on Postural Stability in the Elderly: Preliminary Report." *Changgeng Yi Xue Za Zhi* 23(4):197–204 (April 2000).

Luskin, F. M.; K. A. Newell; M. Griffith; M. Holmes; S. Telles; E. DiNucci; F. F. Marvasti; M. Hill; K. R. Pelletier; and W. L. Haskell. "A Review of Mind/Body Therapies in the Treatment of Musculoskeletal Disorders with Implications for the Elderly." *Alternative Therapies in Health and Medicine* 6(2):46–56 (March 2000).

Hong, Y.; J. X. Li; and P. D. Robinson. "Balance Control, Flexibility, and Cardiorespiratory Fitness Among Older Tai Chi Practitioners." *British Journal of Sports Medicine* 34(1):29–34 (Feb. 2000).

Yocum, D. E.; W. L. Castro; and M. Cornett. "Exercise, Education, and Behavioral Modification as Alternative Therapy for Pain and Stress in Rheumatic Disease." *Rheumatological Discourses in Clinics of North America* 26(1):145–59, x–xi (Feb. 2000).

Yan, J. H. "Tai Chi Practice Reduces Movement Force Variability for Seniors." *Journal of Gerontology in Biological Science and Medical Science* 54(12):M629–34 (Dec. 1999).

Casśaileth, B. R. "Evaluating Complementary and Alternative Therapies for Cancer Patients." *Cancer Journal of Clinics* 49(6):362–75 (Nov.–Dec. 1999).

Hain, T. C.; L. Fuller; L. Weil; and J. Kotsias. "Effects of T'ai Chi on Balance." *Archives of Otolaryngology Head Neck Surgery* 125(11):1191–1195 (Nov. 1999).

Chen, K. M., and M. Snyder. "A Research-Based Use of Tai Chi/Movement Therapy as a Nursing Intervention." *Journal of Holistic Nursing* 17(3):267–79 (Sept. 1999).

Farrell, S. J.; A. D. Ross; and K. V. Sehgal. "Eastern Movement Therapies." *Physical Medicine in Rehabilitation Clinics of North America* 10(3):617–29 (Aug. 1999).

Lan, C.; S. Y. Chen; J. S. Lai; and M. K. Wong. "The Effect of Tai Chi on Cardiorespiratory Function in Patients with Coronary Artery Bypass Surgery." *Medical Science of Sports and Exercise* 31(5):634–8 (May 1999).

Lane, J. M., and M. Nydick. "Osteoporosis: Current Modes of Prevention and Treatment." *Journal of the American Academy of Orthopedic Surgery* 7(1):19–31 (Jan. 1999).

Masley, S. "Tai Chi Chuan." *Archives of Physical and Medical Rehabilitation* 79(11):1483 (Nov. 1998).

Kessenich, C. R. "Tai Chi as a Method of Fall Prevention in the Elderly." *Orthopedic Nursing* 17(4):27–9 (July–Aug. 1998).

Kirsteins, A. "Tai-Chi Chuan." *Archives of Physical and Medical Rehabilitation* 79(4):471 (April 1998).

Achiron, A.; Y. Barak; Y. Stern; and S. Noy. "Electrical Sensation During Tai-Chi Practice as the First Manifestation of Multiple Sclerosis." *Clinical Neurology and Neurosurgery* 99(4):280–1 (Dec. 1997).

Tsai, C. F.; S. A. Chen; C. T. Tai; C. E. Chiang; S. H. Lee; Z. C. Wen; J. L. Huang; and Y. A. Ding. "Exploring the Basis for Tai Chi Chuan as a Therapeutic Exercise Approach." *Archives of Physical and Medical Rehabilitation* 78(8):886–92 (Aug. 1997).

Wolf, S. L.; C. Coogler; and T. Xu. "Exploring the Basis for Tai Chi Chuan as a Therapeutic Exercise Approach." *Archives of Physical and Medical Rehabilitation* 78(8):886–92 (Aug. 1997).

La Forge, R. "Mind-Body Fitness: Encouraging Prospects for Primary and Secondary Prevention." *Journal of Cardiovascular Nursing* 11(3):53–65 (April 1997).

Channer, K. S.; D. Barrow; R. Barrow; M. Osborne; and G. Ives. "Changes in Hemodynamic Parameters Following Tai Chi Chuan and Aerobic Exercise in Patients Recovering from Acute Myocardial Infarction." *Postgraduate Medical Journal* 72(848):349–51 (June 1996).

8. MacCraty, Rollin. *Science of the Heart: Exploring the Role of the Heart in Human Performance*. Boulder Creek, CA: HeartMath, 2001.

9. Becker, R. O. "Evidence for a Primitive DC Electrical Analog System Controlling Brain Function." *Subtle Energies* 2(1):71–88 (1991). See also *The Body Electric* under "New Science" in the Recommended Reading.

10. Nordenstrom, B. E. W. *Biologically Closed Circuits: Clinical, Experimental and Theoretical Evidence for an Additional Circulatory System*. Stockholm: Nordic Medical Publications, 1983.

11. Szent-Györgyi, A. "The Study of Energy Levels in Biochemistry." *Nature* 148: 157–59 (1941).

12. Cho, Z. H.; S. C. Chung; J. P. Jones; et al. "New Findings of the Correlation Between Acupoints and Corresponding Brain Cortices Using Functional MRI." Proceedings of the National Academy of Science 95:2670–73 (March 1998).

13. Jones, J. P.; C. S. So; D. D. Kidney; and T. Sato. "Evaluation of Acupuncture Using MRI and Ultrasonic Imaging." San Diego: Proceedings, Society for Scientific Exploration (http://www. scientificexploration.org), June 2001.

14. For a detailed account of the internal production and circulation of internal water, please see the following: Jahnke, Roger. *The Most Profound Medicine*. Santa Barbara: Health Action Publishing, 1990.

15. Oschman, James. *Energy Medicine: The Scientific Basis*. Edinburgh, London, New York: Churchill Livingstone, 2000.

16. MacCraty; *Science of the Heart.*

17. Burr, H. S., and F. S. C. Northrop. "The Electro-Dynamic Theory of Life." *Quarterly Review of Biology* 8:322–33 (1935).

18. Burr, H. S. *Blueprint for Immortality: The Electric Patterns of Life.* London: Neville Spearman, 1972.

19. Burr, H. S. *Fields of Life.* New York: Ballantine, 1973.

20. Fang, L. Y. *Scientific Investigations into Chinese Qigong.* Edited by Richard Lee. San Clemente, CA: China Healthways Institute, 1999.

21. Zimmerman, J. "Laying on of Hands Healing and Therapeutic Touch: A Testable Theory." *BEMI Currents, Journal of the Bio-Electro-Magnetics Institute* 2:8–17 (1990).

22. Seto, A.; C. Kusaka; S. Nakazato; et al. "Detection of Extraordinary Large Biomagnetic Field Strength from Human Hand." *Acupuncture and Electrotherapeutics Research International Journal* 17:75–94 (1992).

23. Sancier, Kenneth, editor. *Qigong Database.* Menlo Park, CA: Qigong Institute, 2000.

24. Yount, Garret. "Distant Intentionality, Qigong Masters and DNA, Esalen-Noetic Sciences Conference on Subtle Energy and Uncharted Mind." Esalen Center for Theory and Research (http://www.esalenctr.org/display/psi.cfm), 2000.

25. Yount, Garret. "Is It More than a Beautiful Form of Hypnosis?" *Health and Spirituality* (Summer 2001).

26. Jones, J. P.; D. P. O'Hara; and K. Elrod. "Quantitative Evaluation of Pranic Healing Using Radiation of Cells in Culture." San Diego: Proceedings, Society for Scientific Exploration (http://www.scientificexploration.org), June 2001.

27. Tiller; *Science and Human Transformation.*

28. Popp, F. A.; K. S. Li; and W. A. Nagl. "A Thermodynamic Approach to the Temperature Response of Biological Systems as Demonstrated by Low-Level Luminescence of Cucumber Seedlings." *Zeitschrift fur Pflanzenphysiologie* 114:1–13 (1984). (Journal is in English.)

29. Van Wijk, R. "Dead Molecules, Live Organism: Learning about Life Force." Esalen-Noetic Sciences Conference on Subtle Energy and Uncharted Mind. Esalen Center for Theory and Research (http://www.esalenctr.org/display/psi.cfm), 2000.

30. Van Wijk, R.; H. Van Aken; J. E. M. Souren. "An Evaluation of Delayed Luminescence of Mammalian Cells." *Trends in Photochemistry and Photobiology* 4:87–97 (1997).

31. Van Wijk, R.; H. Van Aken; W. Mei; and W. F. A. Popp. "Light-Induced Photon Emission by Mammalian Cells. *Journal of Photochemistry and Photobiology* 75–79, (1993).

32. Clarke, J. "SQUIDs." *Scientific American* (Aug. 1994).

33. Teilhard de Chardin, Pierre. *Activation of Energy.* New York: Harcourt Brace, 1973.

34. Teilhard de Chardin, Pierre. *The Formation of the Noosphere.* New York: Harcourt Brace, 1947.

35. Jahn, R., and B. Dunne. *The Margins of Reality: The Role of Consciousness in the Physical World.* New York: Harcourt Brace, 1987.

36. Nadeau, Robert, and Menas Kafatos. *The Conscious Universe: Parts and Wholes in Physical Reality.* Berlin: Springer Verlag, 2000.

37. Nadeau, Robert, and Menas Kafatos. *The Non-Local Universe: New Physics and Matters of the Mind.* London: Oxford University Press, 1999.

38. Ostriker, J. P., and P. J. Steinhardt. "Quintessential Universe." *Scientific American* (Jan. 2001).

39. Goswami, Amit. *The Visionary Window: A Quantum Physicist's Guide to Enlightenment.* Wheaton, IL: Quest Books, 2000.

40. Jahnke, Roger. "Creating a Field of Healing Qi. Empty Vessel." *Journal of Contemporary Taoism* (Winter 2001).

41. Dossey, Larry. *Re-Inventing Medicine.* San Francisco: HarperCollins, 1999.

42. Dossey, Larry. *Prayer Is Good Medicine: How to Reap the Healing Benefits of Prayer.* San Francisco: HarperSanFrancisco, 1996.

43. Byrd, R. C. "Positive Therapeutic Effects of Intercessory Prayer in a Coronary Care Unit Population." *Southern Medical Journal* 81(7):826–29 (July 1988).

44. Targ, Elizabeth. "New Research in Distant Healing." Esalen-Noetic Sciences Conference on Subtle Energy and Uncharted Mind. Esalen Center for Theory and Research (http://www.esalenctr.org/display/psi.cfm), 2000.

45. Sicher, F.; E. Targ; D. Moore; and H. Smith. "A Randomized Double Blind Study of the Effect of Distant Healing in a Population with Advanced AIDS: Report of a Small Scale Study." *Western Journal of Medicine* 169(6):356–63 (1998).

46. Jahn, R., and B. Dunne. *The Margins of Reality: The Role of Consciousness in the Physical World.* New York: Harcourt Brace, 1987.

47. Nelson, Roger. "The Global Consciousness Project." Esalen-Noetic Sciences Conference on Subtle Energy and Uncharted Mind. Esalen Center for Theory and Research (http://www.esalenctr.org/display/psi.cfm), 2000.

48. Schmidt, Helmut. "The Mysterious Side of Psychokinesis (PK)." Esalen-Noetic Sciences Conference on Subtle Energy and Uncharted Mind. Esalen Center for Theory and Research (http://www.esalenctr.org/display/psi.cfm), 2000.

49. Schmidt, Helmut. "PK Tests in a Pre-Sleep State." *Journal of Parapsychology* 64:317–31 (Sept. 2000).

50. Targ, Russell. "The Scientific and Spiritual Implications of Psychic Abilities." Esalen-Noetic Sciences Conference on Subtle Energy and Uncharted Mind. Esalen Center for Theory and Research (http://www.esalenctr.org/display/psi.cfm), 2000.

51. Targ, Russell. *Miracles of Mind: Exploring Nonlocal Consciousness and Spiritual Healing.* Novato, CA: New World Library, 1999.

52. Radin, Dean. "Time Reversed Human Experience." Esalen-Noetic Sciences Conference on Subtle Energy and Uncharted Mind. Esalen Center for Theory and Research (http://www.esalenctr.org/display/psi.cfm), 2000.

53. Radin, Dean. *The Conscious Universe: The Scientific Truth of Psychic Phenomena.* San Francisco: HarperCollins, 1997.

Recommended Reading

The New Medicine, Mind/Body, Alternative Medicine, Natural Healing

Benson, Herbert. *The Relaxation Response.* New York: Avon Books, 1995.

Benson, Herbert. *Timeless Healing: The Power and Biology of Belief.* New York: Simon & Schuster, 1996.

Borysenko, Joan. *Fire in the Soul: A New Psychology of Spiritual Optimism.* New York: Warner Books, 1994.

Borysenko, Joan. *Minding the Body, Mending the Mind.* New York: Bantam, Doubleday, Dell, 1993.

Brennan, Barbara Ann. *Hands of Light: A Guide to Healing Through the Human Energy Field.* New York: Bantam, Doubleday, Dell, 1993.

Cannon, Walter. *The Way of an Investigator.* New York: W. W. Norton, 1945.

Chopra, Deepak. *Ageless Body, Timeless Mind: The Quantum Alternative to Growing Old.* New York: Harmony Books, 1993.

Chopra, Deepak. *Quantum Healing: Exploring the Frontiers of Mind Body Medicine.* New York: Bantam, Doubleday, Dell, 1990.

Cousins, Norman. *Anatomy of an Illness As Perceived by the Patient: Reflections on Healing and Regeneration.* New York: W. W. Norton & Co, 1979.

Cousins, Norman. *Head First: Biology of Hope and the Healing Power of the Human Spirit.* New York: Penguin, 1990.

Cousins, Norman. *Human Options.* New York: Berkley, 1981.

Covey, Steven. *The Seven Habits of Highly Effective People.* New York: Fireside, 1990.

Dossey, Larry. *Healing Words: The Power of Prayer and the Practice of Medicine.* San Francisco: HarperSanFrancisco, 1995.

Dossey, Larry. *Prayer Is Good Medicine: How to Reap the Healing Benefits of Prayer.* San Francisco: HarperSanFrancisco, 1996.

Dossey, Larry. *Recovering the Soul: A Scientific and Spiritual Approach.* New York: Bantam, Doubleday, Dell, 1989.

Dossey, Larry. *Re-Inventing Medicine.* San Francisco: HarperCollins, 1999.

Dossey, Larry. *Space, Time and Medicine.* Boulder & London: Shambhala, 1982.

Feldenkrais, Moshe. *Awareness Through Movement: Health Exercises for Personal Growth.* New York: Harper and Row, 1972.

Feldenkrais, Moshe. *The Elusive Obvious.* Cupertino, CA: Meta Publications, 1981.

Goleman, Daniel, and Joel Gurin. *Mind Body Medicine.* Yonkers, NY: Consumer Reports Books, 1993.

Gordon, James. *Comprehensive Cancer Care: Integrating Alternative, Complementary and Conventional Therapies.* Cambridge, MA: Perseus, 2000.

Gordon, James. *Manifesto for a New Medicine: Your Guide to Healing Partnerships and the Wise Use of Alternative Therapies.* Reading, MA: Addison-Wesley, 1996.

Green, E. *Beyond Biofeedback.* New York: Delacorte Press, 1977.

Guyton, Arthur C. *Textbook of Medical Physiology.* Philadelphia: Harcourt Brace Jovanovich, 1995.

Krucoff, Mitchell, and Carol Krucoff. *Smart Moves or Health Moves: How to Cure, Relieve, and Prevent Common Ailments with Exercise.* New York: Crown, 2000.

Locke, Steven, and Douglas Colligan. *The Healer Within: The New Medicine of Mind and Body.* New York: Penguin Books, 1986.

Lowen, Alexander. *Bioenergetics.* New York: Penguin, 1986.

McGarey, Gladys. *The Physician Within.* Deerfield Beach, FL: Health Communications, 1997.

McGarey, William. *In Search of Healing: Whole-Body Healing Through the Mind-Body-Spirit Connection.* Walpole, NH: Perigee Press, 1996.

Murphy, Michael. *The Future of the Body: Explorations into the Further Evolution of Human Nature.* Los Angeles: J. P. Tarcher, 1993.

Northrup, Christiane. *Women's Bodies, Women's Wisdom: Creating Physical and Emotional Health and Healing.* New York: Bantam, Doubleday, Dell, 1994.

O'Regan, Brendan, and Caryl Hirshberg. *Spontaneous Remission: An Annotated Bibliography.* San Francisco: Institute of Noetic Sciences Press, 1995.

Ornish, Dean. *Dr. Dean Ornish's Program for Reversing Heart Disease.* New York: Random House, 1990.

Pert, Candace. *Molecules of Emotion.* New York: Scribners, 1997.

Selye, Hans. *The Stress of Life.* New York: McGraw-Hill, 1978.

Shealy, Norman. *The Complete Family Guide to Alternative Medicine: An Illustrated Encyclopedia of Natural Healing.* Dorset, England: Element Books, 1996.

Shealy, Norman. *Miracles Do Happen: A Physician's Experience With Alternative Medicine.* Dorset, England: Element Books, 1996.

Siegel, Bernie. *Love, Medicine and Miracles: Lessons Learned About Self-Healing from a Surgeon's Experience With Exceptional Patients.* New York: HarperCollins, 1990.

Siegel, Bernie. *Peace, Love and Healing: Bodymind Communication and the Path to Self-Healing —An Exploration.* New York: HarperCollins, 1990.

Spiegel, David. *Living Beyond Limits*. New York: Fawcett Columbine Press, 1993.

Sweigard, Lulu. *Human Movement Potential: Its Ideokinetic Facilitation*. New York: Harper and Row, 1974.

Todd, Mabel Elsworth. *The Thinking Body: A Study of the Balancing Forces of the Dynamic Man*. New York: Dance Horizons, 1977.

Trivieri, Larry, and John Anderson, eds. *Alternative Medicine: The Definitive Guide*, second edition. Berkeley, CA: Celestial Arts, 2002.

Weil, Andrew. *8 Weeks to Optimum Health*. New York: Fawcett Books, 1998.

Weil, Andrew. *Natural Health, Natural Medicine: A Comprehensive Manual for Wellness and Self-Care*. New York, Houghton Mifflin Co., 1995.

Weil, Andrew. *Spontaneous Healing: How to Discover and Enhance Your Body's Natural Ability to Maintain and Heal Itself*. New York: Knopf, 1995.

Acupuncture and Chinese Medicine

Beinfield, Harriet, and Efram Korngold. *Between Heaven and Earth—A Guide to Chinese Medicine*. New York: Ballantine Books, 1992.

Chen, Jing. *Anatomical Atlas of Chinese Acupuncture Points*. Jinan, China: Shandong Science and Technology Press, 1982.

Cheng, Xinnong. *Chinese Acupuncture and Moxibustion*. Beijing: Foreign Language Press, 1987.

Conner, J., D. Bensky, and Shanghai College of Traditional Chinese Medicine. *Acupuncture: A Comprehensive Text*. Chicago: Eastland Press, 1981.

Eisenberg, David. *Encounters with Qi: Exploring Chinese Medicine*. New York: W. W. Norton, 1985.

Ellis, A., N. Wiseman, and K. Boss, *Grasping the Wind: An Exploration into the Meaning of the Chinese Acupuncture Point Names*. Brookline, MA: Paradigm Publications, 1989.

Flaws, Bob. *The Dao of Increasing Longevity and Conserving One's Life*. Boulder, CO: Blue Poppy Press, 1991.

Hammer, Leo. *Dragon Rises, Red Bird Flies: Psychology and Chinese Medicine*. Barrytown, NY: Station Hill Press, 1990.

Hui, Jia Li. *Pointing Therapy: A Chinese Traditional Therapeutic Skill*. Shandong, China: Shandong Science and Technology Press, 1990.

Jarret, Lonnie. *Nourishing Destiny: The Inner Tradition of Chinese Medicine*. Boston: Spirit Path Press, 1999.

Kaptchuk, Ted. *The Web That Has No Weaver: Understanding Chinese Medicine*. New York: Congdon & Weed, 1984.

Larre, C., E. Rochat, and S. Stang. *Rooted in Spirit: The Heart of Chinese Medicine*. Barrytown, NY: Station Hill Press, 1993.

Larre, C., J. Schatz, E. Rochat, and S. Stang. *Survey of Traditional Chinese Medicine*. Paris: Institut Ricci, 1986.

Liu, Zheng-cai. *A Study of Daoist Acupuncture*. Boulder, CO: Blue Poppy Press, 1999.

Maciocia, Giovanni. *The Foundations of Chinese Medicine: A Comprehensive Text for Acupuncturists and Herbalists.* Edinburgh, London, New York: Churchill Livingstone, 1989.

Ni, Maoshing. *The Yellow Emperor's Classic of Medicine* (*Huang Di Nei Jing*). Boston and London: Shambhala, 1995.

Seem, Mark. *BodyMind Energetics: Toward a Dynamic Model of Health.* Rochester, VT: Healing Arts Press, 1989.

Unschuld, Paul. *Medicine in China: A History of Ideas.* Berkeley, CA: University of California Press, 1966.

Veith, Ilza. *The Yellow Emperor's Classic of Internal Medicine.* Berkeley, CA: University of California Press, 1949, 1972.

Yan, De-xin. *Aging & Blood Stasis: A New TCM Approach to Geriatrics.* Boulder, CO: Blue Poppy Press, 1995.

Qigong and Tai Chi

Bi, Yongsheng. *Chinese Outgoing-Qi Therapy.* Jinan, China: Shandong Science and Technology Press, 1992.

Chan, Luke. *101 Miracles of Natural Healing.* Cincinnati: Benefactor Press, 1996.

Chang, Stephen. *The Book of Internal Exercises.* San Francisco: Strawberry Hill Press, 1978.

Chen, Yan Feng. *Prenatal Energy Mobilizing Qigong.* Guangzhou, China: Gangdong Science and Technology Press, 1992.

Cheng, Man-Ching. *Cheng Tzu's Thirteen Treatises on T'ai Chi Ch'uan.* Berkeley, CA: North Atlantic Books, 1985.

Cheng, Man-Ching. *Cheng Man-Ching's Advanced Tai-Chi Form Instructions.* Sweet Chi Press, 1985.

Chia, Mantak. *The Inner Structure of Tai Chi: Tai Chi Chi Kung.* Huntington, NY: Healing Tao Publishing, 1998.

China Sports Magazine Staff. *The Wonders of Qigong.* Los Angeles: Wayfarer Publications, 1985.

Chuen, Lam Kam. *The Way of Energy: Mastering the Chinese Art of Internal Strength with Chi Kung Exercise.* New York: Simon and Schuster, 1991.

Cohen, Kenneth. *The Way of Qigong: The Art and Science of Chinese Energy Healing.* New York: Balantine, 1997.

Dong, Y. P. *Still as a Mountain, Powerful as Thunder.* Boston and London: Shambhala Publications, 1993.

Dong, Paul. *Chi Gong: The Ancient Chinese Way to Health.* New York: Paragon House, 1990.

Douglas, Bill. *The Complete Idiot's Guide to T'ai Chi & QiGong.* New York: Macmillan Publishing, 1999.

Garripoli, Francesco. *Qigong: Essence of the Healing Dance.* Deerfield Beach, FL: Health Communications, 1999.

Huang, Alfred. *Complete Tai-Chi: The Definitive Guide to Physical & Emotional Self-Improvement.* Boston: Charles Tuttle, 1993.

Huang, Chungliang Al. *Embrace Tiger, Return to Mountain: The Essence of Tai Ji.* Berkeley, CA: Celestial Arts, 1988.

Huang, Jane. *The Primordial Breath: Ancient Chinese Way of Prolonging Life Through Breath Control.* Torrance, CA: Original Books, 1987.

Huang, We-Shan. *Fundamentals of Tai Chi Chuan: An Exposition of its History, Philosophy, Technique, Practice and Application.* Hong Kong: South Sky Book Company, 1973.

Jahnke, Roger. *Awakening and Mastering the Medicine Within* (instructional video). Santa Barbara, CA: Health Action Publishing, 1995.

Jahnke, Roger. *The Healer Within: Using Traditional Chinese Techniques to Release Your Body's Own Medicine.* San Francisco: HarperCollins, 1997.

Jahnke, Roger. *The Most Profound Medicine.* Santa Barbara, CA: Health Action Publishing, 1990.

Jin, Xiaoguang. *Life More Abundant: The Science of Zhineng Qigong Principles and Practices.* 1999.

Jiao, Guorui. *Qigong: Essentials for Health Promotion.* Beijing: China Reconstructs Press, 1988.

Johnson, Jerry Alan. *Chinese Medical Qigong Therapy: A Comprehensive Text.* Pacific Grove, CA: International Institute of Medical Qigong, 2000.

Johnson, Yanling. *A Woman's Qigong Guide.* Boston: YMAA Publications, 2001.

Jou, Tsung Hwa. *The Tao of Tai Chi Chuan.* Rutland, VT: Charles Tuttle, 1980.

Leonard, George, and Michael Murphy. *The Life We Are Given: A Long-Term Program for Realizing the Potential of Body, Mind, Heart, and Soul.* New York: J. P. Tarcher, 1995.

Liang, Shou-Yu, and Wen-Ching Wu. *Qigong Empowerment: A Guide to Medical, Taoist, Buddhist, Wushu Energy Cultivation.* East Providence, RI: Way of the Dragon Publishing, 1996.

Lin, Zixin. *Qigong: Chinese Medicine or Pseudoscience?* Amhurst, NY: Prometheus Books, 2000.

Liu, Hong. *Mastering Miracles: The Healing Art of Qigong.* New York: Warner Books, 1997.

Liu, Zhengcai. *The Mystery of Longevity.* Beijing: Foreign Language Press, 1990.

Lo, Benjamin Pang Jeng. *The Essence of Tai Chi Chuan.* Richmond, CA: North Atlantic Books, 1979.

Lowenthal, Wolfe. *There Are No Secrets: Professor Cheng Man-Ching and His Tai Chi Chuan.* Berkeley, CA: North Atlantic Books, 1991.

Lu, Kuan Yu. *Taoist Yoga: Alchemy and Immortality.* New York: Samuel Wiser, 1970.

MacRitchie, James. *Chi Kung: Cultivating Personal Energy.* Dorset, England: Element Books, 1993.

MacRitchie, James. *The Chi Kung Way.* San Francisco: HarperCollins, 1997.

McGee, Charles, and E. Poy Yew Chow. *Qigong: Miracle Healing from China.* Coeur d'Alene, ID: MediPress, 1994.

Olsen, Stuart Alve. *The Jade Emperor's Mind Seal Classic: A Taoist Guide to Health, Longevity and Immortality.* St. Paul, MN: Dragon Door Publications, 1992.

Reid, Daniel. *Guarding the Three Treasures: The Chinese Way of Health.* New York: Simon and Schuster, 1993.

Sancier, Kenneth, editor. *Gigong Database.* Menlo Park, CA: Qigong Institute, 2000.

Siou, Lily. *Chi Kung: Mastering the Unseen Life Force.* Honolulu, HI: Tai Hsuan Press, 1973.

Smith, Robert. *Chinese Boxing: Masters and Methods.* New York: Kodansha International, 1980.

Towler, Solala. *A Gathering of Cranes.* Eugene, OR: Abode of the Eternal Tao, 1996.

Wen, Kuan Chu. *Tao and Longevity: Mind Body Transformation.* York Beach, ME: Samuel Wiser, 1984.

Wile, Douglas. *Lost Tai Chi Classics from the Late Ching Dynasty (Chinese Philosophy and Culture).* New York: State University of New York Press, 1995.

Wile, Douglas. *T'ai Chi's Ancestors: The Making of an Internal Art.* Sweet Chi Press, 1999.

Wong, Kew Kit. *The Art of Chi Kung: Making the Most of Your Energy.* Dorset, England: Element Books, 1993.

Yang, Jwing-Ming. *Qigong: The Secret of Youth.* Boston: YMAA Publications, 2000.

Yang, Jwing-Ming. *Taijiquan, Classical Yang Style: The Complete Form and Qigong.* Boston: YMAA Publications, 1999.

Yayama, Toshishiko. *Qi Healing: The Way to a New Mind and Body.* New York: Kodansha International, 1993.

Zhang, Enqin. *Chinese Qigong.* Shanghai: Publishing House of Shanghai College of Traditional Chinese Medicine, 1989.

Zhang, Mingwu. *Chinese Qigong Therapy.* Jinan, China: Shandong Science and Technology Press, 1988.

Sexual Cultivation

Abrams, Douglas, and Mantak Chia. *The Multi-Orgasmic Couple: Sexual Secrets Every Couple Should Know.* San Francisco: HarperSanFrancisco, 2000.

Chang, Jolan. *The Tao of Love and Sex: The Ancient Chinese Way to Ecstacy.* New York: Dutton, 1977.

Chang, Stephen. *The Tao of Sexology: The Book of Infinite Wisdom.* San Francisco: Tao Publishing, 1986.

Chia, Mantak, and Maneewan Chia. *Healing Love through the Tao: Cultivating Female Sexuality.* Huntington, NY: Healing Tao Books, 1986.

Chia, Mantak, and Michael Winn. *Taoist Secrets of Love: Cultivating Male Sexual Energy.* New York: Aurora Press, 1984.

Chu, Valentin. *The Yin-Yang Butterfly: Ancient Chinese Sexual Secrets for Western Lovers.* New York: J. P. Tarcher, 1994.

Cleary, Thomas. *Sex, Health and Long Life: Manuals of Taoist Practice.* Boston and London: Shambhala, 1999.

Johnson, Yanling. *A Woman's Qigong Guide.* Boston: YMAA Publications, 2001.

McNeil, James. *Ancient Lovemaking Secrets: The Journey Toward Immortality.* L9H Publications, 1998.

Wile, Douglas. *Art of the Bedchamber: The Chinese Sexual Yoga Classics Including Women's Solo Meditation Texts.* Albany, NY: State University of New York, 1992.

Translations of Lao Zi and Zhuang Zi

Bynner, Witter. *The Way of Life: According to Lao Tzu.* New York: Perigee Books, 1972.

Cleary, Thomas. *The Essential Tao: An Introduction into the Heart of Taoism through the Authentic Tao Te Ching and the Inner Teachings of Chuan Tzu.* San Francisco: HarperSanFrancisco, 1993.

Feng, Gai-Fu, and Jane English. *Chuang Tsu: Inner Chapters.* New York: Vintage Books, 1974.

Feng, Gai-Fu, and Jane English. *Lao Tsu: Tao Te Ching.* New York: Vintage Books, 1972.

Hamill, S., and J. P. Seaton. *The Essential Chuang Tzu.* Boston and London: Shambhala, 1999.

Lau, D. C. *Lao Tzu: Tao Te Ching.* New York: Penguin Books, 1963.

Legge, James. *Tao Te Ching.* Mineola, NY: Dover Publications, 1997. (Originally published by Oxford University Press, 1891.)

Le Guin, Ursula. *Lao Tzu: Tao Te Ching: A Book About the Way and the Power of the Way.* Boston and London: Shambhala, 1998.

Merton, Thomas. *The Way of Chuang Tzu.* New York: New Directions, 1969.

Mitchell, Stephen. *Tao Te Ching.* New York: Harper and Row, 1988.

Ren, Jiyu. *The Book of Lao Zi: A Modern Chinese Translation.* Beijing: Foreign Language Press, 1993.

Richter, Gregory. *The Gate of all Marvelous Things: A Guide to Reading the Tao Te Ching.* San Francisco: Red Mansions Publishing, 1998.

Star, Jonathan. *Tao Teaching: The Definitive Tradition.* New York: Tarcher-Putnam, 2001.

Chinese Cultivation Traditions, Daoism, Science, and Culture

Bertschinger, Richard. *The Secret of Everlasting Life: The First Translation of the Ancient Chinese Text on Immortality.* Dorset, England: Element Books, 1994.

Blofeld, John. *The Secret and Sublime: Taoist Mysteries and Magic.* New York: Dutton, 1973.

Blofeld, John. *Taoism: Road to Immortality.* Boulder and London: Shambhala, 1978.

Bokenkamp, Stephen. *Early Daoist Scriptures.* Berkeley, CA: University of California Press, 1997.

Chan, Wing Tsit. *A Source Book in Chinese Philosophy.* Princeton, NJ: Princeton University Press, 1963.

Cleary, Thomas. *Book of Balance and Harmony Translated from Master Li, Dao Qun.* New York: North Star Press, 1989.

Cleary, Thomas. *Opening the Dragon Gate: The Making of a Modern Taoist Wizard.* Boston: Charles Tuttle, 1996.

Cleary, Thomas. *Practical Taoism.* Boston and London: Shambhala, 1996.

Cleary, Thomas. *The Secret of the Golden Flower (Tai Yi Jin Hua Zong Zhi).* San Franciso: HarperSanFrancisco, 1991.

Cleary, Thomas. *Vitality, Energy, Spirit: A Taoist Sourcebook.* Boston and London: Shambhala, 1991.

Deng, Ming-Dao. *Seven Bamboo Tablets of the Cloudy Satchel.* New York: Harper and Row, 1987.

Deng, Ming-Dao. *The Wandering Taoist.* New York: Harper and Row 1983.

Hoff, Benjamin. *The Tao of Pooh.* New York: Penguin Books, 1983.

Kaltenmark, Max. *Lao Tzu and Taoism.* Stanford, CA: Stanford University Press, 1969.

Kohn, Livia. *Daoism and Chinese Culture.* Cambridge, MA: Three Pines Press, 2001.

Kohn, Livia. *Early Chinese Mysticism.* Princeton, NJ: Princeton University Press, 1991.

Kohn, Livia. *The Taoist Experience: An Anthology.* New York: State University of New York, 1993.

Kohn, Livia. *Taoist Meditation and Longevity Techniques.* Ann Arbor, MI: Center for Chinese Studies, University of Michigan, 1989.

Kohn, Livia, and Michael Lafargue. *Lao-Tzu and the Tao-Te-Ching.* New York: University of New York Press, 1998.

Lau, D. C., and Roger Ames. *Yuan Dao: Tracing Dao to Its Source.* New York: Ballantine, 1998.

Larfargue, Michael. *The Tao of the Tao Te Ching: A Translation and Commentary.* New York: State University of New York, 1992.

Loy, Ching-Yuen. *The Supreme Way: Inner Teachings of the Southern Mountain Tao.* Berkeley, CA: North Atlantic Books, 1993.

Needham, Joseph, and Robert Temple. *The Genius of China: 3,000 Years of Science, Discovery and Invention.* New York: Simon and Schuster, 1986.

Needham, Joseph, and Colin Ronan. *The Shorter Science and Civilization in China: An Abridgement of Joseph Needham's Original Text.* Cambridge, London, New York: Cambridge University Press, 1978, 1998.

Ni, Hua-Ching. *Life and Teachings of Two Immortals (Volume I): Kou Hong.* Santa Monica, CA: Shrine of the Eternal Breath of Tao, 1992.

Porter, Bill. *Road to Heaven: Encounters with Chinese Hermits.* San Francisco: Mercury House, 1993.

Robinet, Isabelle. *Taoism: Growth of a Religion.* Stanford, CA: Stanford University Press, 1997.

Saso, Michael. *The Gold Pavillion: Taoist Ways to Peace, Healing, and Long Life.* Rutland, VT: Charles Tuttle, 1995.

Saso, Michael. *Taoist Master Chuang.* Sacred Mountain Press, 2000.

Schipper, Kristofer. *The Taoist Body.* Berkeley, CA: University of California Press, 1993.

Towler, Solala. *Embarking on the Way: A Guide to Western Taoism.* Eugene, OR: Abode of the Eternal Tao, 1998.

Ware, James. *Alchemy, Medicine and Religion in the China of A.D. 320.* (Translation of the *Bao Pu Zi,* by Ge Hong. Usually translated as *The Book of the Master Who Embraces Simplicity.*) New York: Dover Publications, 1966.

Wilhelm, Richard. *The Secret of the Golden Flower: A Chinese Book of Life (Tai Yi Jin Hua Zong Zhi).* New York and London: Harcourt Brace Jovanovich, 1962.

Wong, Eva. *Cultivating the Energy of Life.* (Translated from Liu Hua-Yang.) Boston and London: Shambhala, 1998.

Wong, Eva. *Harmonizing Yin & Yang: The Dragon-Tiger Classic.* Boston and London: Shambhala, 1997.

Wong. Eva. *The Shambhala Guide to Taoism.* Boston and London: Shambhala, 1997.

Yates, Robin. *Five Lost Classics: Tao, Huang-Lao and Yin-Yang in Han China.* New York: Ballantine, 1997.

Classic Chinese Works on Cultivation

An asterisk (*) indicates works that have been translated into English and that appear under "Chinese Cultivation Traditions" or "Translations of Lao Zi and Zhuang Zi where the full reference can be found."

* *The Lao Zi or Book on the Integral Way of Life and its Virtue* (*Dao De Jing,* written by Lao Zi). Translated by Gai-Fu Feng and Jane English, Thomas Cleary, Gregory Richter, Ren Jiyu, Witter Bynner, James Legge, D. C. Lau, Ursula Le Guin, Jonathan Star, and Michael Lafargue.

* *The Zhuang Zi* (*Chuang Tzu,* written by Zhuang Zi*)* or *Inner Chapters.* Translated by Gai-Fu Feng and Jane English, Thomas Cleary, Sam Hamill and J. P. Seaton, and Thomas Merton.

* *Book of the Master Who Embraces Simplicity (Bao Pu Zi,* written by Ge Hong). Translated by James Ware.

Book on Precepts (*Zhon Jie Wen,* author unknown), from translated sections in *Taoist Meditation and Longevity Techniques.*

* *Book of Triplex Unity* (*Can Tong Qi,* written by Wei Bo Yang), translated by Richard Bertschinger.

Compendium of Essentials on Nourishing Life (*She Yang Zhen Zhong Fang,* written by Sun Simiao), from translated sections included in Livia Kohn, *Taoist Meditation and Longevity Techniques.* Ann Arbor, MI: Center for Chinese Studies, University of Michigan, 1989.

The Great Clarity Discourse on Protecting Life (author unknown), from translated sections in *Taoist Meditation and Longevity Techniques.*

The Method of Extending One's Years and Increasing Knowing (*Yun Nian Yi Suan Fa,* author unknown), from translated sections in *Taoist Meditation and Longevity Techniques.*

Prescriptions Worth a Thousand Ounces of Gold (*Qian Jin Fang,* written by Sun Simiao) from translated sections in *Taoist Meditation and Longevity Techniques.*

Records of Daoist Essence Preservation—Gathering of Spirit Immortals on Western Mountain (*Dao Zang Jing Hua Ling—Xi Shan Xian Hui Zhen Ji,* author unknown), from translated sections in *Taoist Meditation and Longevity Techniques.*

Record on Nourishing Inner Nature and Extending Life (*Yang Xing Yan Ming Lu,* written by Tao Hong Jing), from translated sections in *Taoist Meditation and Longevity Techniques.*

* *The Secret of the Golden Flower* (*Tai Yi Jin Hua Zong Zhi*), translated by Cleary and Wilhelm.

Scripture of Divine Nature (*Su Ling Jing,* author unknown), from translated sections in *Taoist Meditation and Longevity Techniques.*

Seven Slips of the Cloudy Satchel: Daoist Encyclopedia (*Yun Ji Qi Qian,* author unknown), from translated sections in *Taoist Meditation and Longevity Techniques.*

Application of the Book of Changes to Medicine (*Lei Jing Tu Yi,* unknown Ming Dynasty author), from translated sections in *Taoist Meditation and Longevity Techniques.*

Selections from the Scripture of Great Peace (*Tai Ping Jing Chao,* author unknown), from translated sections in *Taoist Meditation and Longevity Techniques.*

The Visualization of Spirit and Refinement of Qi (*Cun Shen Lian Qi Ming,* Sun Simiao), from translated sections in *Taoist Meditation and Longevity Techniques.*

Yoga, Pranayama, Ayurveda, Chakras

Frawley, David. *Yoga and Ayurveda.* Santa Fe, NM: Lotus Press, 1999.

Hariharananda, Aranya. *Yoga Philosophy of Patanjali.* Calcutta: Calcutta University Press, 1986.

Iyengar, B. K. S. *Light on Pranayama: The Yogic Art of Breathing.* New York: Crossroads, 1989.

Iyengar, B. K. S. *Light on the Yoga Sutras of Patanjali.* London: Thorsons, 1996.

Lad, Vasant. *Ayurveda: Science of Self-Healing.* Santa Fe, NM: Lotus Press, 1984.

RamaCharaka, Yogi. *Science of Breath: The Oriental Breathing Philosophy.* Chicago: Yogi Publication Society, 1904.

Satchidananda, Sri Swami. *The Yoga Sutras of Patanjali.* Buckingham, VA: Integral Yoga Publications, 1997.

Stoler Miller, Barbara. *Yoga Discipline of Freedom: The Yoga Sutra Attributed to Patanjali.* New York: Bantam, Doubleday, Dell, 1998.

Thakkur, Chandrashekhar. *Introduction to Ayurveda: The Science of Life.* New York: ASI Publishers, 1974.

New Science, Quantum, Energetics, and Biofield

Becker, R. O. *The Body Electric: Electromagnetism and the Foundation of Life.* New York: William Morrow and Co., 1985.

Burr, H. S. *Fields of Life.* New York: Ballantine, 1973.

Bohm, David. *The Undivided Universe.* New York: Routledge, 1995.

Bohm, David. *Wholeness and the Implicate Order.* New York: Routledge, 1996.

Capra, Fritjof. *The Tao of Physics: An Exploration of the Parallels Between Modern Physics and Eastern Mysticism.* Boston: Shambhala, 1991.

Capra, Fritjof. *The Turning Point: Science, Society, and the Rising Culture.* New York: Bantam, Doubleday, Dell, 1988.

Capra, Fritjof. *The Web of Life: A New Scientific Understanding of Living Systems.* New York: Anchor Books Doubleday, 1996.

Goswami, Amit. *The Visionary Window: A Quantum Physicist's Guide to Enlightenment.* Wheaton, IL: Quest Books, 2000.

Hawking, Stephen. *A Brief History of Time: From the Big Bang to Black Holes.* New York: Bantam, 1988.

Jahn, R., and B. Dunne. *The Margins of Reality: The Role of Consciousness in the Physical World.* New York: Harcourt, Brace, Jovanovich Publishers, 1987.

Kuhn, T. S. *The Structure of Scientific Revolutions.* Chicago: University of Chicago Press, 1970.

MacCraty, Rollin. *Science of the Heart: Exploring the Role of the Heart in Human Performance.* Boulder Creek, CA: HeartMath, 2001.

Nadeau, Robert, and Menas Kafatos. *The Conscious Universe: Parts and Wholes in Physical Reality.* Berlin: Springer Verlag, 2000.

Nadeau, Robert, and Menas Kafatos. *The Non-Local Universe: New Physics and Matters of the Mind.* London: Oxford University Press, 1999.

Nordenstrom, B. E. W. *Biologically Closed Circuits: Clinical, Experimental and Theoretical Evidence for an Additional Circulatory System.* Stockholm: Nordic Medical Publications, 1983.

Oschman, James. *Energy Medicine: The Scientific Basis.* Edinburgh, London, New York: Churchill Livingstone, 2000.

Radin, Dean. *The Conscious Universe: The Scientific Truth of Psychic Phenomena.* San Francisco: HarperCollins, 1997.

Sheldrake, Rupert. *A New Science of Life.* Los Angeles: J. P. Tarcher, 1981.

Targ, Russell. *Miracles of Mind: Exploring Nonlocal Consciousness and Spiritual Healing.* Novato, CA: New World Library, 1999.

Tiller, William. *Science and Human Transformation: Subtle Energies, Intentionality and Consciousness.* Walnut Creek, CA: Pavior Publishing, 1997.

Wolf, Fred. *The Spiritual Universe.* New York: Simon and Schuster, 1996.

Zohar, Danah. *The Quantum Self.* New York: William Morrow, 1990.

Zohar, Danah, and Ian Marshall. *The Quantum Society: Mind, Physics and a New Social Vision.* New York: William Morrow–Quill Publishing, 1994.

Zukov, Gary. *The Dancing Wu Li Masters: An Overview of the New Physics.* New York: Bantam, 1994.

Resources

Organizations and Associations

National Qigong (Chi Kung) Association, USA (NQA)
http://www.NQA.org
The umbrella organization in the United States for all schools and styles of Qigong and Tai Chi, membership includes practitioners of Tai Chi and Qigong from all walks of life as well as instructors. Internet site includes a directory of members and instructors.

Qigong Institute (QI)
http://www.qigonginstitute.org
Looks at Qigong and Tai Chi from the perspective of research, has a database of abstracts of scientific investigation from around the world. Internet site includes a directory of instructors.

American Qigong Association
http://www.eastwestqi.com/aqa
A nationwide association devoted to Qigong.

Qigong Association of America
http://www.qi.org
Informative and balanced website.

World Tai Chi and Qigong Association
http://www.worldtaichiqigongassn.org
Fosters access to Qigong and Tai Chi and sponsors World Tai Chi and Qigong Day.

National Commission for the Certification of Acupuncture and Oriental Medicine
http://www.nccaom.org
The national organization that certifies practitioners of Chinese medicine in the United States.

National Center for Complementary and Alternative Medicine (NCCAM)
http://nccam.nih.gov
The aspect of the National Institutes of Health (NIH) devoted to Complementary and Alternative Medicine with numerous research projects on Qigong and Tai Chi.

American Organization for the Body Therapies of Asia (AOBTA)
http://www.aobta.org
The professional organization for health-care providers who practice Asian methods of body therapy.

American Association of Oriental Medicine (AAOM)
http://www.aaom.org
National membership organization for practitioners of Oriental Medicine.

Acupuncture and Oriental Medicine Alliance
http://acuall.org
Practitioners and consumers who support access to Asian health-care practices.

Internet Sites

The Healer Within—http://www.HealerWithin.com
Dr. Jahnke's Tai Chi and Qigong site—http://www.Qigong-ChiKung.com
Breathe Deep newsletter—http://www.wujiproductions.com
Open Directory Project—
   http://dmoz.org/Health/Alternative/Acupuncture_and_Chinese_Medicine/Qigong
Health World—http://www.Healthy.Net/Qigong
ChiLel Qigong—http://www.chilel.com

Chinese Language
Zhong wen—http://zhongwen.com
An amazing site for studying Chinese characters, includes the *Dao De Jing* (*Tao Te Ching*).

Daoism (Taoism)
Daoism (Taoism) Philosophy—http://www.daoism.net
World Organization of Daoism—http://www.daoism.org
Daoist (Taoist)Depot—http://www.edepot.com/taoism.shtml
Excellent Daoism Resource—http://www.daoiststudies.org
Excellent scholarly site of Dr. Fabrizio Pregadio—http://helios.unive.it/~pregadio/home.html

Health Organizations
Enter Tai Chi or Qigong at the internet site search or look under exercise and fitness.
Arthritis Foundation—http://www.arthritis.org
American Cancer Society—http://www.cancer.org
The YMCA—http://www.ymca.net
American Diabetes Association—http://www.diabetes.org
American Heart Association—http://www.americanheart.org

Books, Journals, and Magazines

Redwing Books
http://www.redwingbooks.com
Wide variety of books on Qigong, Tai Chi, and Chinese medicine.

Empty Vessel: A Journal of Contemporary Taoism
http://www.abodetao.com
Explores Chinese arts with a focus on Daoism (Taoism) including Qigong and Tai Chi;
  contains a catalog of books and videos.

Qi: The Journal of Traditional Eastern Health and Fitness
http://www.qi-journal.com
Explores Chinese arts with a focus on health and fitness including Qigong and Tai Chi,
  catalog of books and videos.

Tai Chi Magazine
http://www.tai-chi.com
Explores Tai Chi and Qigong; contains a catalog of books and videos.

Kung Fu Magazine
http://www.kungfumagazine.com
Explores Kung Fu and Qigong, traditional Chinese martial arts and healing.

Blue Poppy
http://www.bluepoppy.com
Excellent resource on Chinese traditions of health, longevity, and medicine.

Retreats and Training Centers

Omega Institute
http://www.eomega.org
Rhinebeck, New York—Catskills Retreat Center, plus urban conferences in major cities,
  retreats in Carribean and Costa Rica.

Esalen Institute
http://www.esalen.org
Big Sur, California—beautiful retreat center, plus the Esalen Center for Theory and
  Research.

Naropa University—Continuing Education
http://www.naropa.edu/conted
Transpersonal and contemplative psychology, Buddhist studies, gerontology, somatic
  psychology.

Kripalu Center
http://www.kripalu.com
Lovely retreat center in western Massachusetts.

The California Institute of Integral Studies
http://www.ciis.org
A graduate school for training in body, mind, and spirit.

The Fetzer Institute
http://www.fetzer.org
Research exploring the integral relationships among body, mind, and spirit.

The Institute of Noetic Sciences
http://www.ions.org
Research, conferences, world travel.

Association for Research and Enlightenment
http://www.are-cayce.com
The work of Edgar Cayce on health, intuition, and spirituality.

Dr. Jahnke's Training Materials

Further Study with the Institute of Integral Qigong and Tai Chi

The amount of need for healing and empowerment in our hospitals, clinics, community centers, social service agencies, schools, churches, and businesses is immense. Through workshops and trainings we inform and inspire people in the practice of Qigong and Tai Chi. To help fill the need to mobilize the Qi cultivation arts throughout our communities we train instructors at beginning as well as more advanced levels.

Qigong (Chi Kung) and Tai Chi (Taiji) Training

Workshops for students and practitioners—weekend, week long:
Wellness, Health Promotion, and Stress Mastery
Healer Within
Walking Qigong
The Healing Promise of Qi
The Ten Levels of Qi Cultivation and Mastery
Tai Chi Easy: Tai Chi Three and Tai Chi Ten
Integral Tai Chi Qigong
Integral Tai Chi—Short Form
Vitality Medical Qigong
Standing Qigong Meditation
Connective Tissue, Tendon Changing Qigong
Marrow Bathing Qigong
Seven Precious Gestures
Spontaneous Qigong
Inner Alchemy
Primordial Qigong—Wuji
Trainings for teachers, mentors, and health professionals—weekend, week long, month long
Wellness and health promotion programs
Healing journeys and immersion study retreats to China, Santa Barbara, Oregon, and Hawaii

Lectures and Keynotes for Conferences and Retreats

Hospitals
Medical Organizations
Corporate Human Resources
Professional Associations
Schools and Colleges
Faith Organizations
Social Service Agencies

The Circle of Life and PHASES training
Training for health-care professionals
Workshops for agencies and communities

Dr. Jahnke's Books and Videos

The Healer Within—book and video
Awakening and Mastering the Medicine Within—video
The Most Profound Medicine—book
Tai Chi Qigong, Tai Chi Three, and Tai Chi Ten—video
Healing Promise of Qi—video
Qi Cultivation Reminder Chime—Qigong practice aid
To order direct please call 800-824-4325.

Internet Resources

http://www.FeelTheQi.com
http://www.HealerWithin.com
http://www.Qigong-ChiKung.com

To contact Roger Jahnke and the Institute of Integral Qigong and Tai Chi, please write
243 Pebble Beach, Santa Barbara, CA 93117.

Index